Law and Professional Issues in Nursing

Sara Miller McCune founded SAGE Publishing in 1965 to support the dissemination of usable knowledge and educate a global community. SAGE publishes more than 1000 journals and over 800 new books each year, spanning a wide range of subject areas. Our growing selection of library products includes archives, data, case studies and video. SAGE remains majority owned by our founder and after her lifetime will become owned by a charitable trust that secures the company's continued independence.

Los Angeles | London | New Delhi | Singapore | Washington DC | Melbourne

Fourth Edition

Law and Professional Issues in Nursing

Richard Griffith
Cassam Tengnah

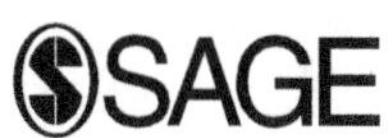

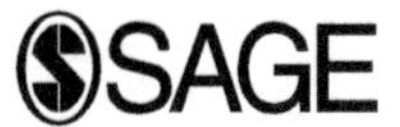

Learning Matters
An imprint of SAGE Publications Ltd
1 Oliver's Yard
55 City Road
London EC1Y 1SP

SAGE Publications Inc.
2455 Teller Road
Thousand Oaks, California 91320

SAGE Publications India Pvt Ltd
B 1/I 1 Mohan Cooperative Industrial Area
Mathura Road
New Delhi 110 044

SAGE Publications Asia-Pacific Pte Ltd
3 Church Street
#10-04 Samsung Hub
Singapore 049483

Editor: Alex Clabburn
Production controller: Chris Marke
Project management: Swales & Willis Ltd, Exeter, Devon
Marketing manager: Tamara Navaratnam
Cover design: Wendy Scott
Typeset by: C&M Digitals (P) Ltd, Chennai, India
Printed by CPI Group (UK) Ltd, Croydon, CR0 4YY

First edition published 2008
Second edition published 2010
Third edition published 2014
Fourth edition published 2017

Library of Congress Control Number: 2016954954

British Library Cataloguing in Publication data

A catalogue record for this book is available from the British Library

ISBN 978-1-4739-6941-4
ISBN 978-1-4739-6942-1 (pbk)

Contents

TRANSFORMING NURSING PRACTICE TNP

Transforming Nursing Practice is a series tailor-made for pre-registration student nurses. Each book in the series is:

- Affordable
- Mapped to the NMC Standards and Essential Skills Clusters
- Full of active learning features
- Focused on applying theory to practice

Each book addresses a core topic and has been carefully developed to be simple to use, quick to read and written in clear language.

> "An invaluable series of books that explicitly relates to the NMC standards. Each book covers a different topic that students need to explore in order to develop into a qualified nurse... I would recommend this series to all pre-registration nursing students whatever their field or year of study.
>
> **Linda Robson**
> **Senior Lecturer, Edge Hill University**
>
> The set of books is an excellent resource for students. The series is small, easily portable and valuable. I use the whole set on a regular basis.
>
> **Fiona Davies**
> **Senior Nurse Lecturer, University of Derby**
>
> I recommend the SAGE/Learning Matters series to all my students as they are relevant and concise. Please keep up the good work.
>
> **Thomas Beary**
> **Senior Lecturer in Mental Health Nursing, University of Hertfordshire**"

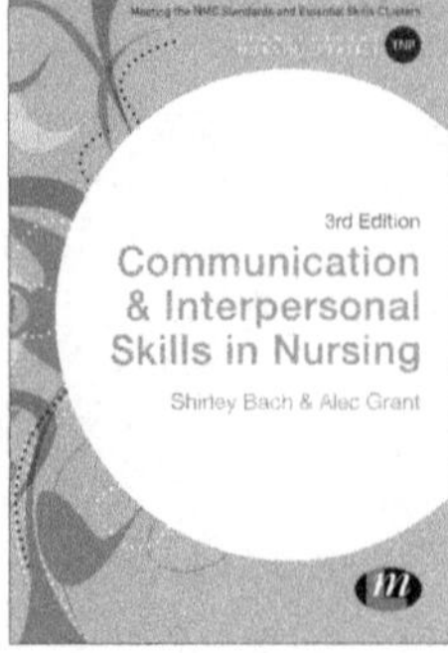

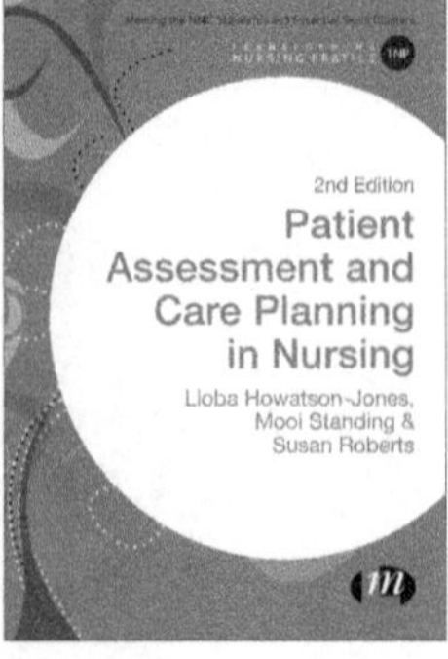

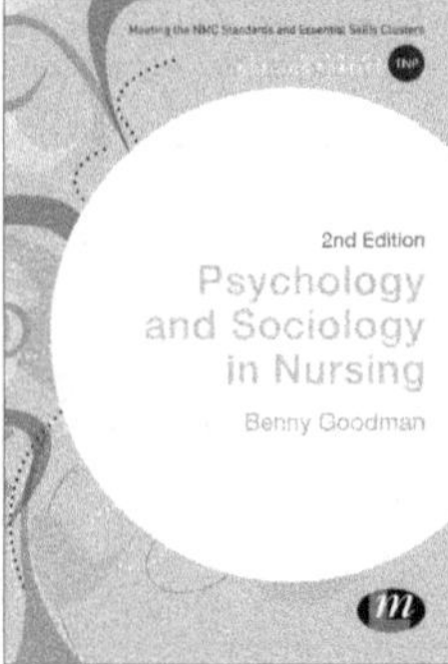

ABOUT THE SERIES EDITORS

Dr Mooi Standing is an Independent Academic Consultant (UK and International) and responsible for the personal and professional learning skills titles. She is an accredited NMC Quality Assurance Reviewer of educational programmes and a Professional Regulator Panellist on the NMC Practice Committee.

Sandra Walker is Senior Teaching Fellow in Mental Health at the University of Southampton and responsible for the mental health nursing titles. She is a Qualified Mental Health Nurse with a wide range of clinical experience spanning more than 20 years.

CORE KNOWLEDGE TITLES:

Becoming a Registered Nurse: Making the Transition to Practice
Communication and Interpersonal Skills in Nursing (3rd Ed)
Contexts of Contemporary Nursing (2nd Ed)
Getting into Nursing (2nd Ed)
Health Promotion and Public Health for Nursing Students (3rd Ed)
Introduction to Medicines Management in Nursing
Law and Professional Issues in Nursing (4th Ed)
Leadership, Management and Team Working in Nursing (2nd Ed)
Learning Skills for Nursing Students
Medicines Management in Children's Nursing
Microbiology and Infection Prevention and Control for Nursing Students
Nursing and Collaborative Practice (2nd Ed)
Nursing and Mental Health Care
Nursing in Partnership with Patients and Carers
Palliative and End of Life Care in Nursing
Passing Calculations Tests for Nursing Students (3rd Ed)
Pathophysiology and Pharmacology for Nursing Students
Patient Assessment and Care Planning in Nursing (2nd Ed)
Patient Safety and Managing Risk in Nursing
Psychology and Sociology in Nursing (2nd Ed)
Successful Practice Learning for Nursing Students (2nd Ed)
Understanding Ethics for Nursing Students (2nd Ed)
Understanding Psychology for Nursing Students
Using Health Policy in Nursing Practice
What is Nursing? Exploring Theory and Practice (3rd Ed)

PERSONAL AND PROFESSIONAL LEARNING SKILLS TITLES:

Clinical Judgement and Decision Making for Nursing Students (3rd Ed)
Critical Thinking and Writing for Nursing Students (3rd Ed)
Evidence-based Practice in Nursing (3rd Ed)
Information Skills for Nursing Students
Reflective Practice in Nursing (3rd Ed)
Succeeding in Essays, Exams and OSCEs for Nursing Students
Succeeding in Literature Reviews and Research Project Plans for Nursing Students (3rd Ed)
Successful Professional Portfolios for Nursing Students (2nd Ed)
Understanding Research for Nursing Students (3rd Ed)

MENTAL HEALTH NURSING TITLES:

Assessment and Decision Making in Mental Health Nursing
Engagement and Therapeutic Communication in Mental Health Nursing
Medicines Management in Mental Health Nursing (2nd Ed)
Mental Health Law in Nursing
Physical Healthcare and Promotion in Mental Health Nursing
Promoting Recovery in Mental Health Nursing
Psychosocial Interventions in Mental Health Nursing

ADULT NURSING TITLES:

Acute and Critical Care in Adult Nursing (2nd Ed)
Caring for Older People in Nursing
Dementia Care in Nursing
Medicines Management in Adult Nursing
Nursing Adults with Long Term Conditions (2nd Ed)
Safeguarding Adults in Nursing Practice (2nd Ed)

You can find more information on each of these titles and our other learning resources at **www.sagepub.co.uk**. Many of these titles are also available in various e-book formats, please visit our website for more information.

Foreword

Here is a text that will provide you with excellent guidance for your years as a student and as a qualified practitioner. The authors have revised this edition and brought together in a sensible format all you need to know about the law and how it protects and guides us for safe practice. People have different reactions to laws. Some people see them as a protection for themselves, and others, against harm. Others see them as barriers or constraints hidden within dense levels of bureaucracy. Another view is that they are a baffling labyrinth of unfamiliar terms that date back to archaic times and are represented by a medieval dress code – picture the lawyer in gown and wig! After reading this book you will see that they provide the conditions from which we can pursue our professional, and personal, lives in a manner that safeguards our patients and those for whom we care.

In the text there is an emphasis on the law, but it is grounded in the principles of the Human Rights Act 1998. It is this ethos that, in turn, shapes how we manage sometimes difficult moral and ethical dilemmas; always with a view to practising within the principles of the NMC *Code: Professional standards of practice and behaviour for nurses and midwives.* There are very detailed explanations of concepts such as accountability, responsibility, discrimination, disability and equality. You will find chapters dedicated to mental health and children's rights. Difficult issues such as gaining consent from vulnerable groups are explained with examples to illustrate how the laws can be understood and applied.

The concluding chapters on record keeping, confidentiality and health and safety provide up-to-date information on aspects of professional care that are integral to our activities. Yet, they are often so ingrained that we neglect the significance of the laws that are designed to protect our patients and provide professional safeguards. These chapters provide essential, practical guidance to achieve good practice and meet legal requirements. A particularly useful addition is the section on using social networking sites in Chapter 12.

In each chapter the relevant NMC *Standards for Pre-registration Nursing Education* are stated, a feature of the Transforming Nursing Practice series. This ensures nursing students will see exactly how the information in the book relates to achieving their competencies and be ready to practise in the contemporary world of nursing we know today.

Professor Shirley Bach

Legislation

Table of cases

A v United Kingdom [1998] 2 FLR 959.
A&D v B&E [2003] EWHC 1376 (FAM).
Aintree University Hospitals Foundation Trust v James [2013] UKSC 67.
Aintree University Hospitals NHS Foundation Trust v David James [2013] EWCA Civ 65.
Airedale NHS Trust v Bland [1993] AC 789.
Association X v United Kingdom (7154/75) [1978] European Commission on Human Rights.
Attorney General v Guardian Newspapers Ltd [1987] 1 WLR 1248.
Attorney General v Mulholland [1963] 2 QB 477.
B v B (A Minor) (Residence Order) [1992] 2 FLR 327.
B v B (Minors) (Residence and Care Disputes) [1994] 2 FLR 489.
B v Croydon HA [1995] 2 WLR 294.
B v United Kingdom (36536/02) [2005] All ER D 63.
Barnado v McHugh [1891] AC 388 (CA).
Barnett v Chelsea and Kensington Hospital Management Committee [1969] 1 QB 428 (QBD).
Blyth v Birmingham Waterworks [1856] 11 Exch. 781.
Blyth v Bloomsbury HA [1993] 4 Med LR 151.
Bolam v Friern HMC [1957] 1 WLR 582.
Bolitho v City and Hackney HA [1998] AC 232.
Bolton v Stone [1951] AC 850.
British Home Stores Ltd v Burchell [1980] ICR 303 (EAT).
Burke v GMC & others [2005] EWCA Civ 1003 (CA).
C and B (Children) (Care Order: Future Harm) [2000] 2 FCR 614.
C v C [1946] 1 All ER 562.
Camden LBC v R (A Minor) (Blood Transfusion) [1993] 2 FLR 757.
Canterbury v Spence, 464 F. 2d 772 – Court of Appeals, Dist. of Columbia Circuit 1972.
Caparo Industries Plc v Dickman [1992] 2 AC 605 (HL).
Centre for Reproductive Medicine v U [2002] EWCA Civ 565.
Chatterton v Gerson [1981] 1 All ER 257.
Cheshire West and Chester Council v P [2014] UKSC 19.
Chester v Afshar [2002] EWCA 724.
Ciarlariello v Schacter [1991] 2 Med. LR 391.
Ciarlariello v Schacter [1993] 2 SCR 119.
Coleman v Attridge Law [2008] ALL ER (EC) 1105.
Cornelius v De Taranto [2001] EWCA Civ 1511.
Council for the Regulation of Health Care Professionals v (1) The Nursing and Midwifery Council (2) Steven Truscott [2004] EWCA Civ 1356.
D v National Society for the Prevention of Cruelty to Children [1977] 2 WLR 201.
D v United Kingdom [1997] 24 EHRR 423.
Deacon v McVicar [1984] (Unreported Queens Bench Division 7th June).
Devi v West Midlands RHA [1981] EWHC 1980.
Dewen v Barnet Healthcare Trust and Barnet London Borough Council [2000] 2 FLR 848.
Donoghue v Stevenson [1932] AC 562.
Dugmore v Swansea NHS Trust [2002] EWCA Civ 1689.
Edwards v National Coal Board [1949] 1 KB 701.
F v West Berkshire HA [1990] 2 AC 1 (HL).
French v Chief Constable of Sussex [2006] EWCA Civ 312.
G V G (Minors: Custody Appeal) [1985] 1 WLR 647 (HL).
Gaskin v UK [1990] 1 FLR 167.
Gauntlett v Northampton HA [1985] 134 NLJ 623.
Gillick v West Norfolk and Wisbech AHA [1986] AC 112 (HL).
Glass v United Kingdom [2004] 1 FLR 1019.
Gold v Haringey HA [1987] 1 FLR 125.
Hall v Brooklands Auto Racing Club [1933] 1 KB 205.
Herczegfalvy v Austria [1993] (A/242B) 15 EHRR 437.
Hills v Potter [1983] 3 All ER 716.
HL v United Kingdom (45508/99) [2005] 40 EHRR 32.
Hucks v Cole [1968] 112 SJ 483 (CA).
Humberside County Council v B [1993] 1 FLR 257.
In the Estate of Park [1953] 2 All ER 1411.
J (A Minor) (Child in Care: Medical Treatment) [1993] Fam 15.
J (A Minor) (Prohibited Steps Order: Circumcision) [2000] 1 FLR 571.
J v C [1970] AC 668.
JD v East Berkshire Community Health NHS Trust [2003] EWCA Civ 1151.
John v Central Manchester and Manchester Children's University Hospitals NHS Foundation Trust [2016] EWHC 407 (QB).
KD (A Minor) (Ward: Termination of Access) [1988] AC 806 (HL).
Kent v Griffiths and Others [2000] 3 CLL Rep 98.

King v Sussex Ambulance NHS Trust [2002] EWCA Civ 953.
Knott v Newham Healthcare Trust [2003] EWCA Civ 771.
Lancashire County Council v W (A Child) (Care Orders: Significant Harm) [2000] 2 AC 147.
Lister v Romford Ice and Cold Storage Co Ltd [1957] AC 555.
London and Westcliff Properties v Minister of Housing and Local Government [1961] 1 All ER 610.
Margaret, Duchess of Argyll v Duke of Argyll [1967] Ch 302.
Marriott v West Midlands HA [1999] Lloyd's Rep Med 23.
Maynard v West Midlands RHA [1984] 1 WLR 634 (HL).
McLennan v Newcastle HA [1992] 3 Med LR 215.
Mohr v Williams [1905] 104 NW 12 (Minn).
Montgomery v Lanarkshire Health Board [2015] UKSC 11.
MS v UK 24527/08 [2012] ECHR 804 [2012] MHLO 46.
Nettleship v Weston [1971] QB 691 (CA).
Newcastle upon Tyne Hospitals Foundation Trust v LM [2014] EWHC 454 (COP).
NHS Trust A v M [2001] Fam 348.
A NHS Trust v MB and Mr & Mrs B [2006] EWHC 507.
An NHS Trust v Mr and Mrs H [2012] EWHC B18 (Fam).
Northamptonshire County Council v S [1993] Fam 136.
O'Brien v Cunard SS Co [1891] 28 NE 266.
P&Q (by their litigation friend, the Official Solicitor) v Surrey County Council [2014] UKSC 19.
Palmer v Tees HA [1999] Lloyds Medical Reports 151.
Pearce ex parte Pearce v United Bristol Healthcare NHS Trust CA [1996] EWCA Civ 878.
Potts v NWRHA [1983] QB 348.
Prendergast v Sam and Dee [1989] 1 Med LR 36.
Pretty v DPP [2001] UKHL 61.
Pretty v United Kingdom [2002] 2 FLR 45.
Prince Albert v Strange [1849] EWHC Ch J 20.
R (adult: medical treatment) [1996] 2 FLR 99.
R (Axon) v Secretary of State for Health [2006] EWHC 37.
R (Burke) v GMC and Others [2004] EWHC 1879 (Admin).
R (Burke) v GMC [2005] EWCA 1003.
R (H) v Mental Health Review Tribunal for North East London Region [2001] EWCA Civ 415.
R (Mahmood) v Secretary of State for the Home Department [2001] 1 WLR 840.
R (on the application of A and Others) v East Sussex County Council and Another [2003] EWHC 167.
R (on the application of C) v Secretary of State for the Home Department [2002] EWCA Civ 647.
R (on the application of N) v M [2002] EWCA Civ 1789.
R (on the application of Nicklinson) v Ministry of Justice [2014] UKSC 38.
R (on the application of Oliver Leslie Burke) (Respondent) v General Medical Council (Appellant) and The Disability Rights Commission and 8 Others (Interveners) [2005] EWCA Civ 1003.
R (on the application of PS) v RMO (DR G) and SOAD (DR W) [2003] EWHC 2335 QBD.
R (on the application of Purdy) v Director of Public Prosecutions [2009] UKHL 45.
R (on the application of S) v Plymouth City Council [2002] EWCA Civ 388.
R (on the application of SSG) v Liverpool City Council (1), Secretary of State for Health (2) and LS (Interested Party) [2002] (EWHC 22nd October).
R (on the application of Stennett) v Manchester City Council [2002] UKHL 34.
R (Philips) v NMC [2008] EWC 1698.
R (Robertson) v City of Wakefield Metropolitan Council [2002] 2 WLR 889.
R (Tagoe-Thompson) v Central and North West London Mental Health NHS Trust [2002] EWHC 2803 (Admin).
R v Adomako [1995] 1 AC 171 (HL).
R v Amaro [2015] (Nottingham Crown Court, 2 November).
R v B [2001] 1 Cr App R (S) 412.
R v Banu [1995] 16 Cr App R (S) 656.
R v Barraclough [1992] 13 Cr App R (S) 604.
R v Bateman [1925] Cr App R 8.
R v Bell [2001] 1 Cr App R 108.
R v Bigwood [2000] (Unreported July 24, 2000).
R v Bodkin Adams [1957] Crim LR 365.
R v Bourne [1939] 1 KB 687.
R v Collard [2002] EWCA Crim 2219.
R v Cox [1992] 12 BMLR 38.
R v Department of Health Ex p. Source Informatics Ltd (No. 1) [2001] QB 424.
R v Ealing District HA Exp. Fox [1993] 1 WLR 373.
R v G [1999] 2 Cr App R (S) 395.
R v Hampshire County Council [1999] 2 WLR 359.
R v Hinks [2001] 2 AC 241.
R v McShane [1977] Crim LR 737.
R v Mental Health Review Tribunal for South Thames Region Exp. Smith [1998] EGCS 55 (CA).
R v Misra and Srivastava [2004] EWCA Crim 2375.
R v Moor 2000 Crim LR 41.
R v Nicholson [2012] EWCA Crim 1568.
R v O [2005] EWCA Crim 3082.
R v Patel [2013] EWCA Crim 965.
R v Salisbury [2005] EWCA Crim 3107 (CA).
R v Smith [1979] Crim LR 251.
R v Stone & Dobinson [1977] QB 354.

R v Tabassum [2000] 2 Cr App R 328.
R v Williams [2004] (Unreported Llanelli Magistrates Court 24th November).
R v Woollin [1999] 1 AC 82 ((HL)).
Re AK (Adult Patient) (Medical Treatment: Consent) [2001] 1 FLR 129 (Fam Div).
Re B (A Child) [2003] EWCA Civ 1148 (CA).
Re B (A Minor) (Care Order: Criteria) [1993] 1 FLR 815.
Re B (A Minor) (Treatment and Secure Accommodation) [1997] 1 FLR 767.
Re B (A Minor) (Wardship: Medical Treatment) [1981] 1 WLR 1421.
Re B (Children) (Emotional Welfare: Interim Care Order) [2002] EWCA Civ 1225.
Re B (Minors) (Residence Order) [1992] Fam 162.
Re B (Consent to Treatment: Capacity) [2002] EWHC 429.
Re C (Adult: Refusal of Treatment) [1994] 1 WLR 290.
Re DH (A Minor) (Child Abuse) [1994] 1 FLR 679.
Re E (Children) (Care Proceedings: Social Work Practice) [2000] 2 FLR 254.
Re G (Children) (Same Sex Partner) [2006] EWCA Civ 372.
Re H (Minors) (Sexual Abuse: Standard of Proof) [1996] 1 FLR 80.
Re J [2000] 1 FLR 571 (Fam).
Re L (Care Proceedings: Disclosure to Third Party) [2000] 1 FLR 913.
Re L (Medical Treatment: Gillick Competence) [1998] 2 FLR 810.
Re M (A Child) (Refusal of Medical Treatment) [1999] 2 FLR 1097 (CA).
Re M (A Minor) (Care Order: Threshold Conditions) [1994] 2 FLR 577 (HL).
Re M (A Minor) (Medical Treatment) [1997] 2 FLR 1097.
Re MB (Caesarean Section) [1997] 2 FLR 426 (CA).
Re O (A Child) (Supervision Order: Future Harm) [2001] EWCA Civ 16.
Re O (A Minor) (Care Order: Education Procedure) [1992] 2 FLR 7.
Re P (A Minor) (1981) 80 LGR 301.
Re P (Adoption: Parental Agreement) [1985] FLR 365.
Re R (A Minor) (Wardship Consent to Treatment) [1992] Fam 1.
Re S (A Minor) (Custody) [1991] 2 FLR 388.
Re S (A Minor) (Representation) [1993] 2 WLR 801.
Re SKR [1994] CLY 1583.
Re T [1994] Times Law Report, 5 May.
Re T (Adult: Refusal of Treatment) [1992] 3 WLR.
Re T (A Minor) (Wardship: Medical Treatment) [1997] 1 WLR 242 (CA).
Re W (A Minor) (Medical Treatment Court's Jurisdiction) [1992] 3 WLR 758.
Re W (A Minor) (Residence Order) [1992] 2 FLR 332.
Re Wyatt (A Child) (Medical Treatment: Continuation of Order) [2005] EWCA Civ 1181.
Reibl v Hughes [1980] 2 S.C.R. 880.
Reid v United Kingdom [2003] 37 EHRR 9.
Reynolds v North Tyneside HA [2002] Lloyd's Rep Med 459.
Richards v Swansea NHS Trust [2007] EWHC 487.
Roe v Ministry of Health [1954] 2 QB 66 (CA).
Rogers v Whitaker [1992] HCA 58; 175 CLR 479.
Ross v Ryanair Ltd [2004] EWCA 1751.
S (A Child) v Newcastle and North Tyneside HA [2001] EWCA Civ 1868.
S (Children) (Care Order: Implementation of Care Plan) [2002] UKHL 10.
St George's Healthcare NHS Trust v S [1998] 3 WLR 936 (CA).
Saunders v Leeds Western HA [1993] 4 Med LR 355.
Schloendroff v Society of New York Hospitals [1914] 211 NY 125.
Selmouni v France [1998] 29 EHRR.
Sidaway v Bethlem Royal Hospital [1985] AC 871.
Smith v Brighton and Lewes Hospital Management Committee [1958] Times Law Reports, 2 May.
Stephens v Avery [1988] 2 WLR 1280.
Sutton v Population Services Family Planning Programme [1981] Times Law Report, 8 November (CA).
Tand v United Kingdom [1999] 7 BHRC 659.
Tanko v Finland [1994] 18 EHRR CD 179.
Tarasoff v Regents of the University of California [1976] 17 Cal 3d 425.
Tracey v Cambridge Uni Hospital NHS Foundation Trust and others [2014] EWCA Civ 822.
Tudor v Spen Corner Veterinary Centre [2006] Case No. 2404211/05 Employment Tribunal.
W v Egdell [1990] 2 WLR 471.
Williamson v East London and City HA [1998] Lloyd's Rep Med.
Wilsher v Essex HA [1988] AC 1074 (HL).
Wilson v Swanson [1956] 5 DLR (2d) 113 (Canadian Supreme Court).
Winspear v City Hospitals Sunderland NHSFT [2015] EWHC 3250.
Winterwerp v The Netherlands [1979] 2 EHRR 387.
Woolgar v Chief Constable of Sussex [2000] 1 WLR 25.
X v Liverpool City Council and the Chief Constable of Merseyside Police [2005] EWCA Civ 1173.
X *v Y and Others* [1988] 2 All ER 648.
Z v United Kingdom [2001] 2 FLR 612 (29392/95).

Table of statutes

Custody of Infants Act 1839
Matrimonial Causes Act 1857
Offences Against the Person Act 1861
Birth and Deaths Registration Act 1875

Lunacy Act 1890
Easter Act 1928
Mines and Quarries Act 1954
Agriculture (Safety, Health and Welfare Provisions) Act 1956
Housing Act 1957
Public Records Act 1958
Marriage Act 1960
Factories Act 1961
Suicide Act 1961
Offices, Shops and Railway Premises Act 1963
Nuclear Installations Act 1965
Abortion Act 1967
Theft Act 1968
Medicine Act 1968
Family Law Reform Act 1969
Mines and Quarries (Tips) Act 1969
European Community Act 1972
Health and Safety at Work etc., Act 1974
Sex Discrimination Act 1975
Race Relations Act 1976
Road Traffic Act 1981
Mental Health Act 1983
Representation of the People Act 1983
Public Health (Control of Disease) Act 1984
Valerie Mary Hill and Alan Monk (Marriage Enabling) Act 1985
Family Law Reform Act 1987
Road Traffic Act 1988
Children Act 1989
Access to Health Records Act 1990
NHS and Community Care Act 1990
Death With Dignity Act 1995 (ORS 127.800-995)
Disability Discrimination Act 1995
Nurses, Midwives and Health Visitors Act 1997
Data Protection Act 1998
Human Rights Act 1998
Crime and Disorder Act 1998
Public Interest Disclosure Act 1998
Health Act 1999
Adults with Incapacity (Scotland) Act 2000
Race Relations Amendment Act 2000
House of Lords Reform Act 2001
Anti-Terrorism, Crime and Security Act 2001
National Health Service Reform and Health Care Professions Act 2002
Children Act 2004
Mental Capacity Act 2005
Disability Discrimination Act 2005
Safeguarding Vulnerable Groups Act 2006
Mental Health Act 2007
Protection of Vulnerable Groups (Scotland) Act 2007
Health and Social Care Act 2008
Equality Act 2010
Protection of Freedoms Act 2012

Table of secondary legislation

Health and Safety (First Aid) Regulations 1981 (1981/917).
United Nations (1989) Convention on the Rights of the Child adopted under General Assembly Resolution 44/25.
Health and Safety (Display Screen Equipment) Regulations 1992 (1992/2792).
Manual Handling Operations Regulations 1992 (1992/2793).
Personal Protective Equipment at Work Regulations 1992 (1992/2966).
Workplace (Health, Safety and Welfare) Regulations 1992 (1992/3004).
Reporting of Injuries, Diseases and Dangerous Occurrences Regulations 1995 (1995/3163).
Health and Safety (Consultation with Employees) Regulations 1996 (1996/1513).
Health and Safety (Safety Signs and Signals) Regulations 1996 (1996/0341).
Fire Precautions (Workplaces) Regulations 1997 (1997/1840).
Safety Representatives and Safety Committee Regulations 1977 (1997/500).
Provision and Use of Work Equipment Regulations 1998 (1998/2306).
Health Service Commissioner (1999) *Inappropriate Response to Deterioration in the Condition of a Patient over the Weekend against Hastings and Rother NHS Trust – Case No. E.2291/98–99.*
Management of Health and Safety at Work Regulations 1999 (SI 1999/3242).
Control of Substances Hazardous to Health Regulations 2002 (SI 2002/2677).
Health Service (Control of Patient Information) Regulations 2002 (SI 2002/1438).
Nursing and Midwifery Order 2001 (SI 2002/253).
Police Act 1997 (Enhanced Criminal Record Certificates) (Protection of Vulnerable Adults) Regulations 2002 (SI 2002/446).
Medicines for Human Use (Clinical Trials) Regulations 2004 (SI 2004/1031).
Hazardous Waste (England and Wales) Regulations 2005 (SI 2005/894).
Medicines for Human Use (Prescribing) (Miscellaneous Amendments) Order 2006 (SI 2006/915).
Mental Health (Nurses) (England) Order 2008 (SI 2008/1207).

Adults With Incapacity (Scotland) Act 2000 Code Of Practice For Continuing And Welfare Attorneys SE/2001/90 2001.

The Adults with Incapacity (Supervision of Welfare Guardians etc. by Local Authorities) (Scotland) Regulations (2002/95) 2002.

Health and Social Care Act 2008 (Regulated Activities) Regulations 2014 (SI 2014/2936).

The Mental Capacity (Deprivation of Liberty: Standard Authorisations, Assessments and Ordinary Residence) Regulations 2008 (2008/100).

Health and Social Care Act 2008 (Regulated Activities) Regulations 2010.

The Mental Health (Wales) Measure 2010.

National Health Service (Concerns, Complaints and Redress Arrangements) (Wales) Regulations 2011 (SI 2011/704(W108)).

The Mental Health (Independent Mental Health Advocates) (Wales) Regulations 2011.

Health and Safety (Sharp Instruments in Healthcare) Regulations 2013.

Introduction

The position of the patient in healthcare is now more legalised than ever before. About a billion pounds are paid in compensation to patients for the harm they suffered when under the care of the National Health Service. In 2014–15 the regulatory body for nursing, the Nursing and Midwifery Council (NMC, 2015b), removed some 493 nurses and midwives from the professional register because their fitness to practise was impaired. A wide range of laws regulate the relationship between the nurse and patient and that relationship is changing. The law now places greater emphasis on partnership working with patients which is replacing the paternalistic nurse knows best approach. Laws are in place to ensure public trust and confidence in the profession. To maintain that confidence new laws and regulations continue to be introduced by the government in response to a changing health service and to ensure maximum protection for the patients in your care.

The NMC has established standards of competence to be met by applicants to different parts of the register, and these are the standards it considers necessary for safe and effective practice. This book is structured so that it will help you to understand and meet the competencies required for entry to the NMC register. The relevant competencies are presented at the start of each chapter so that you can clearly see which ones the chapter addresses.

Chapter 1 introduces you to the legal system and provides you with the essential building blocks for understanding where laws come from, how laws develop through cases that come before the courts and how to locate, read and interpret the different types of law that affect your future role as a registered nurse. By closely reading and following the activities in this chapter you will begin to develop a legal awareness that will underpin your nurse education.

Mere knowledge of the law is not enough to enable you to practise safely as a registered nurse. As a student nurse you must also learn how to apply the law in an ethical and principled way. During your time as a student nurse you will face dilemmas that affect your practice, such as when, if ever, it is right to disclose information about a patient to another person. Chapter 2 considers principled decision-making in nursing and provides you with a framework to enable you to make decisions that are morally acceptable and ethically right while highlighting when it might be necessary to seek the approval of the court for your actions.

These two chapters cover fundamental topics that underpin a registered nurse's relationship with their patients, profession and society, making them essential reading for you and all student nurses. The legal and professional principles considered in these chapters will guide you through the complex legal problems you are likely to encounter in your career as a registered nurse. For example, you will see how a legal standard of care is imposed on you through the law of negligence; how laws such as the Human Rights Act 1998, Mental Health Act 1983 and Mental Capacity Act 2005 protect vulnerable adults; and how the Children Act 1989 safeguards children. You are given the opportunity to apply the laws discussed in these chapters to your own practice through guided activities designed to consolidate your knowledge and assist you with assignment preparation and writing.

Chapter 3: Professionalism is a fundamental concept crucial to the protection of the public and individual patients, particularly where they are vulnerable adults or children. It is essential that the term is clearly understood by student nurses as it is the means by which the law imposes standards and boundaries on professional practice. This chapter highlights how nurses are answerable and accountable for their actions by elements of criminal, civil and contract law. The chapter then considers the role of professional regulation in protecting the public from nurses whose fitness to practise is called into question.

Understanding the concept of professionalism is essential for student nurses who must demonstrate their fitness to practise in order to become registered nurses subject to *The Code: Professional standards of practice and behaviour for nurses and midwives* (NMC, 2015a).

Chapter 4: Equality and human rights. Student nurses must ensure their practice respects the rights, dignity and freedoms of others and recognises the health needs of the diverse cultures that make up the population of the United Kingdom. This chapter considers how the law promotes equality and human rights in the health service and emphasises the duty of registered nurses to ensure that they do not discriminate on the grounds of race or disability when caring for patients.

The chapter stresses the important role of human rights in healthcare and how it underpins the dignity and compassion that lie at the heart of your practice as a student nurse.

Chapter 5: Consent to treatment. Nursing care is delivered in a very hands-on way and, as a student nurse, you will regularly need to touch your patients in order to examine them or provide treatment. Student nurses must ensure that any touching is lawful and appropriate, and the chapter considers how the law promotes the autonomy of an adult patient and what constitutes a real consent. It then discusses how the provisions of the Mental Capacity Act 2005 protect vulnerable adults and young persons by regulating how decisions can be made for those who lack capacity to make a decision about the care and treatment they require. The chapter ends by considering when it is lawful to withdraw or withhold treatment from a patient and your duty to support patients through end of life care.

Chapter 6: Mental health. The position of the patient with mental health problems is now regulated by a number of laws that seek to protect those adults and children considered to be vulnerable in our society.

You will care for people with mental health problems regardless of the branch speciality you have chosen to follow. It is essential, then, that as a student nurse you understand the key provisions of the Mental Health Act 1983 as amended by the Mental Health Act 2007, and the strong body of case law that has developed from it dealing with fundamental issues of liberty, autonomy and respect.

This chapter emphasises that when caring for a person with mental health problems it is essential that, as a nurse, you not only apply the requirements of the legislation accurately but do so ethically and with due regard for the rights of the vulnerable patients in your care.

Chapter 7: Protecting the vulnerable adult. As a student nurse you will learn to provide nursing care to people in hospital and the community with disability and illness and who, by reason of mental or other disability, age or illness, are unable to take care of themselves or protect themselves from significant harm or serious exploitation.

It is vital that you are able to identify such vulnerable adults and are able to recognise signs of abuse and what action to take if you suspect abuse.

Chapter 8: Consent and children. This chapter focuses on the issue of consent to examination and treatment in relation to children, and follows the law as it changes to take account of the development of the child to adulthood. Consent is considered in relation to a child of tender years, a Gillick-competent child and the 16- and 17-year-old child. As with adult patients, a nurse who provides care or treatment without consent will be held accountable, so it is essential that as a student nurse you are familiar with the requirements for a lawful consent from a child.

Chapter 9: Safeguarding children. Nurses have a key role in the identification of children who may have been abused or who are at risk of abuse. Nurses are also well placed to recognise when parents or other adults have problems that might affect their capacity to fulfil their roles with children safely. It is vital, therefore, that student nurses develop a sound working knowledge of the Children Acts of 1989 and 2004 and know when to refer a child for help as a 'child in need' and how to act on concerns that a child is at risk of significant harm through abuse or neglect.

Chapter 10: Negligence. Negligence is the civil law's way of imposing a standard of care on nurses, requiring them to be careful when caring for patients.

This chapter considers the extent of a nurse's duty of care towards their patients and why it is essential for student nurses to provide care and treatment that is evidence based and research driven in order to meet their legal duty.

It goes on to discuss negligence as a criminal act through a discussion of the offence of gross negligence manslaughter.

Chapter 11: Record keeping is a fundamental skill that must be developed to a consistently high standard by student nurses. Records outline the care given to patients and must be sufficiently detailed to show that students and nurses have discharged their legal and professional obligations. This chapter considers the importance of record keeping and how student nurses should write records to ensure that the legal requirements are met. By drawing on case law it also highlights the consequences for nurses of failing to meet those requirements.

Chapter 12: Confidentiality. Maintaining the confidentiality of a patient's health information is a fundamental element of professional conduct for all registered nurses and is one of the key standards imposed on student nurses by the NMC through their student guide to professional conduct. This is because the relationship between nurse and patient is essential for proper assessment and care that is largely based on a patient's personal history of their health problem. Patients pass on sensitive information in confidence and expect you to respect their privacy by ensuring the confidentiality of the information they give. The dilemma you face is that the duty of confidentiality is not absolute and there are exceptions to the rule. It is essential that as a student nurse you learn when the general requirement to maintain the confidentiality of patient information can be overridden and information about a person can be properly disclosed to another.

Social media has given rise to new challenges relating to confidentiality, and a new section on this topic has been added for this edition.

Chapter 13: Health and safety. From the very outset of your nurse education your safety and the safety of the patients in your care will be the major concern of your university and clinical placement area. They have obligations under the law to protect your health and safety, and you have a duty to look after your health and safety and that of your patients. You must be able to apply in practice the legal duties imposed on nurses under the Health and Safety at Work Act 1974 and its regulations.

Throughout the book you will find activities in the text that will help you to make sense of, and learn about, the material being presented by the authors. Some activities ask you to reflect on aspects of practice, or your experience of it, or the people or situations you encounter. *Reflection* is an essential skill in nursing, and it helps you to understand the world around you and often to identify how things might be improved. Other activities will help you develop key skills, such as your ability to *think critically* about a topic in order to challenge received wisdom, or your ability to *research a topic and find appropriate information and evidence*, and to be able to make decisions using that evidence in situations that are often difficult and time-pressured. Finally, communication and working as part of a team are core to all nursing practice, and some activities will ask you to carry out *group activities* or think about *communication skills* to help develop these.

All the activities require you to take a break from reading the text, think through the issues presented and carry out some independent study, possibly using the internet. Where appropriate, there are sample answers presented at the end of each chapter, and these will help you to understand more fully your own reflections and independent study. Remember, academic study will always require independent work; attending lectures will never be enough to be successful on your programme, and these activities will help to deepen your knowledge and understanding of the issues under scrutiny and give you practice at working on your own.

You might want to think about completing the activities as part of your personal development plan (PDP) or portfolio. After completing each activity, write it up in your PDP or portfolio in a section devoted to that particular skill, then look back over time to see how far you have developed. You can also do more of the activities for a key skill that you have identified a weakness in, which will increase your skill and confidence in this area.

Chapter 1
Introduction to law in nursing

NMC Standards for Pre-registration Nursing Education

This chapter will address the following competencies:

Domain 1: Professional values

1. All nurses must practise with confidence according to *The Code: Professional standards of practice and behaviour for nurses and midwives* (NMC, 2015a), and within other recognised ethical and legal codes frameworks.

Chapter aims

By the end of this chapter you will be able to:

- define the term law;
- identify primary and secondary sources of legal material;
- outline the role of Acts of Parliament;
- state the role of precedent at common law;
- list the key features of a published Act, Statutory Instrument and Case Report;
- describe the relevance of law to healthcare.

Introduction

This chapter examines how the law influences nursing. It begins by highlighting that the Nursing and Midwifery Council's (NMC) *Code* (2015a), which sets out the standards for professional practice, is underpinned by the law. The chapter then defines the term 'law' and considers how laws are made by looking at the role of Parliament and the courts. You are then introduced to the published forms of law and are encouraged to become familiar with the main features of an Act of Parliament, a Statutory Instrument and a Case Report. Finally, the chapter highlights the benefits of legal awareness to a student nurse.

A book on law and professional issues in nursing may seem an unusual collection of topics for a course of study that will largely focus on meeting the needs of individuals with various health problems. Why is it necessary for you to study law and ethics when you want to devote your time to the study of nursing and caring for patients?

The reality is that law is now fundamental to the study of nursing and underpins your relationship with the profession and with your patients. It seeks to provide maximum protection for patients by setting the standards for care, punishing unprofessional behaviour and providing redress to patients who have suffered as a result of a nurse's acts or omissions. The law informs nursing at every stage and it is essential that you understand and are able to critically reflect on the legal issues relevant to nursing practice.

You will see in Chapter 3 that the concept of professionalism requires you to be law abiding, of good character and to apply the knowledge, skills and values expected of a registered nurse. Failing to discharge that professionalism will result in legal sanctions being applied to protect the public and maintain confidence in the nursing profession.

The professional practitioner

Case study 1.1: Professionalism in action

A children's nurse who stole insulin and injected herself when she was meant to be looking after sick babies was struck off the NMC's register and prosecuted for theft as a result of her unprofessional behaviour. The nurse fell so ill after taking the insulin that she had to be treated at the emergency department and was kept overnight for observation.

(Scottish Star, *2013)*

To maintain public confidence in the profession of nursing all registered nurses are legally and professionally answerable for their actions, irrespective of whether they are following the instructions of another or using their own initiative. Healthcare litigation is growing and patients are increasingly prepared to assert their legal rights. Compensation payments for clinical negligence in the National Health Service (NHS) are currently running at some £1.23 billion a year (NHS LA, 2015).

Whilst the financial burden of compensation on the NHS is considerable the cost of unprofessional behaviour in human terms has been even greater.

A public inquiry into the care of patients at Mid Staffordshire NHS Foundation Trust found that up to 1200 patients had died needlessly as a result of staff and management failings between January 2005 and March 2009. The inquiry report (known as the Francis report) found that:

- Patients were left in excrement in soiled bed clothes for lengthy periods.
- Assistance was not provided with feeding for patients who could not eat without help.

- Water was left out of reach.
- In spite of persistent requests for help, patients were not assisted in their toileting.
- Wards and toilet facilities were left in a filthy condition.
- Privacy and dignity, even in death, were denied.
- Triage in A&E was undertaken by untrained staff.
- Staff treated patients and those close to them with callous indifference.

(House of Commons, 2013)

The recommendations of the Francis report (2013) and of three further inquiries into how unprofessional behaviour resulted in poor care and unnecessary patient deaths (Andrews and Butler, 2014; National Advisory Group on the Safety of Patients in England, 2013; DH, 2012b) have resulted in fundamental changes to the statutory regulation of health services, the professional regulation of nurses and law protecting patients.

It is little wonder that the NMC insists that student nurses are able to practise in accordance with an ethical and legal framework that ensures that the interests of patients are paramount (NMC, 2010). A thorough and critical appreciation of the legal, ethical and professional issues affecting nursing practice is essential if you are to develop the professional awareness necessary to satisfy the NMC that you are an accountable practitioner, competent to practise as a registered nurse.

Activity 1.1 — *Professional standards of behaviour*

The standards imposed on registered nurses by the NMC are contained in *The Code: Professional standards of practice and behaviour for nurses and midwives* (NMC, 2015a).

Read *The Code,* which can be downloaded from the NMC website at **www.nmc-uk.org**, and identify the standards that apply to:

- your relationship with patients;
- your relationship with colleagues;
- your relationship with the profession;
- your relationship with society generally.

The Code highlights how the law and legal system underpins the professional standards imposed on nurses. Keep it with you as you work through this book.

The Code requires registered nurses to discharge their professionalism by keeping to and upholding the standards and values set out in *The Code,* acting with honesty and integrity at all times and keeping to the laws of the country in which they are practising (NMC 2015a, standard 20). To achieve that standard student nurses must be able to define and apply the law as it relates to their practice.

Defining law

Activity 1.2 *Reflection*

Before reading on, think about the laws you are aware of and what their role is; then write down what you believe the term 'law' means.

Now read the following for further guidance.

A typical dictionary would define law as

> *a rule enacted or customary in a community and recognised as commanding or forbidding certain actions;*

or

> *a body of such rules.*

A key characteristic of law is that it is perceived as binding upon the community The English word 'law' is derived from the Old Norse *lagu* meaning 'laid down' or 'fixed'. The definition suggests that law is made up of rules, but is it the case that all rules have legal force?

Activity 1.3 *Reflection*

Consider the following rules – which of these rules do you think are laws?

- Honour your mother and father.
- Do not steal.
- Be truthful in all circumstances.
- Do not kill other people.
- Rescue your neighbour's drowning child.
- Register a child's birth.
- Do not park on double yellow lines.

See below for an explanation of the rules.

Positive rules

Positive rules impose a legal obligation to do or refrain from doing something. If a positive rule is breached, a sanction may be imposed for breaking the law.

Normative rules

Normative rules set out what a person should do, or what they should refrain from doing. Note the word *should* – the individual is not compelled to abide by normative rules, they simply ought to. Normative rules are based on values that highlight a desired form of conduct but they do not carry legal force.

In the last activity the positive rules were as follows:

- Do not kill other people – it is a common law offence to kill other people; that is the offence of murder.
- Do not park on double yellow lines – parking on double yellow lines constitutes a road traffic offence.
- Do not steal – stealing is an offence under the Theft Act 1968.
- Register a child's birth – an example of the law requiring a particular action, in this case under the Birth and Deaths Registration Act 1875.

The normative rules were as follows:

- Honour your mother and father – this is established through religious teachings and reflects the fifth commandment of the Ten Commandments. It is not a requirement of the law in the UK.
- Be truthful in all circumstances – veracity is a moral or ethical issue. The need to be truthful in law occurs in specific circumstances such as when giving evidence under oath.
- Rescue your neighbour's drowning child – there is generally no duty of simple rescue in the UK. If you had a professional duty such as being a lifeguard at a swimming pool, you would be legally obliged to rescue the child.

In some cases the law requires that a person take action, for example the requirement that a child's birth be registered. However, in most cases the law requires a person to refrain from doing something, for example from killing others, parking on double yellow lines or stealing.

Relevance to healthcare

In healthcare we see a drawing together of normative and positive rules. The law imposes a minimum standard of acceptable care and behaviour on you as a registered nurse. Patients, however, deserve the highest possible standard of care and behaviour, so the health and social care organisations where you work and the profession, through *The Code* (2015), require a standard that is higher than the law expects.

The Code is underpinned by a shared set of values common to all United Kingdom (UK) healthcare regulatory bodies. In a clear drawing together of both normative and positive rules, it requires that as a registered nurse you:

- prioritise people;
- practise effectively;
- preserve safety;
- promote professionalism and trust.

During your training as a student nurse you will be expected to live up to the standards of the NMC's *Code* and the law and professional issues that underpin them. Higher education institutions have fitness to practise panels where students who are accused of falling below the standards required of them are held to account. The decisions of the panels are based on the fitness to practise guidance espoused by *The Code* and includes academic integrity.

Case study 1.2: Plagerism leads to six-month suspension from the professional register

A nurse who copied, verbatim, whole passages from a published article and passed it off as his own work in an assignment as part of a nursing degree accepted a six-month suspension from the professional register after admitting that his actions were unprofessional and dishonest.

(NMC, 2015b)

Criminal and civil law

The same unlawful action can be dealt with in different ways by the law. For example, touching a person without permission – that is, without consent – can be both a crime and a *tort* – a civil wrong.

The crime might be charged under the Offences Against the Person Act 1861. This very old statute is still very much in force today and forbids many forms of unlawful touching, such as actual bodily harm (section 47), wounding (sections 18 and 20) or even procuring a miscarriage (section 58). A crime is an act that is capable of being followed by criminal proceedings and with an outcome, an acquittal or a conviction that is criminal in nature.

Unlawful touching can also be pursued through the civil courts as the tort of trespass to the person. The law of tort is primarily concerned with providing a remedy, by way of compensation, to persons who have been harmed by the conduct of others.

The nature of law

From our discussion of the law we can define law as

> *a rule of human conduct imposed upon and enforced among the members of a given state.*

Two ideas underpin this notion of the law:

- **order**, in the sense that there is a method or legal system that underpins the creation and implementation of the law; and
- **compulsion**, or the enforcement of obedience to the rules that are laid down by the law.

Sources of legal material

In your study of the law as it applies to healthcare and nursing, you will use a range of primary and secondary sources of law to inform your practice and your studies. Figure 1.1 highlights the typical sources of primary and secondary legal material that you can use in your studies.

Sources of primary legal material

Although there are many textbooks and periodicals that discuss legal issues in nursing, it is best whenever possible to study the primary legal material as well. This will give you a detailed understanding of the law as it relates to nursing.

There are three major sources of primary legal material, as follows.

1. Legislation

- Acts of Parliament that may also be referred to as statute law or *lex scripta* (written law).
- Secondary legislation:
    - Statutory Instruments, which are also known as delegated legislation and subordinate legislation.

2. Judicial decisions

These are decisions from cases decided in court, and are also known as the common law or *lex non scripta* (unwritten law from judges).

3. European Community and Human Rights law

Parliament has allowed these areas to be sources of law by incorporating them through Acts of Parliament (the European Community Act 1972 and the Human Rights Act 1998).

Other sources of law and influences on judges are as follows.

Royal Prerogative

The Royal Prerogative used to be the main source of law before the development of the parliamentary system in the UK. It now describes the powers, handed down direct from monarchs to ministers over many years, that allow governments, among other things, to go to war, regulate the Civil Service, issue passports and grant honours, all without any need for approval from Parliament. As these powers have been handed down over many centuries new powers cannot be created.

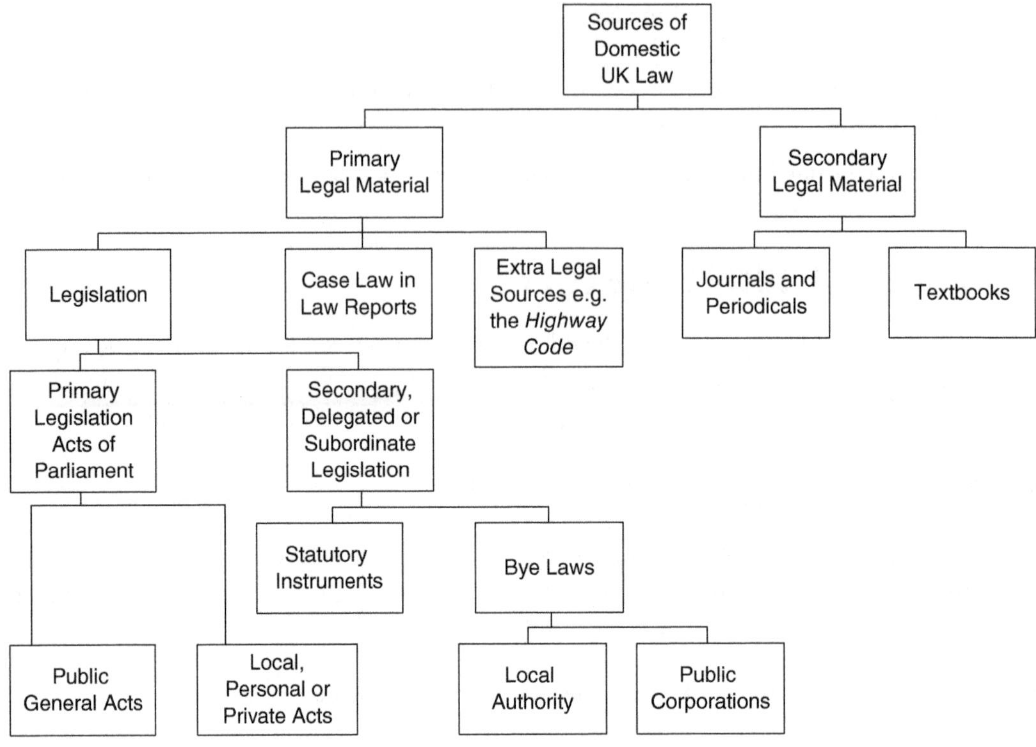

Figure 1.1: Sources of legal material.

When having to consider a novel dispute or how to apply an ancient law to a modern situation, judges may take account of extra legal sources to assist them.

Received wisdom

- Legal writers: The law is extensively analysed and tested by academics and practitioners, and judges often resort to such analysis to assist them when having to decide a novel or complex case.
- Public opinion: In *Gillick v West Norfolk and Wisbech AHA* [1986], a case concerning the lawfulness of giving contraceptive treatment to girls under the age of 16, the House of Lords heard an appeal from the Court of Appeal, which had made a decision relying on a seventeenth-century precedent. Lord Scarman, in his opinion, said that part of the court's function was to reflect public opinion and to bring the law kicking and screaming into the twentieth century.

Codes and best practice

Judges will also refer to extra legal sources of law that bring together normative and positive rules and signal best practice in a particular area. For example, where a judge has to decide if a nurse's conduct is acceptable, then he or she will refer to the NMC's *Code* (2015). In a road traffic case the judge will refer to the *Highway Code.* These sources are only ever persuasive on a judge, who is not bound by them.

Case study 1.3: The definition of a patient

In R (Phillips) v NMC *[2008], a nurse who had been struck off for an inappropriate relationship with a client argued that, once a personal relationship had begun to form, he arranged for a colleague to take on the woman's case and so she was no longer a client of his.*

When considering the definition of a patient in this case the court relied on the best practice guidance issued by the United Kingdom Central Council for Nursing and Midwifery in a booklet entitled Practitioner–client relationships and the prevention of abuse *(NMC, 2002). This stated that the term 'client' was used throughout the document and referred to all groups and individuals who have direct or indirect contact with registered nurses, midwives or health visitors in a professional capacity.*

From this definition the court was satisfied that the woman remained a client as she was being cared for by the same team and so had indirect contact with the nurse. The court upheld the striking off order.

Legislation

The UK is a parliamentary democracy and the laws of the country are created and amended through the Queen in Parliament. That is, a new law or bill is considered, debated and scrutinised by the elected House of Commons and appointed House of Lords before receiving Royal Assent and becoming an Act of Parliament.

The Acts you are concerned with in your studies are *public general Acts*. These apply to classes or sub-classes of people. For example, the Mental Health Act 1983 (as amended) concerns the care and treatment of people with mental disorder; the Children Act 1989 is concerned with the welfare of children.

You will not be concerned with *private Acts*, which have a much narrower application and concern local issues and persons. For example, a private Act of Parliament, the Valerie Mary Hill and Alan Monk (Marriage Enabling) Act 1985, was passed to allow a man to marry his ex-wife's mother (his mother-in-law) – an action that was generally forbidden by the Marriage Act 1960.

The function of Acts

Acts of Parliament are generally created to fulfil one of five main purposes.

Revision of substantive rules of law

The laws of the UK need to be kept up to date and Acts are created to modernise existing law in order to bring it into line with modern society. A body known as the Law Commission keeps law under review and makes suggestions for reform. These are not always acted upon in a timely manner, however. For example, a Law Commission report (Law Commission, 1993) into decision-making for incapable adults, submitted in 1993, eventually resulted in the Mental Capacity Act 2005.

Consolidation of Acts

Laws build up in a piecemeal fashion over many years and there is often a need to consolidate different parts of a law into one Act of Parliament. For example, the Health and Safety at Work etc. Act 1974 consolidated several other Acts concerning safety in the workplace, including the Mines and Quarries Act 1954, the Agriculture (Safety, Health and Welfare Provisions) Act 1956, the Factories Act 1961, the Offices, Shops and Railway Premises Act 1963, the Nuclear Installations Act 1965 and the Mines and Quarries (Tips) Act 1969.

Codification

Codification means putting a rule of the common law into statute law. Where a decision in a case is considered fundamental or very important, Parliament will codify it by making the rule part of an Act. For example, in *R v Bourne* [1939], a surgeon was acquitted of procuring a miscarriage by abortion when a jury decided that doing so to preserve the mental and physical health of the mother was lawful. When the Abortion Act 1967 was enacted, Parliament codified that decision under section 1(1) of the 1967 Act.

Collection of revenue

Taxation is a function of Acts. Each year the government presents its budget to Parliament, which allows the raising of revenue through taxation.

Social legislation

This is a broad category that covers the many facets of running the country. It is the main area of party political differences and the main source of debate in Parliament.

How a bill becomes an Act of Parliament

There are many stages that a bill has to go through before it can become an Act of Parliament (see Figure 1.2).

Manifesto

All political parties have a manifesto, which is their promise to the electorate of the actions they will take and the laws they will pass if they become the government. It is these promises that persuade us to vote for a party.

Not all such promises become law, because when a party takes office they are supplied with detailed information by senior civil servants and may discover that the reforms are not realistic, or are too expensive.

Other laws enacted during a government's term of office will be a reaction to an event, such as a war, or a ruling by the courts. In 2005, a man argued that having to ask for a private Act to

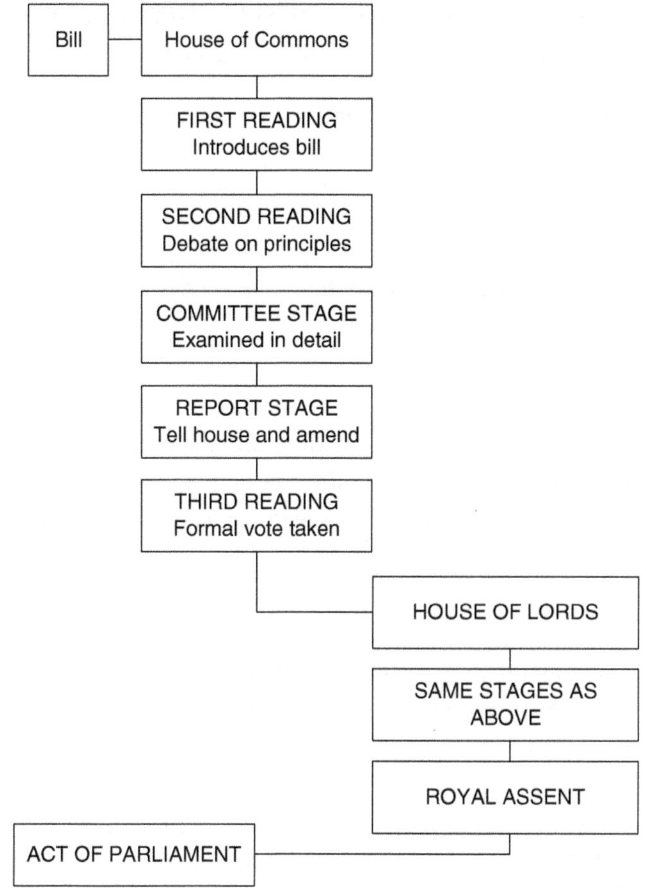

Figure 1.2: Stages of a bill.

be allowed to marry his former daughter-in-law was a violation of his human rights and the government was forced to change the law to bring it into line with the Human Rights Act 1998 (*B v United Kingdom (36536/02)* [2005]).

Queen's Speech

The Queen's Speech at the State Opening of Parliament in November announces the main bills constituting the government's legislative programme. The government actually writes the speech for the Queen to read.

Green Papers and White Papers

Green Papers are consultation papers that seek comments from the public. The importance of consultation was seen when Tony Blair attempted to abolish the role of the Lord Chancellor without first consulting anyone. He then discovered that this could not happen without first changing over 500 statutes that referred to the functions of the Lord Chancellor.

Following the Green Paper, the government will present to Parliament a White Paper, which is a statement of policy and contains definite proposals for legislation.

After consultation, Parliamentary Counsel (Draftsmen) will draft a bill into the form of words necessary for a bill.

Bills

In order to become an Act of Parliament, a bill must be passed by both Houses of Parliament and receive Royal Assent (collectively known as 'the Queen in Parliament').

First reading

The first reading of a bill involves a member reading the title of the bill. The first reading takes place without debate and is essentially an announcement that the bill has been introduced, after which copies of the bill are made available for members to read and are placed on the Parliament website.

Second reading

The second reading provides the first occasion for debate on the general principles of a bill, and then detailed discussion takes place during the committee stage.

Committee stage

When a bill has passed its second reading in the House of Commons, it is then referred to a General Committee. The Committee examines the clauses of the bill line by line, word by word, and detailed amendments are considered.

Report stage

Any amendments made during the committee stage must be approved or rejected by the whole House during the report stage, which is a detailed debate where further amendments may be moved.

Third reading

The third reading of a bill often follows on immediately after the report stage. The bill is reviewed in its final form, including amendments made at earlier stages. Then the final version of the bill is approved and passed by hand – bound in green ribbon – to the Lords. When the Lords return the bill it is bound in red ribbon.

In the House of Lords, broadly the same procedure is followed.

Once all stages have been completed the bill receives Royal Assent and becomes an Act (see Figure 1.3). The date of Royal Assent is not necessarily the date the Act comes into force. Many Acts begin at a later date with the issuing of a commencement order. For example, the part of the NHS and Community Care Act 1990 that introduced the notion of the NHS Trust did not commence until 1993. The Easter Act 1928, which sets Easter on a specific date, has never come into force.

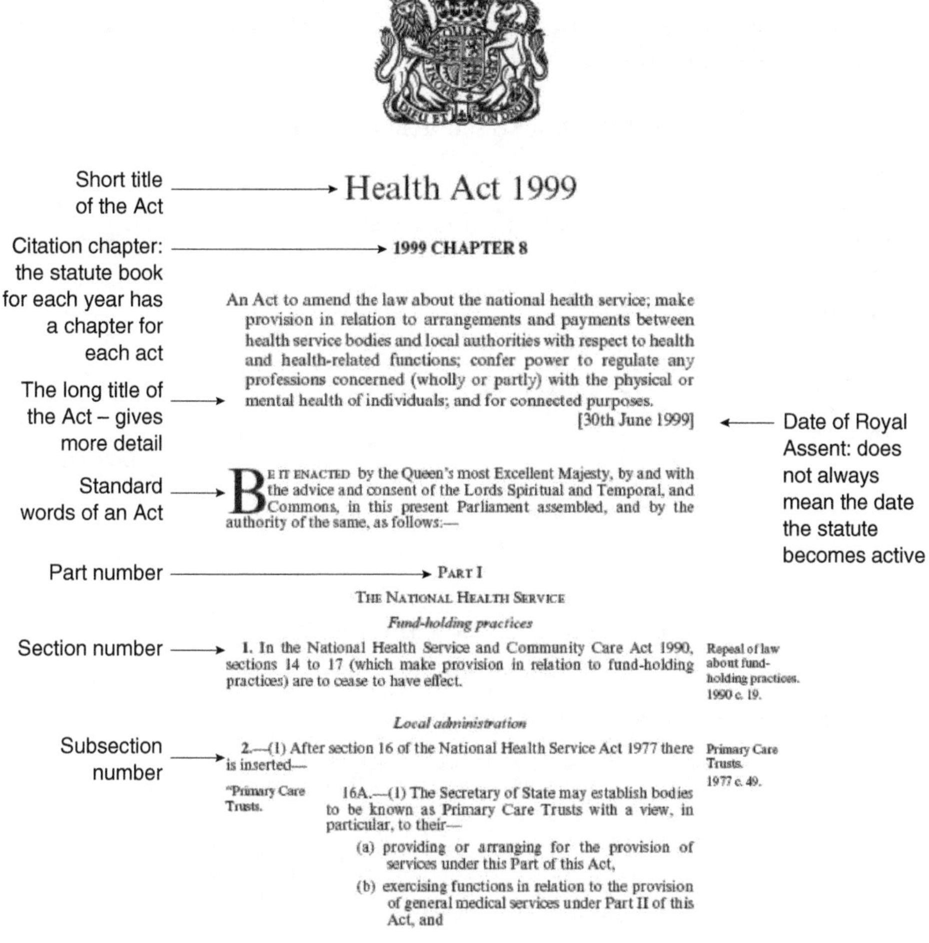
ELIZABETH II c. 8

Health Act 1999

1999 CHAPTER 8

An Act to amend the law about the national health service; make provision in relation to arrangements and payments between health service bodies and local authorities with respect to health and health-related functions; confer power to regulate any professions concerned (wholly or partly) with the physical or mental health of individuals; and for connected purposes.
[30th June 1999]

BE IT ENACTED by the Queen's most Excellent Majesty, by and with the advice and consent of the Lords Spiritual and Temporal, and Commons, in this present Parliament assembled, and by the authority of the same, as follows:—

PART I

THE NATIONAL HEALTH SERVICE

Fund-holding practices

1. In the National Health Service and Community Care Act 1990, sections 14 to 17 (which make provision in relation to fund-holding practices) are to cease to have effect. Repeal of law about fund-holding practices. 1990 c. 19.

Local administration

2.—(1) After section 16 of the National Health Service Act 1977 there is inserted— Primary Care Trusts. 1977 c. 49.

"Primary Care Trusts. 16A.—(1) The Secretary of State may establish bodies to be known as Primary Care Trusts with a view, in particular, to their—

(a) providing or arranging for the provision of services under this Part of this Act,

(b) exercising functions in relation to the provision of general medical services under Part II of this Act, and

Figure 1.3: The first page of a public general Act, with its constituent parts labelled.

Secondary legislation

With the rigorous scrutiny that bills must undergo, only some 50 Acts are passed by Parliament each year. It is therefore not uncommon for an Act to give powers to government ministers and other public bodies to introduce secondary legislation that enables general updating of the law. Secondary legislation, also sometimes called subordinate legislation, is generally in the form of a *Statutory Instrument* and includes regulations and orders. For example, the Medicines for Human Use (Clinical Trials) Regulations 2004 set the requirements for testing new medicines, while the Medicines for Human Use (Prescribing) (Miscellaneous Amendments) Order 2006 introduced independent and supplementary prescribing of medicines by nurses and other health professionals.

Some 5,000 Statutory Instruments are approved by Parliament each year. An important Statutory Instrument affecting nursing is the Nursing and Midwifery Order 2001, which established the NMC. The order was created under powers given by section 60 of the Health Act 1999. Where a minister or public body acts contrary to the powers bestowed by an Act, their decision can be challenged as *ultra vires*. For example, in *London and Westcliff Properties v Minister of Housing and Local Government* [1961], a council compulsorily purchased a property, then sold it to a company at a reduced cost. The court held that this was *ultra vires*, as the Housing Act 1957 required councils to obtain the best possible price for a property.

The annotated first page of the 2001 Order is shown in Figure 1.4.

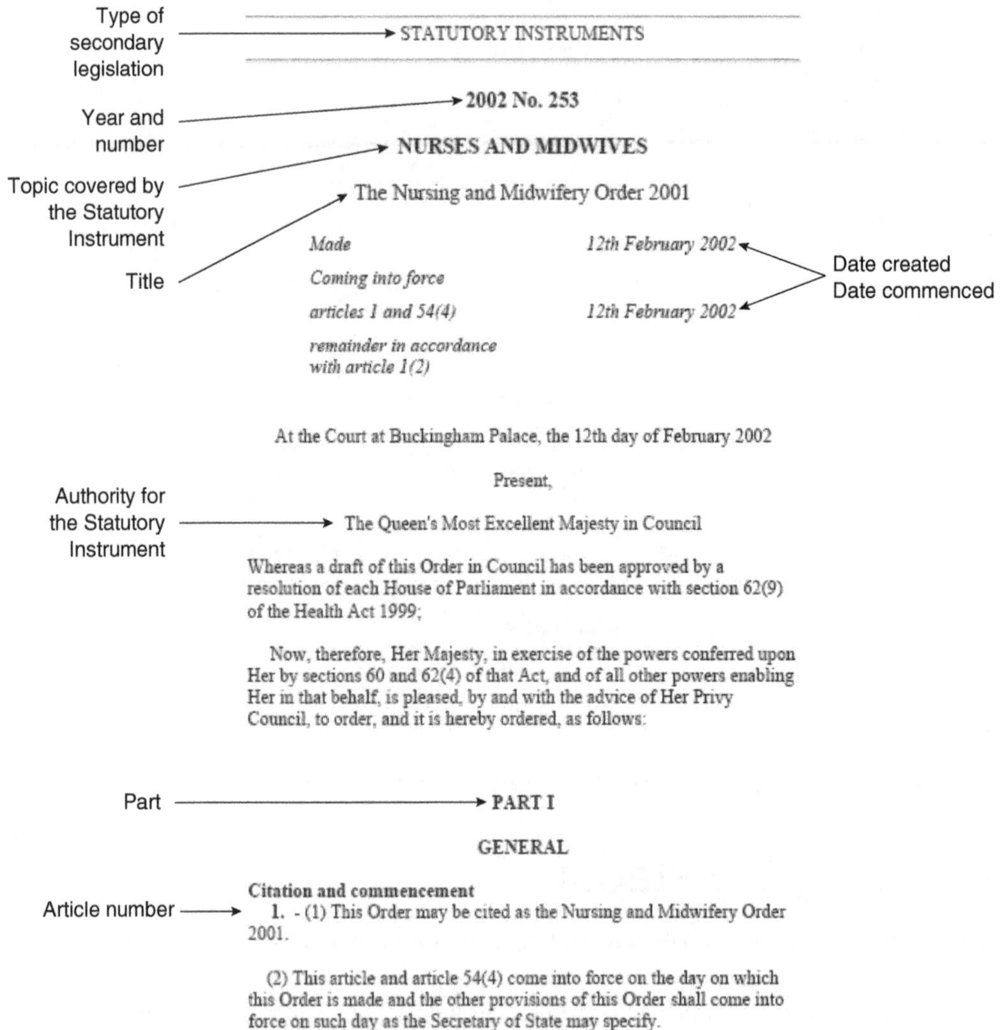

STATUTORY INSTRUMENTS

2002 No. 253

NURSES AND MIDWIVES

The Nursing and Midwifery Order 2001

Made — *12th February 2002*

Coming into force

articles 1 and 54(4) — *12th February 2002*

remainder in accordance with article 1(2)

At the Court at Buckingham Palace, the 12th day of February 2002

Present,

The Queen's Most Excellent Majesty in Council

Whereas a draft of this Order in Council has been approved by a resolution of each House of Parliament in accordance with section 62(9) of the Health Act 1999;

Now, therefore, Her Majesty, in exercise of the powers conferred upon Her by sections 60 and 62(4) of that Act, and of all other powers enabling Her in that behalf, is pleased, by and with the advice of Her Privy Council, to order, and it is hereby ordered, as follows:

PART I

GENERAL

Citation and commencement

1. - (1) This Order may be cited as the Nursing and Midwifery Order 2001.

(2) This article and article 54(4) come into force on the day on which this Order is made and the other provisions of this Order shall come into force on such day as the Secretary of State may specify.

(3) Different days may be specified under paragraph (2) for different

Figure 1.4: First page of the Nursing and Midwifery Order 2001, with its constituent parts labelled.

Devolution in Scotland, Wales and Northern Ireland

Devolution is the granting of powers from the central United Kingdom government to the governments of Scotland, England and Wales. Devolved governments were created following referenda in Wales and Scotland in 1997, and the Scottish Parliament, National Assembly for Wales and Northern Ireland Assembly were established a year later.

The Scottish Parliament has powers to make primary legislation in certain devolved areas of policy that includes health policy. Law and policy relating to health in Scotland is now for the Scottish Parliament to decide and legislate, and there are many examples of how health policy in Scotland differs from the rest of the United Kingdom. For example, the law concerning adults who lack the ability to make decisions comes under the Adults with Incapacity (Scotland) Act 2000 in Scotland but is dealt with under the provisions of the Mental Capacity Act 2005 in England and Wales.

The powers of the Northern Ireland Assembly are not as wide-ranging as those of Scotland and Wales. In Wales, following a referendum in 2011, the Assembly can now make primary legislation in twenty devolved areas, including health, social welfare and education. The Assembly also has the power to make secondary legislation relating to Wales.

It is essential that you ensure that the policies and laws you apply in your nursing practice relate to the country you work in.

Activity 1.4 *Research*

Mental health law in England, Scotland, Wales and Northern Ireland

Using your university library and learning resource centre, list the laws that regulate the care and treatment of people with mental health problems in England, Scotland, Wales and Northern Ireland.

An outline answer is given at the end of the chapter.

Judicial interpretation of statutes

Once an Act has completed its parliamentary stages and becomes law, the authoritative and compelling interpretation of that statute is for judges and no one else. When it comes to a dispute only the judges' views count. Governance in the UK is structured to prevent tyranny by attempting to ensure that no one person or body has an over-dominant role. The system sees three components of governance come together but as separate entities, with different roles as illustrated in Figure 1.5.

Judicial function

The role of the courts is to give force to the intention of Parliament as expressed in the words of the Act, and to make decisions between disputing parties. The courts cannot question statutes as Parliament is supreme and an Act of Parliament is our supreme source of law. Judges must apply the statute to the particular facts before them and to do this they need to interpret the words in an Act.

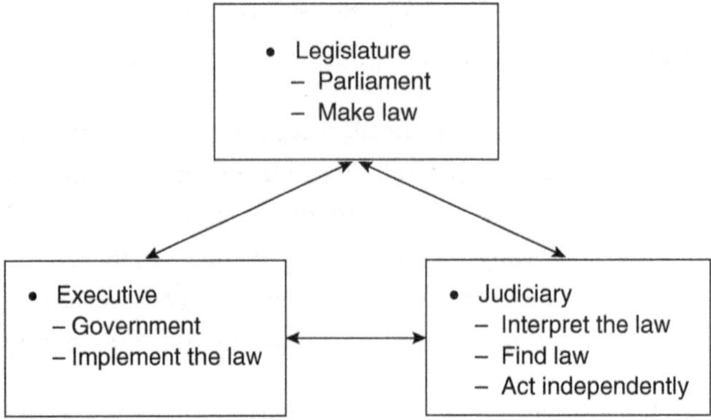

Figure 1.5: Three components of governance.

Parliament makes law, judges interpret and apply the law, and they have a great deal of discretion in how they do this.

Judicial decisions, the common law

The common law consists of laws that arise from cases decided by the courts. It works on a system of precedent and is often referred to in Latin as *stare decisis* or 'let the decision stand'. When a judge decides a case, he or she must refer to decisions in previous similar cases in the higher courts and keep to the rulings in those cases. If the previous case was about a similar set of facts and the same legal rules, then the current case has to be decided in the same way.

Activity 1.5 — *Critical thinking*

Precedent in action: The case of the snail in the ginger beer

In *Donoghue v Stevenson* [1932] two friends have a drink in a Paisley café. Mrs Donoghue has a ginger beer, which she gradually pours and drinks from an earthenware bottle from the bottom of which comes a green sludge, the remains of a decomposing snail. This causes her gastroenteritis and nervous shock, so she sues the manufacturer and the court awards her damages. The court finds that the manufacturer owes her a duty of care, which they have breached, causing her harm, because through their carelessness a snail entered the bottle in the manufacturing process.

Does precedent apply? Consider the following situations and decide whether the judge in the cases would be bound by the precedent set in the *Donoghue v Stevenson* [1932] case.

1. A woman buys a bottle of lemonade from a supermarket. Before she opens it she sees that it contains a dead wasp. Can she sue in negligence?
2. Utilities contractors dig a hole in a pavement and mark it with an upturned sledge hammer. Most people see the hazard and avoid it but a blind man falls in and breaks a leg. Can he sue in negligence?

3. A child is eating fish fingers for school dinner when he chokes on a one-inch piece of bone that needs surgery to remove. His mother sues the manufacturers, who say they are not to blame as there is a warning on the package. Are they right?
4. A woman has a sterilisation but it is poorly done and she has a healthy child. Can she sue in negligence?

An outline answer is given at the end of the chapter.

The structure of the courts

The use of precedent is seen as:

- giving certainty to the law;
- preventing arbitrary decisions;
- maintaining equality;
- providing a rational basis for decision-making.

A court is bound by precedent where the decision of a higher court is materially similar to a case being considered in a lower court. Senior judges ensure this rule is rigidly enforced.

The courts are structured on a hierarchical system (see Figure 1.6) that allows a series of appeals in the same case.

It is essential in your study of law and nursing to look carefully at which courts the case has been heard in and inform your practice by reference to the decision in the most senior court. For example, in *Gillick v West Norfolk and Wisbech AHA* [1986], the case began in the High Court, which decided that advice to doctors that girls under the age of 16 could be given contraceptive advice and treatment without parental consent was lawful if the girl was sufficiently mature and intelligent to make the decision herself. The Court of Appeal overruled the decision of the High Court and declared the advice unlawful. In the House of Lords the decision of the Court of Appeal was reversed and the advice was declared lawful.

The House of Lords was replaced by the Supreme Court in October 2009. As the most senior court, the justices of the Supreme Court now set out guidance that, in their opinion, will bind future cases. Opinions in cases from the House of Lords and the newly established Supreme Court can be reliably used to inform your practice as a nurse.

To assist with the application of the system of precedent, significant decisions of judges in cases are set out in law reports, which lawyers and those studying the law can use to inform their practice. There is a large number of commercial law reports available and some cases are even reported in the broadsheet newspapers. Case Reports contain a lot of detail about the facts and law of a case. Many are now freely available from the websites of organisations such as the British

United Kingdom Supreme Court
The most senior domestic court
12 members of the Supreme Court sit in benches of up to nine judges
The members are known as Justices of the Supreme Court
Hear Appeals from the Court of Appeal and in exceptional circumstances the High Court

Court of Appeal

32 Lord Justices of Appeal

Criminal Division	Civil Division
Hears appeals from the Crown Court	Hears appeals from the High Court, tribunals and certain cases from county courts

The High Court

92 Justices or Puisne Judges

Queen's Bench Division	Family Division	Chancery Division
Contract and tort Administrative Court Supervises the legality of decisions of inferior courts, tribunals, local authorities, Ministers of the Crown, and other public bodies and officials	Divisional Court Hears appeals from the magistrates' courts	Divisional Court Hears appeals from the county courts on bankruptcy and land law

Crown Court
Trials of indictable offences, appeals from magistrates' courts, cases for sentence

County Courts
Majority of civil litigation subject to nature of the claim

Magistrates' Courts
Trials of summary offences, committals to the Crown Court, family proceedings courts and youth courts

Tribunals
Hear appeals from decisions on: immigration, social security, child support, pensions, tax and land

Figure 1.6: The structure of the courts.

and Irish Legal Information Institute (**www.bailii.org**) and they are an excellent source of primary law. Your university law library will have a wide range of law reports with cases relevant to nursing and healthcare, many of which will be mentioned in this book. Figure 1.7 shows the layout of a typical law report.

Case law is a particularly relevant source of law in healthcare as the sensitive nature of the disputes inevitably gives rise to decisions that have an impact on how you conduct your nursing practice.

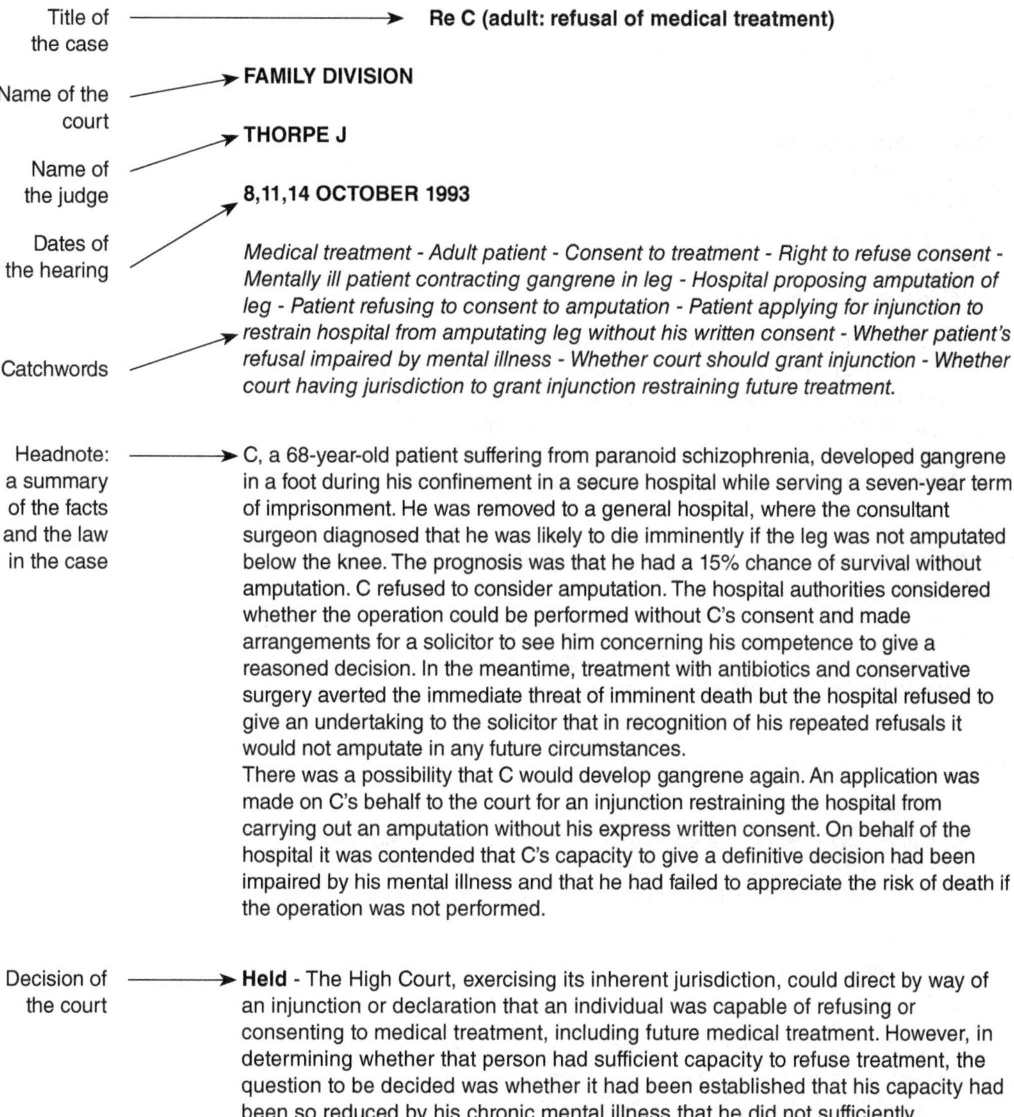
Law report citation
[1994] 1 All ER 819
Title of the case
Re C (adult: refusal of medical treatment)
Name of the court
FAMILY DIVISION
Name of the judge
THORPE J
Dates of the hearing
8,11,14 OCTOBER 1993
Catchwords
Medical treatment - Adult patient - Consent to treatment - Right to refuse consent - Mentally ill patient contracting gangrene in leg - Hospital proposing amputation of leg - Patient refusing to consent to amputation - Patient applying for injunction to restrain hospital from amputating leg without his written consent - Whether patient's refusal impaired by mental illness - Whether court should grant injunction - Whether court having jurisdiction to grant injunction restraining future treatment.
Headnote: a summary of the facts and the law in the case
C, a 68-year-old patient suffering from paranoid schizophrenia, developed gangrene in a foot during his confinement in a secure hospital while serving a seven-year term of imprisonment. He was removed to a general hospital, where the consultant surgeon diagnosed that he was likely to die imminently if the leg was not amputated below the knee. The prognosis was that he had a 15% chance of survival without amputation. C refused to consider amputation. The hospital authorities considered whether the operation could be performed without C's consent and made arrangements for a solicitor to see him concerning his competence to give a reasoned decision. In the meantime, treatment with antibiotics and conservative surgery averted the immediate threat of imminent death but the hospital refused to give an undertaking to the solicitor that in recognition of his repeated refusals it would not amputate in any future circumstances.
There was a possibility that C would develop gangrene again. An application was made on C's behalf to the court for an injunction restraining the hospital from carrying out an amputation without his express written consent. On behalf of the hospital it was contended that C's capacity to give a definitive decision had been impaired by his mental illness and that he had failed to appreciate the risk of death if the operation was not performed.

Decision of the court	**Held** - The High Court, exercising its inherent jurisdiction, could direct by way of an injunction or declaration that an individual was capable of refusing or consenting to medical treatment, including future medical treatment. However, in determining whether that person had sufficient capacity to refuse treatment, the question to be decided was whether it had been established that his capacity had been so reduced by his chronic mental illness that he did not sufficiently understand the nature, purpose and effects of the proffered medical treatment. That in turn depended on whether he had comprehended and retained information as to the proposed treatment, had believed it and had weighed it in the balance when making a choice. Although C's general capacity to make a decision had been impaired by schizophrenia, the evidence failed to establish that he lacked sufficient understanding of the nature, purpose and effects of the proposed treatment, but instead showed that he had understood and retained the relevant treatment information, believed it and had arrived at a clear choice. It followed that the presumption in favour of his right to self-determination had not been displaced. A declaration would be made accordingly (see p 822 *a* and p 824 *f* to p 825 *a d* to *f*, post).

Figure 1.7: (Continued)

Re T (Adult: Refusal of Medical Treatment) [1992] 4 All ER 649 and *Airedale NHS Trust* v *Bland* [1993] 1 All ER 821 applied.

Notes

For consent to medical treatment, see 30 *Halsbury's Laws* (4th edn reissue) para 39, and for cases on the subject, see 33 *Digest* (Reissue) 273-275, *2242-2246*.

Cases referred to in judgment

Airedale NHS Trust v *Bland* [1993] 1 All ER 821, [1993] AC 789, [1993] 2 WLR 316, HL. ← Law cases discussed in the judgment

T (adult: refusal of medical treatment), Re [1992] 4 All ER 649, [1993] Fam 95, [1992] 3 WLR 782, CA.

Originating summons

By an originating summons issued on 4 October 1993, C, a patient confined to Broadmoor Hospital, sought an injunction restraining the defendants, Heatherwood Hospital, Ascot, from amputating his right leg in the present and future without his express written consent. The summons was heard in chambers but judgment was given by Thrope J in open court. The facts are set out in the judgment.

Richard Gordon and Craig Barlow (instructed by Scott-Moncrieff & Harbour, Brighton) for the plaintiff.

← The lawyers arguing the case

Adrian Hopkins (instructed by J Tickle & Co) for the defendants. P A B Jackson (instructed by the Official Solicitor) as amicus curiae.

THORPE J.

This originating summons was issued on 4 October 1993 by C. It seeks under the court's inherent jurisdiction an injunction restraining Heatherwood Hospital, Ascot from amputating his right leg without his express written consent.

The plaintiff is 68 and of Jamaican origin. He came to England in 1956, his passage being paid by the woman with whom he had lived since 1949. In 1961 she left him, and in 1962 he accosted her at work and after an altercation stabbed her. He was sentenced at the Old Bailey to seven years' imprisonment. While serving that sentence he was diagnosed as mentally ill and transferred from Brixton to Broadmoor. On admission he was diagnosed as suffering from chronic paranoid schizophrenia. He was treated both with drugs and ECT. Over the years he has mellowed and has been accommodated for the past six years on an open ward of the parole house. He is described as neat and tidy, becoming more sociable with staff and other patients in the past two years. ← The judgment of the court in detail

Figure 1.7: Annotated law report.

Table 1.1: The advantages of legal awareness to a student nurse

The legally aware student nurse:

- **Realises that many aspects of daily life are governed by law**

Most aspects of life are regulated by law. Legal awareness helps you appreciate the importance of the legal framework which supports the structure of society. It also allows you to appreciate that personal and social problems may have a legal dimension.

- **Knowingly acts in accordance with certain legal principles**

Many parts of the law are necessarily complex and difficult to understand. However, the underlying principles are quite simple. These affect everyone on a day-to-day basis and therefore an understanding of them is important. Indeed, ignorance of the law can bring very serious consequences.

- **Understands the key elements of the legal system**

Knowledge of the law is of limited value unless you understand the various ways in which the legal system works to enforce the law. It is important to understand the role of those agencies that have powers to enforce the law and of the mechanisms by which you can seek legal help and advice.

- **Knows when and where to seek appropriate advice**

The law is vast and constantly changing. You need to develop a sense of:

  - when the law can help or hinder;
  - what you can find out for yourself and where;
  - when you should seek expert help;
  - how to get the appropriate help or advice.

- **Understands the nature of law**

Even though many day-to-day situations have a legal dimension, there are some problems that the law can do little about, even when in theory this should not be the case.

Chapter summary

- A thorough and critical appreciation of the legal and professional issues affecting nursing practice is essential if you are to develop the professional awareness necessary to become a registered nurse.
- Positive rules impose a legal obligation to do or refrain from doing something. If a positive rule is breached a sanction may be imposed for breaking the law.
- Normative rules set out what a person should do.
- Healthcare sees a drawing together of normative and positive rules.

continued . . .

- Law is defined as a rule of human conduct imposed upon and enforced among the members of a given state.
- The United Kingdom is a parliamentary democracy and the laws of the country are created and amended through the Queen in Parliament.
- Once an Act has completed its parliamentary stages and becomes law, the authoritative and compelling interpretation of that statute is for judges and no one else.
- An Act of Parliament is our supreme source of law.
- The common law is derived from decided cases and works through a system of precedent that ensures that materially similar cases are decided in the same way, creating a degree of certainty in the law.

Activities: Brief outline answers

Activity 1.4: Research (page 19)

Mental health law is a good example of how the devolved administrations in England, Scotland, Wales and Northern Ireland have introduced laws that specifically apply to their areas.

The Mental Health Act 1983 (as amended) regulates the care and treatment of people with mental disorder in England.

The Mental Health Act 1983 (as amended) also regulates the care and treatment of people with mental disorder in Wales but the Welsh government has passed the Mental Health (Wales) Measure 2010 that extends the rights of patients to access mental health services, advocacy services and statutory care and treatment planning.

The Mental Health (Care and Treatment) (Scotland) Act 2003 (as amended) sets out the powers for the admission, treatment and aftercare of people with mental disorder in Scotland.

In a radical, and many argue and enlightened, approach to mental healthcare the Northern Ireland Assembly has enacted the Mental Capacity (Northern Ireland) Act 2016 that gives physical and mental disorders equal status in terms of the need for consent to treatment. Admission and treatment for people 16 and older with a mental disorder will no longer be subject to compulsory detention and treatment provisions of the Mental Health (Northern Ireland) Order 1986. Instead the consent of a capable patient will be required before admission and treatment can begin. In common with physical disorders, where a person with a mental disorder lacks capacity to make a decision then care and treatment will only proceed if it is in their best interests to do so.

Activity 1.5: Critical thinking (pages 20–1)

1. The woman in the first case cannot sue in negligence as she has not suffered a personal injury. She discovered the wasp before drinking the lemonade.
2. Although the facts in this case seem very different, the case is still materially similar to the *Donoghue v Stevenson* [1932] case. The contractor owes a duty of care to other users of the footpath. They have failed to take adequate precautions to prevent a fall. It is reasonably foreseeable that a person with a visual impairment might come along the road. Harm has been caused by the contractor breaching its duty of care and so a claim in negligence is possible.
3. The facts and rules in this example appear similar but the manufacturer is arguing that the warning absolves them of their duty of care. You might argue, however, that as the fillet fish fingers are marketed towards children the manufacturer should take greater care. Should consumers be expected to mash each finger to check for bones? This case was settled out of court with a compensation payment.

4. At first glance this again appears to be a case of carelessness, but to be actionable, as in *Donoghue v Stevenson* [1932], there must be harm to the individual. The courts consider a healthy child as an economic loss not a personal injury. Mrs Donoghue would not have been able to sue in negligence if her bottle had contained water instead of a snail. Similarly, no claim for negligence would succeed for carelessness that resulted in the birth of a healthy baby.

Further reading

To understand the law and how it applies it is essential to have some knowledge of legal method. One of the following will help.

Hanson, S (2015) *Learning Legal Skills and Reasoning*, 4th edn. London: Routledge-Cavendish.

Holland, J and Webb, J (2016) *Learning Legal Rules: A student's guide to legal method and reasoning*. London: Blackstone Press.

To understand health law in context it is useful to have an understanding of health policy and the following can be recommended.

Crinson, I (2008) *Health Policy: A critical perspective*. London: Sage.

Ham, C (2009) *Health Policy in Britain*, 6th edn. London: Palgrave Macmillan.

Useful websites

To keep up to date with changes in health law we recommend the following.

www.bailii.org The British and Irish Legal Information Institute provides free access to law reports from the UK courts.

www.dh.gov.uk Outlines government policy on health in England.

www.justice.gov.uk/government/news/welcome-to-the-new-home-on-the-web-for-the-ministry-of-justice Ministry of Justice information and updates.

www.opsi.gov.uk/ legislation/uk.htm Full text of legislation and Statutory Instruments.

www.parliament.uk/about/how UK Parliament website, where you can find information about how a bill becomes law.

www.scotland.gov.uk/ Topics/Health Scottish government health policy and publications.

www.wales.gov.uk/topics/health/ Welsh Assembly health policy and documents.

Chapter 2
Principled decision-making in nursing

NMC Standards for Pre-registration Nursing Education

This chapter will address the following competencies:

Domain 1: Professional values

1. All nurses must practise with confidence according to *The Code: Professional standards of practice and behaviour for nurses and midwives* (NMC, 2015a), and within other recognised ethical and legal frameworks. They must be able to recognise and address ethical challenges relating to people's choices and decision-making about their care, and act within the law to help them and their families and carers find acceptable solutions.

Domain 3: Nursing practice and decision-making

6. All nurses must practise safely by being aware of the correct use, limitations and hazards of common interventions, including nursing activities, treatments, and the use of medical devices and equipment. The nurse must be able to evaluate their use, report any concerns promptly through appropriate channels and modify care where necessary to maintain safety. They must contribute to the collection of local and national data and formulation of policy on risks, hazards and adverse outcomes.

Chapter aims

By the end of this chapter you will be able to:

- describe the terms 'morals' and 'ethics';
- outline the principle-based approach;
- explain how the principle-based approach can be used when considering a moral problem relating to practice.

Introduction

In Chapter 1 we saw that nurses are required to practise in a way that discharges their professionalism by abiding by the law and their professional *Code* of standards (NMC, 2015a). However, you will also find during the course of your practice that the law does not always provide the answer to the complex dilemmas you will face as a nurse. These situations give rise to questions about whether a nursing intervention is morally acceptable and ethically right. This chapter will explore the notion of morals as they apply to nursing. Here we will consider what is meant by morals and ethics, and discuss some of the common dilemmas that have arisen in nursing. Leading on from this the chapter suggests a framework for a principle-based approach to decision-making in nursing and how it may be necessary to go to court to resolve disagreements arising from an ethical dilemma.

By reading this chapter and completing the activities you will develop a principle-based approach to resolving the dilemmas you will encounter as a nurse, and ensure that your stance is ethically based and acceptable under the law and your code of professional standards.

Moral dilemmas in nursing

Situations will arise in nursing where no clear conclusion can be immediately drawn from your understanding of the law or from the professional *Code*. For example, a nurse may believe that a doctor's decision not to resuscitate a patient with a terminal and painful illness is wrong. The nurse may believe the patient's life should be sustained and is suddenly faced with a dilemma about what is right or wrong. Both the doctor's decision to withhold resuscitation and the nurse's desire to continue treatment to preserve life are lawful. Neither is proposing to act unlawfully and so the decision is one of morality.

Morals are influenced not only by the law but by our culture, religion, beliefs, values and experience. As a nurse you will find that some clinical decisions are morally acceptable to you while others are not.

To develop an understanding of ethics and morality it is essential that these dilemmas are explored and analysed to provide clarity where there is conflict. This will help you judge whether a decision is right or wrong and inform your practice.

Moral issues and ethical approaches

Before we move on to consider what moral issues are and how they may be addressed, read Activity 2.1.

Activity 2.1 *Reflection*

A moral dilemma

A couple, both in their eighties, have been living in a residential home for about seven years. They have been married for 60 years and have rarely been apart from each other. The wife is totally blind and hard of hearing, and uses a wheelchair. When the husband's

continued . . .

health started to deteriorate they both asked the nurses to ensure that the wife is present during the last hours of his life. They both said that they would like to hold each other's hands before being separated.

One day, at about 5 a.m., the husband's health started to deteriorate very rapidly. The nurses decided to bring the wife to his bedside and allow them to spend some precious time together. This was their expressed wish. While a nurse was trying to take the wife to her husband's room, the wheelchair broke. The nurse had to look for another one and by that time the husband had already died. All the nurses on duty became very concerned about what to tell the wife. They knew that if the wife was told the truth, that is, her husband had died, she would be very upset at not being with him at the time of his death. Or they could lie to her, let her believe that her husband was still alive, let her hold her husband's hands for a while and then tell her that he had just passed away.

What would you do in this situation? Write down what you believe should be the decisions made to deal with this situation and give the reasons for whatever you decide. The aim of this exercise is to allow you to think about what you believe is right or wrong.

Now read below for further information.

You have probably considered many issues when deciding what you believe is the right decision and best course of action in this situation. For example, you may believe that the wife has a right to be told the truth. That it is wrong to tell a lie whatever the circumstances and it is your duty to tell the truth. This belief may be based on factors such as your culture, your upbringing, your experience or your religion. You may also have considered what would happen if the wife found out that she had not been told the truth. Would she report you to someone in authority? Would disciplinary action be taken against you? Would she lose trust and confidence in you and the nursing profession?

On the other hand, you might consider that the truth will hurt deeply and she might be unhappy for some considerable time. You may believe that you have a duty not to hurt her, emotionally in this case, but to ensure her happiness and well-being. As such, you feel it to be in her best interest if she is not told the truth. At least she will be happy and will have fond memories of being with her husband when he died.

Many different issues have emerged from this activity. You have had to judge what you believe is right and in doing so you have applied some key ethical principles to this moral conundrum. It is likely that you have at least considered the principles of:

- **rights** – the right of the wife to be told the truth;
- **duty** – your duty not to lie to the wife;
- **veracity** – telling the truth about what has happened;
- **consequence** – the consequence of being truthful or lying to the patient;

- **beneficence** – doing good to the wife;
- **non-maleficence** – doing no harm to the wife.

Activity 2.2 — *Critical thinking*

Ethical principles

The examples above are some of the principles that you are likely to have considered when addressing the moral dilemma in Activity 2.1.

Look again at what you have written and tick any issues that are more or less similar to those highlighted above.

As this is for your own observation and experience, there is no outline answer at the end of the chapter.

These are examples of ethical approaches that can be used to judge the rights or wrongs of a decision in a situation where there is a moral dilemma. The approaches do not provide you with an answer; rather, they help you decide whether a course of action is right or wrong. They enhance your ability to analyse situations and make a decision based on the moral principles underpinning nursing practice.

Activity 2.3 — *Reflection*

Morals and ethics

Now that you have some understanding about moral issues and ethical theories, it is important to have a clearer understanding of the terms 'morals' and 'ethics'.

Write down your understanding of the terms 'morals' and 'ethics'. You can relate to the discussion above as well as your own understanding of these terms.

There are some suggested definitions at the end of the chapter.

Morals and ethics

According to Thompson et al. (2000) 'morals' and 'ethics' are terms used to refer to social customs regarding the rights and wrongs, in theory and practice, of human behaviour. 'Moral' refers to what a person believes is right or wrong based on their culture, experience, upbringing, education and religion.

For example, you may believe that the sanctity of human life should always be respected and all patients should be treated even if they refuse to give consent. Others may believe that the sanctity of human life should not be respected where it merely prolongs the suffering of the person, such as in cases of patients with terminal illness in intractable pain. A person's morals are founded on their beliefs and values. Decisions made by that individual will be influenced by their beliefs and values. As a nurse you will have your own set of beliefs and values, your own moral background that will influence your decisions when caring for a person.

Activity 2.4 *Critical thinking*

Should we treat the patient?

A patient has been admitted to the accident and emergency department after a road traffic accident. He has sustained some severe injuries and requires a blood transfusion. He is conscious and understands the nature of his injuries and the need for a life-saving blood transfusion. However, he refuses to consent to such treatment despite being fully aware that his life is at risk. In about an hour he will lapse into unconsciousness and eventually die. His wife and two children have arrived at the hospital and they are all begging the doctor in charge of his treatment to save his life. They are obviously very distressed at the thought of possibly losing someone they all love. However, the doctor decides not to administer the blood transfusion even if this will lead to the patient's death.

Write down what moral issues may arise from this scenario. Then write down what you believe should be done in this situation and why.

As this is for your own observation and experience, there is no outline answer at the end of the chapter.

You may think that it is morally wrong not to treat a patient who has refused a life-saving blood transfusion. This may well be based on the belief that the sanctity of life should be respected at all times. The decision in allowing the patient to die may be uncomfortable for you. You may want to force your views and beliefs about the sanctity of life on to the patient and doctor. You may even consider ways of forcing the patient to have the blood transfusion. You may consider his wife and children, and feel that their wishes should be respected. All these are what you believe are the right things to consider and act upon. However, what you consider to be right could in itself be immoral. It could be argued that the patient has a right to refuse treatment and that his autonomy should be respected. As such, a patient must not be forced to accept treatment just because others believe it is right. Such coercion may be viewed as unprofessional, unlawful and immoral. This gives rise to a moral dilemma that needs to be considered. A moral dilemma, according to Thompson et al. (2000), is a choice between two equally unsatisfactory alternatives. For example, you may believe that a patient is capable of making a decision to refuse treatment and this should be respected (respect for autonomy). Another nurse may believe that one must always act in a way that promotes the well-being of others and decide to treat him despite his refusal to consent to that treatment.

This is where ethics and the application of ethical principles will help you to judge the right or wrong of a decision.

According to Edwards (2009), ethics may be described as the enquiry into moral situations and the language employed to describe them. Therefore, ethics involves the application of principles to a moral problem in order to help judge if an action is right or wrong.

A principle-based approach to ethical decision-making

A common approach to the ethics of healthcare was developed by the American philosophers Beauchamp and Childress (1989), and is based on four prima facie moral principles and attention to their application.

The four principles approach argues that, whatever our personal philosophy, politics, religion, moral theory or life stance, we will be able to commit ourselves to these four prima facie moral principles. The four principles are considered to encompass most of the moral issues that arise in healthcare.

'Prima facie' means that the principle is binding unless it conflicts with another moral principle – if it does you will have to choose between them. The four principles approach does not provide a method for choosing the right answer to a moral dilemma, but it will provide a common set of moral commitments, a common moral language and a common set of moral issues (Gillon, 1994).

The four moral principles are as follows:

- *Respect for autonomy – respect for the right of an individual to decide for himself or herself.*
- *Non-maleficence – obligation not to harm others.*
- *Beneficence – act in ways that promote the well being of others.*
- *Justice – obligation to treat others fairly.*
  (Beauchamp and Childress, 1989)

Autonomy

The first principle, respect for autonomy, requires respect for the choice made by an individual. In a healthcare context, this means that a patient has a right to decide whether or not to undergo any healthcare intervention, even if the refusal will lead to harm or death. The term 'autonomy' is derived from the Greek meaning 'self-governing'. It refers to the capacity of an individual to make an informed and uncoerced decision about their future. Autonomy is about self-rule with no control, undue influence or interference from others. It respects an individual's choice based on their own values and beliefs.

Gillon (1994) referred to three concepts of autonomy:

- **Autonomy of thought** involves deciding for oneself using all available information and weighing this information.
- **Autonomy of will** involves the intention to do something as a result of a decision.
- **Autonomy of action** involves doing something based on one's decision, such as refusing to consent to treatment.

Scenario: The right to self-determination

Hannah, 13, was found to have leukaemia at the age of four. After chemotherapy, she was diagnosed with a heart muscle disease called cardiomyopathy: a hole in her heart caused by a high-strength drug she had been given to kill off an infection. She now needed a heart transplant, but turned it down to return home to die in the company of her parents and siblings because she had had enough of hospitals.

Hannah's wish to [illegible] uthorities, but a child protection office [illegible] allowing Hannah to remain at home.

Eight months lat [illegible] e transplant list after she suffered parti [illegible] ay.

Beneficence

Gillon (1994) argue [illegible] hers they inevitably risk harming them. Nurs [illegible] ce and non-maleficence together with the ai [illegible]

The NMC's *Code* (20 [illegible] to provide overall benefit to patients with n [illegible] icence. To achieve this, nurses are committed to a wide range of obligations. Nurses must ensure that they are able to deliver competent safe care, and so they need rigorous and effective education and training both before and during their professional careers. They must also ensure that nursing care is of benefit to the patient. In doing this, nurses must respect the patient's autonomy. What constitutes benefit for one patient may be harm for another. For example, a mastectomy may constitute an overall benefit for one woman with breast cancer, while for another the destruction of part of her femininity may be so harmful that it cannot be outweighed by the prospect of extended life expectancy.

Case study 2.1: Beneficence conflicts with non-maleficence

A nurse was so concerned about poor care in the hospital where she worked that she agreed to participate in a television documentary.

The nurse secretly filmed the neglect of elderly patients. She was hailed as a hero for her actions by patients' groups and fellow nurses, and received awards for bringing her concerns to the public's attention.

The NMC, however, took a dim view of her actions as the filming was without the consent of her patients and was a breach of confidentiality. She was initially struck off the nursing register for

continued . . .

misconduct in April 2009 after admitting breaching patient confidentiality, but said she had agreed to film at the hospital to highlight terrible conditions there.

Following a public outcry and threat of court action, the striking-off order was replaced by a one-year caution.

Justice

The fourth principle is justice – that is, an obligation to treat others fairly. Justice includes the principles of fairness, equity and an entitlement to what is deserved. Gillon (1994) suggests the principle can be divided into three categories.

- Fair distribution of scarce resources (**distributive justice**).
- Respect for people's rights (**rights-based justice**).
- Respect for morally acceptable laws (**legal justice**).

Equality is at the heart of justice; it is important to treat equals equally and to treat unequals unequally in proportion to the inequalities. In the context of the allocation of resources, conflicts exist between moral concerns such as:

- providing sufficient healthcare to meet the needs of all who need it;
- when this is not possible, to distribute healthcare resources in proportion to the need for healthcare;
- allowing nurses to give priority to the needs of their patients;
- providing equal access to healthcare for all;
- allowing people as much choice as possible in selecting their healthcare;
- maximising the benefit produced by the available resources;
- respecting the autonomy of those who provide resources by limiting the cost to taxpayers.

All these criteria for allocating healthcare resources can be morally justified but not all can be fully met simultaneously.

Rights-based justice requires respect for patients' rights. Nurses have no special privilege as health workers to create rights for patients or decide which rights should apply. For example, a nurse's disapproval of a patient's lifestyle will not provide a morally defensible justification for refusing to care for a person with AIDS. The principle of justice also requires nurses to obey morally acceptable laws. Even though you may disapprove of the law, you are morally obliged to obey it.

Case study 2.2: Justice for all

A hospital spent £20,000 creating a private ward to provide dialysis treatment for a patient, a convicted rapist, who had conducted a reign of terror at hospital where he received life-saving dialysis treatment three times a week. The hospital had to take out a court order barring him from attacking staff and spent £18,000 a year to pay for security guards to escort him during his visits. It paid a further £2,000 annually for taxis to take him to and from the hospital to ensure he did not loiter around the building. This is because the hospital felt his human rights would be violated if they refused to treat him.

Applying the four principles

Activity 2.5 *Critical thinking*

An expectant mother refuses to have an injection

MB, a patient, is 40 weeks pregnant and the baby is in a breech position. She is told that a vaginal delivery would pose serious risks to the child and that a caesarean section will improve the child's chances of survival. She has consented on more than one occasion to the operation but has subsequently withdrawn her consent on each occasion due to her irrational fear of needles. The patient is now in labour. She continues to refuse consent for the injection.

In a group, apply the four principles to this situation and consider if the caesarean should proceed despite MB's objections.

As the answer depends on your observations, there is no outline answer at the end of the chapter.

Respect for autonomy

The principle of respect for autonomy entails taking into account and giving consideration to the patient's views on treatment. Autonomy is not an all-or-nothing concept. MB may not be fully autonomous and so not legally competent to refuse treatment, but this does not mean that ethically her views should not be considered and respected as far as possible. She has expressed her wishes clearly; she does not want a needle inserted for the anaesthetic. An autonomous decision does not have to be the correct decision otherwise individual needs and values would not be respected. However, an autonomous decision is one that is informed. Has MB been given information about the consequences of refusing treatment in a manner that she can understand? Has she been supported to weigh values and beliefs against the consequences of having or refusing treatment?

Beneficence

Nurses must act to benefit their patients. This principle may clash with the principle of autonomy when the patient makes a decision that you do not think will benefit the patient – that it is not in her best interests. Here we should consider both the long-term and short-term effects of overriding MB's views. In the short term, MB will be frightened to have a needle inserted in her arm and of being in hospital – this may lead her to distrust healthcare professionals in the future and to be reluctant to seek medical help. In the long term, there will be a benefit to MB in having her autonomy overridden on this occasion. Without treatment she may die, along with her unborn child.

The benefits of acting in her best interests would need to be weighed against the dis-benefits of failing to respect MB's autonomy. From a legal point of view, the wishes of a competent patient cannot be overridden in their best interests.

Non-maleficence

Non-maleficence means doing no harm to the patient. MB would be harmed by forcibly restraining her in order to insert the needle for anaesthesia, but if she is not treated immediately she will die along with her child.

Which course of action would result in the greatest harm? The assessment relies on assumptions: how successful is the operation likely to be; how likely will MB be willing and able to care for her child?

Justice

It would be relevant to consider cost-effectiveness of the treatment options for MB, and the impact the decision about her treatment would have on her child. However, if she is a competent adult who refuses treatment despite acknowledging the risk to her life and that of her child, you are morally and legally obliged to respect her rights and obey the law. Where there is a conflict between a mother and unborn child, the law resolves it in favour of the mother. You would have to obey the law even though you may believe that an unborn child should have a right to be born alive.

Disagreement on resolving a dilemma

Disagreements over the best way to resolve an ethical dilemma can usually be resolved following discussions with other members of the healthcare team, the patient and their relatives. Where the disagreement persists then it will be necessary, in the most serious cases, to seek a declaration from a court (*Airedale NHS Trust v Bland* [1993]).

A declaration, as the name suggests, is an order from the court declaring that a proposed course of action is lawful. The declaration is binding on the parties in court so does not create a precedent and every case is considered on its unique facts and merits.

Case study 2.3: Declaration upholding the right to refuse treatment

A woman with a long history of depression and schizophrenia and who had been a Jehovah's Witness for some 40 years was admitted to hospital after being found wandering and confused. Significant internal bleeding was discovered and she was adamant that she would not want treatment with any blood products. The emergency care team felt she had the capacity to make that decision, and that she was aware the consequences might be that she would die. The next day her condition deteriorated significantly. The emergency care team sought a declaration form the Court of Protection that they had acted correctly in not giving a blood transfusion in accordance with the woman's wishes.

The court accepted that on the evidence the care team had acted correctly, there was no evidence that her decision was influenced by her mental disorder and her wishes and beliefs carried great weight in this case. The court declared that it was lawful to accede to those wishes and not give the blood. Sadly, some 8 days later she died.

(Newcastle upon Tyne Hospitals Foundation Trust v LM *[2014] EWHC 454 (COP))*

In *Newcastle upon Tyne Hospitals Foundation Trust v LM* [2014], set out in the case study above, it can be seen that the emergency care team wanted to respect the woman's autonomy by agreeing to her wish not to have a life-sustaining blood transfusion. The dilemma for the team was that respecting autonomy would violate her right to life and the principles of non-maleficence and justice and so they took their dilemma to court for a declaration. The court declared that while the right to life was fundamental it was not absolute. Autonomy should prevail in this case by respecting the woman's wishes and beliefs even though it led to her death.

Where applications for a declaration concern a critically ill child the court is obliged to consider the best interests of the welfare of the child as paramount (Children Act 1989, section 1). The test for establishing the best interests of the welfare of a child has been developed by the courts as cases have been brought for judgment over the last 30 years. Over that time the courts have had the opportunity to consider each aspect of the care of critically ill children and the test for best interests has become ever more sophisticated and extends beyond a mere balancing of the risks and benefits of continued treatment.

In the early cases the notion of a best interest adopted by the courts was limited to the likely life expectancy of the child if life-sustaining treatment were to be given (*Re B (A Minor) (Wardship: Medical Treatment)* [1981]). Some ten years later the court refined the determination of a best interest to include the pain and suffering the child would have to endure.

Case study 2.4: Pain and suffering

In J (A Minor) (Child in Care: Medical Treatment) *[1993] a profoundly brain damaged child with a very short life expectancy was not thought to be benefitting from treatment and both the parents and medical team sought an order allowing them to curtail treatment. The court held that*

continued . . .

denial of treatment to prolong life could only be sanctioned when in the best interests of the child. The test that applied was based on an assessment of the quality of life of the child and their future pain and suffering in relation to the life-saving treatment. The court declared that it was not in the child's best interests to continue with treatment and the child died shortly after.

No absolutist test

In *J (A Minor) (Child in Care: Medical Treatment)* [1993] it was argued that in the case of critically ill children an absolutist test should be applied. That is, doctors and nurses should have a duty to continue life-sustaining treatment right up to the death of the child. The court, however, found that even where the patient was a critically ill child it was never the case that doctors and nurses had to continue giving treatment even where it was clearly futile. What the court called the absolutist test would never apply.

Case study 2.5: Application of broader welfare, family and non-medical factors to the best interests test

In Re T (A Minor) (Wardship: Medical Treatment) *[1997] a child born with a life-threatening liver defect required a liver transplant if he was to live beyond his second birthday. His mother refused consent as she considered it was in her son's best interests not to suffer stressful and painful invasive surgery. The judge in the High Court considered medical evidence that the chances of success were good and declared that the mother's refusal to accept the unanimous advice of the doctors was not the conduct of a reasonable parent.*

The Court of Appeal declared the judge's decision was flawed as the paramount consideration of the court was not the reasonableness of the mother's decision but the child's best interests, taking into account all factors, not just medical considerations. The Court of Appeal declared that it was in the child's best interests that decisions as to his future treatment be left to his parents.

In *A NHS Trust v MB and Mr & Mrs B* [2006] similar grounds were used to justify the continuation of treatment in the case of a terminally ill child who was unable to breathe unaided since birth and required positive pressure ventilation. The NHS trust argued that his quality of life was so low and the burdens of living so great that it was in his best interests to withdraw all forms of ventilation. His parents however, argued that a tracheostomy should be performed to enable long term ventilation.

In common with all cases concerning children the court held that the child's welfare was their paramount consideration (Children Act 1989 section 1). The court considered the quality and value to the child of his relationship with his family and found it was not in his best interests to discontinue ventilation with the inevitable result that he would die. He had age-appropriate cognition, a relationship of value with his family and other pleasures from sight, touch and sound. Those benefits were precious and real and the routine discomfort, distress and pain did not outweigh those benefits.

However, the court also held that to undergo procedures that went beyond ventilation such as cardiopulmonary resuscitation, administration of intravenous antibiotics and blood sampling should not be provided unless the medical team thought it clinically appropriate.

A decision on a critically sick child's best interests must be determined on wider grounds than benefits and risks of continued treatment. To make this determination it is necessary to discuss the child's best interests with the parents.

Referring the matter to court

Where parents strongly oppose the giving or withholding of treatment then, unless the situation is urgent, the matter will need to be referred to the court for a declaration. Failing to seek the courts approval in these circumstances would be a breach of the child's right to respect for a private and family life under article 8 of the European Convention on Human Rights.

Case study 2.6: Failure to seek High Court approval for a treatment opposed by parents

In Glass v United Kingdom *[2004] a severely physically and mentally disabled baby argued, through his mother as his litigation friend, that his right to physical integrity under the European Convention on Human Rights 1950, article 8 had been breached when on his readmission with respiratory failure, the hospital insisted that he was dying and that diamorphine should be given to relieve his distress. His mother disagreed and objected to the proposed treatment in the belief that it would harm his chances of recovery. Despite her objection diamorphine was administered but his condition improved and he returned home.*

The European Court of Human Rights found that treatment contrary to his mother's wishes breached the baby's right to physical integrity under article 8 as the hospital had failed to seek the High Court's approval for the proposed treatment.

Permissive declarations

When the court's approval for a plan of care is sought the method used to authorise treatment is by way of a declaration where the court declares that the proposed treatment is lawful. A declaration is binding on the parties before the court and doctors and nurses are bound by their terms.

The courts are aware that a declaration may restrict a health professional's ability to exercise their clinical judgement. To avoid such a situation the court resorts to the use of a permissive declaration (*A NHS Trust v MB and Mr & Mrs B* [2006]). In a permissive declaration the court authorises the withholding of treatment at the discretion of the care team.

Case study 2.7: Permissive declaration

In Re Wyatt (A Child) (Medical Treatment: Continuation of Order) *[2005] the intervention of the court was sought in respect of the medical treatment of a critically ill child who had also developed an intermittent rasping cough and a viral infection. The only intervention would be intubation and ventilation but the doctors argued that it would not be in her best interests as essentially it would be futile. The parents were of the view that if she were ventilated she would recover.*

The court made it clear that in the best interests of the child the care team should be able to refrain from having to intervene by way of intubation and ventilation. The authority was granted by way of a permissive not mandatory declaration so that at the moment the decision arose the care team could exercise their clinical judgement, in the child's best interests, as to whether to withhold the treatment or not.

When seeking a declaration for the court to resolve a moral dilemma in relation to the care of a critically sick child the court will take into account the specific facts of each case and will consider factors that go beyond a blinkered clinical assessment of the benefits and risks of treatment. The courts now adopt a more sophisticated consideration of the child's life expectancy, pain and suffering weighed against the views of the parents, their relationship with their child and what other pleasures the child is able to enjoy. Where nurses and doctors cannot come to a consensus on limiting or withdrawing life-sustaining treatment with parents then it will be necessary to seek court approval to comply with the child's rights under the European Convention on Human Rights, article 8 (Council of Europe, 1950).

Chapter summary

- Many situations in healthcare practice give rise to questions about whether such practice is morally acceptable and ethically right.
- 'Moral' refers to what we believe is right or wrong and this is based on our culture, experience, upbringing, education and religion.
- 'Ethics' refers to the application of certain principles or theories to a moral problem in order to judge if an action is right or wrong.
- The application of ethical principles to a moral problem will enable you to judge if an action is right or wrong.
- The principle-based approach is a framework that acts as a tool for considering moral problems.
- When considering a moral dilemma each principle must be taken into account unless one conflicts with another.
- The application of the principles will depend on their relevance to the moral conflicts being judged.

continued . . .

- A declaration is an order from the court declaring that a proposed course of action is lawful.
- A declaration is binding on the parties in court so does not create a precedent.
- Where there is strong opposition over the giving or withholding of treatment then, unless the situation is urgent, the matter will need to be referred to the court for a declaration.

Activity: Brief outline answers

Activity 2.3 Reflection (page 31)

Morality is our seemingly instinctive sense of right and wrong. However, as you will see as you work through the chapter, morality is not based on instinct but is a product of our learning or socialisation. It is therefore often subjective and unexamined.

Immoral is usually used to mean deliberately doing something obviously wrong.

Ethics is the reflective study of good, and how, as a registered nurse, you make the right choices even when doing right may also involve doing harm or wrong. It is a learned process that even immoral people can use to their own evil ends, but it can help moral people in their pursuit of good.

Unethical is often used to mean immoral.

Further reading

To further explore the notion of a principle-based approach to decision-making we recommend:

Edwards, S (2009) *Nursing Ethics*, 2nd edn. London: Palgrave Macmillan.

To appreciate the range of dilemmas you are likely to encounter as student nurses and the need for a decision-making framework we recommend:

Mallik, M, Hall, C and Howard, D (2009) *Nursing Knowledge and Practice: Foundations for Decision-Making*, 3rd edn. London: Bailliere Tindall.

Useful website

It is essential that you inform your decision-making with up-to-date professional advice and information from the NMC at **www.nmc-uk.org**.

Chapter 3
Professionalism

NMC Standards for Pre-registration Nursing Education

This chapter will address the following competencies:

Domain 1: Professional values

1. All nurses must practise with confidence according to *The Code: Professional standards of practice and behaviour for nurses and midwives* (NMC, 2015a), and within other recognised ethical and legal frameworks.
7. All nurses must be responsible and accountable for keeping their knowledge and skills up to date through continuing professional development. They must aim to improve their performance and enhance the safety and quality of care through evaluation, supervision and appraisal.
8. All nurses must practise independently, recognising the limits of their competence and knowledge. They must reflect on these limits and seek advice from, or refer to, other professionals where necessary.

Chapter aims

By the end of this chapter you will be able to:

- define the terms 'professionalism' and 'accountability';
- state the four spheres of accountability in nursing practice;
- outline the conduct required to avoid liability in each of the four spheres of accountability in nursing practice;
- determine whether accountability can be exercised;
- evaluate the role of accountability in nursing.

Introduction

This chapter draws together the principles introduced in Chapters 1 and 2 and highlights that from your first day as a student nurse you will be working toward the competencies and skills required of a registered nurse. As a registered nurse the need for professionalism means that you will be answerable for what you do and what you fail to do. The chapter begins by considering definitions of the terms 'professionalism' and 'accountability' and how they apply in nursing. Then the four spheres of accountability and the standards of professionalism they impose through the law are introduced. The chapter concludes by looking in some detail at the role of the profession's regulatory body, the NMC, in maintaining public confidence in nursing.

Professionalism and accountability are words that are familiar to nurses, as they are in almost daily use in professional practice with their inclusion in many nursing texts and trust policies. The terms underpin the NMC's *Code* (2015a). Professionalism and accountability are fundamental concepts crucial to the protection of the public and individual patients. It is therefore essential that the terms are clearly understood by student nurses as they represent the means by which the law imposes standards and boundaries on professional practice.

Activity 3.1 *Reflection*

Defining professionalism and accountability

- Write down your understanding of the terms 'professionalism' and 'accountability'.
- In a group discuss the meanings of 'professionalism' and 'accountability' with an emphasis on nursing practice.

Now read the following for further guidance.

Defining professionalism

Professionalism may be defined as the competence, skills and values expected of a professional. In relation to nursing a key theme of the NMC *Code* (2015a) emphasises the need to promote professionalism and trust. Registered nurses are required to uphold the reputation of the profession at all times by displaying a personal commitment to the standards of practice and behaviour set out in the *Code*, be law abiding and of good character. Registered nurses must be a model of integrity and leadership for others, such as student nurses, to aspire to. This should then lead to trust and confidence in the profession from patients, people receiving care, other healthcare professionals and the public.

Defining accountability

Registered nurses who fall below the legal or professional requirements of a registered nurse will be held to account for their acts and omissions.

Lewis and Batey (1982) defined accountability as

> *the fulfilment of a formal obligation to disclose to relevant others the purposes, principles, procedures, relationships, results, income and expenditures for which one has authority.*

An analysis of this definition reveals the fundamental nature of accountability. The 'fulfilment of a formal obligation' suggests that it has basis in law. There is a formal or legal relationship between the practitioner and the 'reverent others', or higher authorities, that hold you to account. The extent of their scrutiny is illustrated by the inclusion of 'the purposes, principles, procedures, relationships, results, income and expenditures for which one has authority' in the definition. It is not just your conduct but your competence and integrity, your professionalism that can be called to account. Put more concisely, to be accountable is to be answerable for your acts and omissions.

Accountability is therefore defined as being answerable for your personal acts or omissions to a higher authority with whom you have a legal relationship.

Case study 3.1: Nurse forgot to give child medicine

A nurse was struck off the professional register after forgetting to give a child his medication. An NMC fitness to practise panel heard how the boy suffered because of the mistake. The nurse was then found to have forged a signature to claim she had given him the drugs at a later date.

The NMC said that the unprofessional behaviour arose from the nurse's attitude rather than any lack of knowledge. She was an experienced nurse and should have known not to depart from the standards of a registered nurse.

(Sunday Mercury, *2013)*

Activity 3.2 — *Critical thinking*

The role of professionalism and accountability

Having considered the definition and nature of professionalism and accountability in nursing practice, write down what role they fulfil in nursing. There are at least four key roles that they fulfil; see if you can think of more.

Now read the following for further information.

The purpose of professionalism and accountability

The principle aim of holding nurses accountable for their actions is to ensure that nurses behave professionally at all times and this ensures that the public and patients are not harmed by their acts and omissions, and to provide redress to those who have been harmed. To achieve that aim professionalism and accountability have the following functions.

- **A protective function** – By requiring registered nursing to act professionally and to hold to account those who fail to discharge their professionalism the public are protected from the acts or omissions of nurses that might cause harm. You can be called to account for your conduct and competence if it is thought that you have fallen below the standards required of you in law.
- **A deterrent function** – The sanctions available to the authorities that hold you to account protect the public and patients by discouraging you from acting in a way that would be considered unprofessional or unlawful. A registered nurse must act at all times in a manner worthy of a nurse – in work, in public and in their private lives.
- **A regulatory function** – By imposing professionalism and making you accountable to a range of higher authorities, the law regulates your behaviour. The regulatory framework makes it clear what standards you are required to comply with as a registered nurse.
- **An educative function** – Nurses who are called to account and asked to justify their actions have their cases heard in public with a view to reassuring patients that only the highest standards of professionalism will be tolerated. This public scrutiny of a nurse allows other members of the profession to learn from the mistakes and misconduct of others.

Case study 3.2: Nurse struck off after poor catheter fitting

A registered nurse was struck off the NMC's register after an incompetent catheter fitting left a patient needing hospital treatment.

The experienced nurse made a number of mistakes while performing the procedure on the older man, and the catheter was not inserted into the bladder. She then failed to ensure that urine was discharged after its insertion and made a number of failings over making notes for the procedure in the man's records.

The patient was left in significant distress and he had to be admitted to hospital for treatment.

The NMC found the nurse's fitness to practise to be impaired and removed her name from the register.

(Lancashire Telegraph, *2013*)

Holding nurses to account for unprofessional behaviour

From Lewis and Batey's (1982) definition of accountability you have seen that, as a nurse, you have a formal obligation to answer for your actions to a range of higher authorities, which have a legal relationship with you that enables them to demand that you justify your actions.

If you fail to satisfy those requirements, sanctions may be applied against you. For example, during your training, the university and the NHS Trust have legal authority over you. They can hold you to account through reasonable disciplinary measures. The sanctions they can impose could lead to dismissal from your course.

Activity 3.3 — *Critical thinking*

Accountability to higher authorities

List the authorities that can hold you to account in your role as a nurse. To help you with this exercise, think of the authorities that offer protection to the public, including your patients.

See Figure 3.1 for the answers.

In order to provide maximum protection to the public and patients against the lack of professionalism from registered nurses, four areas of law are drawn together and can individually or collectively hold you to account.

Figure 3.1 depicts these four areas of accountability and highlights the authorities that can hold you to account as a registered nurse. In each case a legal relationship exists that allows you to be called to account for your actions.

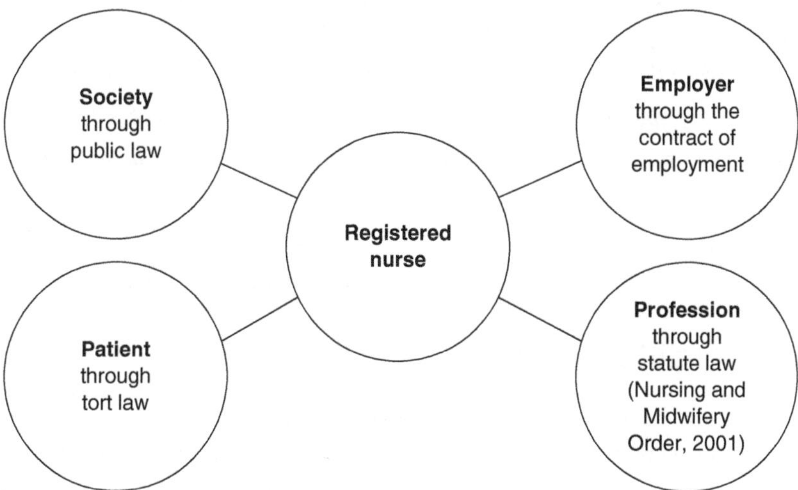

Figure 3.1: Four areas of accountability.

Activity 3.4 — *Evidence-based practice and research*

The drugs overdose

A nurse has administered overdoses of diamorphine to hasten the death of two patients under her care. Both patients survive but suffer irreversible brain damage.

Using Figure 3.1, list the authorities that may hold the nurse to account and the possible sanctions they might bestow.

An outline answer is given at the end of the chapter.

Accountability to oneself

Very often nurses argue that they are accountable to themselves for their acts and omissions. Such an argument is characteristic of the altruistic nature of the profession. A nurse who harms a patient through their acts or omissions will often feel remorse and will reflect on their practice to prevent a recurrence. However, this cannot be regarded as a nurse truly holding themselves to account as they cannot apply sanctions or provide redress for the person who has been wronged.

The authorities mentioned in Figure 3.1 protect the public through the powers conferred on them by the law and can apply sanctions to the nurse who fails to meet the standard imposed by the law.

The areas of accountability are not mutually exclusive. They can individually impose sanctions on nurses who fail to meet the required legal standard. Where misconduct is particularly serious, all four areas of accountability will impose sanctions against the nurse.

Case study 3.3: Nurse who stole drugs jailed

A former care home manager who stole drugs from residents to feed her addiction was jailed for killing an elderly patient. The registered nurse gave the 97-year-old patient a lethal dose of a drug she had not been prescribed because of a desire to control the patient's death. She also stole around 8,000 doses of medication to feed her addiction to prescription drugs and altered records to hide the thefts.

A jury agreed she had substituted the patient's diamorphine with a fatal dose of Tramadol. She also pleaded guilty to ten counts of possessing class A and C drugs, and one of perverting the course of justice by altering records.

(Daily Mail, *2010)*

Being answerable to society

As individuals working in the UK, nurses are subject to the same laws as any other member of society. There is nothing about your status as a nurse that exempts you from these laws. If you are suspected of committing a crime during the course of your practice or otherwise, you can be called to account for your actions.

Case study 3.4: Accountability to society

In R v Hinks *[2001], a care worker was convicted of theft under section 1 of the Theft Act 1968, when a jury decided that accepting gifts of sums of money from a patient in her care who had limited intelligence was a dishonest thing to do.*

The patient she cared for was grateful for the way the care worker looked after him and would give Hinks gifts of money as a sign of appreciation.

However, a jury decided that accepting such gifts from a vulnerable adult was a dishonest act and convicted her of theft.

Increase in prosecutions of nurses

Following the public outcry arising from the findings of the inquiries into poor care and avoidable deaths of patients in Mid Staffordshire and south Wales (House of Commons, 2013; Andrews and Butler, 2014) the government has sought to restore public confidence in their supervision and management of the NHS by making it a criminal offence to ill treat or wilfully neglect a patient in your care (Criminal Justice and Courts Act 2015, section 20).

Case study 3.5: Nurse convicted for ill-treatment

A nurse who was filmed by a concerned relative shouting at a vulnerable patient to shut up and causing bruising by poking her in the face was given a four-month prison sentence after admitting ill-treatment of the patient.

More detail on the use of the criminal law to protect patients from harm by nurses can be found in Chapter 7 of this book.

Accountability to the patient

As well as being accountable to society in general, nurses are also accountable to the individual patients under their care. The tort or civil law system allows a patient to seek redress, usually in the form of compensation, if they believe that harm has been caused to them through nurses' negligence.

In the NHS, clinical negligence claims have a potential value of some £4 billion. In 2014–15 alone some £1.22 billion was paid out in connection with clinical negligence claims (NHS LA, 2015).

Case study 3.6: Health board pays compensation for negligent care

The family of a patient received a four-figure pay-out after a health board accepted its care was negligent in the last weeks of her life.

The health board admitted that it had not followed NICE guidelines requiring patients to receive an initial and ongoing risk assessment of pressure sore ulceration. As a result the patient acquired a pressure sore but was still not referred to a tissue viability nurse for advice on the management of the pressure sore.

(South Wales Argus, *2013)*

Accountability to the employer

A nurse who is employed by the NHS, or other organisation, is accountable to their employer through the contract of employment. The contract sets out the terms and conditions of employment and the standard of work expected of the employee (Rideout, 1983). Many of these terms are written in the contract, such as salary, holiday entitlement, hours of work, etc. and are known as 'express contract terms'. In addition, many conditions that regulate the relationship between employer and employee are not expressly written into the contract but are there by virtue of decided cases or employment-related legislation. These are known as 'implied contract terms' and include a warranty from the employee to the employer that they will carry out their duties with due care and diligence.

An employer is vicariously liable for the actions of its employees. That is, if an employee commits a civil wrong in the course of their employment, it is the employer who is liable to pay any compensation. Employers will wish to minimise the likelihood of that liability arising and are entitled under contract law to hold their employees to account through reasonable disciplinary procedures.

For nurses, their employer is the most likely authority to hold them to account. There are two reasons why this is the case. First, a patient with a grievance against a nurse is more likely to complain to their employer than take legal action. Second, employment law allows a lower burden of proof when deciding whether an employee is guilty of misconduct. Employment law only requires that an employer hold an honest and genuine belief that the employee is guilty of misconduct based on the outcome of a reasonable investigation (*British Home Stores Ltd v Burchell* [1980]).

Case study 3.7: An honest and genuine belief

A support worker who was suspended then sacked over allegations of mistreating residents was fairly dismissed, according to an employment appeal tribunal.

The tribunal did not make any conclusions on the allegations of assault on 12 residents, but decided that the employer had conducted a reasonable investigation, as a result of which they held an honest and genuine belief that the care assistant had probably committed the alleged abuse.

(This is Worcestershire, *2004)*

As well as being accountable to their employer through reasonable disciplinary procedures, nurses also owe a contractual duty of care to their employers. A breach of that duty allows an action for damages for breach of contract (*Lister v Romford Ice and Cold Storage Co Ltd* [1957]). Therefore, if an employing trust pays compensation for the negligence of one of their employees, they may seek to reclaim that compensation by suing the employee for a breach of their contractual duty of care.

Professional accountability

Registered nurses are accountable to the profession through the provisions of the Health Act 1999, and the Nursing and Midwifery Order 2001. The NMC was established under these provisions in 2002 to protect the public by establishing standards of education, training, conduct and performance for nurses to ensure that those standards are maintained (Nursing and Midwifery Order 2001, article 3(2)). As the regulatory body for the profession, the NMC is concerned with protecting the public.

The key to the NMC's role is the professional register, where the names of those entitled to be called registered nurses are maintained. An active registration is required if a nurse intends to practise. The NMC protects the public by controlling entry on to the register through standards of training and education, and regulating a practitioner's right to remain on the register by imposing professional standards.

'Fitness to practise' is the term used by the NMC to describe a registrant's suitability to be on the register without restrictions. The NMC has the power to hold a registered practitioner to account if it is alleged that their fitness to practise is impaired. Article 22 of the Nursing and Midwifery Order 2001 states that fitness to practise may be impaired by:

- misconduct;
- lack of competence;
- a conviction or caution (including a finding of guilt by a court martial);
- physical or mental ill health;
- a finding by any other health or social care regulator or licensing body that a registrant's fitness to practise is impaired;
- a fraudulent or incorrect entry in the NMC's register.

The standards by which practitioners are judged, and which the NMC considers the public are entitled to expect, are set out in the NMC's *The Code: Professional standards of practice and behaviour for nurses and midwives* (NMC, 2015a). Practitioners who appear before the NMC's fitness to practise panels are held to account against those standards.

The Code

A revised code of professional conduct was issued by the NMC in March 2015. Although titled *The Code: Professional standards of practice and behaviour for nurses and midwives* (NMC, 2015a) it is referred to simply as *The Code.* To make full use of *The Code* it is essential to read its clauses in conjunction with fuller guidance from the NMC in the form of advice sheets. For example, *The Code* requires that registered nurses respect people's confidentiality and fuller information on the extent of this duty is given in the NMC's Confidentiality Advice Sheet. Both *The Code* and the advice sheets are available from the NMC's website at **www.nmc-uk.org**.

The standards of practice and behaviour expected by the NMC is that of the average practitioner, not the highest possible level of practice. This approach is similar to that adopted by the civil law when judging a skilled practitioner under the *Bolam* test to determine whether liability in negligence has arisen (see Chapter 9). The key difference between the law of negligence and professional accountability is that no action in negligence can occur without harm to the patient.

A breach of *The Code* can occur and a practitioner can be held to account even though there has been no harm to a patient. Failing to meet the requirements of *The Code* and the resulting lack of professionalism is enough for the NMC to hold the registered nurse to account.

Case study 3.8: Lack of professionalism

A nurse who helped herself to a patient's chips and curry sauce was struck off the nursing register. The patient had bought the food with a support worker at a local chip shop and brought it back to the hospital dining room. The nurse asked for a chip and took one anyway when the patient didn't answer. She then asked for some sauce before pouring curry sauce over the chips and eating them.

She was initially suspended for four months then stuck off when a panel of the NMC's conduct and competency committee found that her actions amounted to misconduct.

(Rudgard, 2015)

The revised *Code* is based on four themes that require registered nurses to:

- prioritise people;
- practise effectively;
- preserve safety;
- promote professionalism and trust.

The revised *Code* has updated the standards of practice and behaviour required of registered nurses to reflect changes in professional nursing practice. The primary role of the NMC is to protect the public and the focus of *The Code* is on improving the quality and safety of care. The standards in this revision of *The Code* now include:

- a professional duty of candour;
- ensuring the fundamentals of care are delivered effectively during all stages of life (see Chapter 5);
- using all forms of communication, including social media (see Chapter 12);
- guidance on effective record keeping (see Chapter 11).

Duty of candour

Activity 3.5 *Critical thinking*

Before you read on write down what you consider candour to mean.

The inclusion of a professional duty of candour in *The Code* arose from the government accepting a recommendation from the Francis report for such a duty to encourage openness and transparency in health services, including nursing services, in an attempt to prevent a repeat of the deliberate concealment of poor care and negligence found in the Mid Staffordshire Hospital scandal (DH, 2014).

The Francis report (House of Commons, 2013) defines candour as the volunteering of relevant information to persons who have been harmed by the provision of services, whether or not the information has been requested and whether or not a complaint has been made. The duty places a legal obligation on nurses to report poor practice where patients have been harmed.

In order to ensure that both care workers, such as nurses, and care providers, such as NHS trusts, health boards and other health services, are open and honest with patients about their care, two different duties of candour apply to nurses:

- an organisational duty that is imposed on the employing trust and
- a professional duty imposed on registered nurses through *The Code*.

Statutory organisational duty of candour

The organisational duty of candour imposed on nurses working in England falls under the provisions of the Health and Social Care Act 2008 and the Health and Social Care Act 2008 (Regulated Activities) Regulations 2014. It applies to all health service bodies regulated by the Care Quality Commission (CQC), the statutory regulator for health services in England.

The 2014 regulations introduce revised fundamental standards for health bodies registered with the CQC and include a duty of candour. The Health and Social Care Act 2008 (Regulated Activities) Regulations 2014, regulation 20 requires nursing services to act in an open and transparent way with patients in relation to their care and treatment. It imposes a general duty to be candid with patients whether or not there has been a complaint and seeks to encourage an open honest culture.

In practice, the organisational duty of candour requires a nurse to tell the patient or their representative about a notifiable patient safety incident as soon as is reasonably practicable after the incident.

Notifiable patient safety incident

A notifiable safety incident is defined as one where a patient suffered or could suffer unintended harm resulting in:

- death;
- severe harm;

- moderate harm; or
- prolonged psychological harm.

The definition of these terms is derived from the National Patient Safety Agency's *Seven Steps to Patient Safety* (2004). These define harm as:

- injury;
- suffering;
- disability; or
- death.

Prolonged psychological harms is one that must be experienced continuously for 28 days or more.

To meet the threshold for disclosure under the duty of candour the harm must be moderate or severe as set out in Box 3.1.

Box 3.1: National Patient Safety Agency terms and definitions

No harm

Impact prevented – Any patient safety incident that had the potential to cause harm but was prevented, resulting in no harm.

Impact not prevented – Any patient safety incident that ran to completion but no harm occurred to people receiving care.

Low harm: Any patient safety incident that required extra observation or minor treatment and caused minimal harm, to one or more persons receiving care.

Moderate harm: Any patient safety incident that resulted in a moderate increase in treatment and which caused significant but not permanent harm, to one or more persons receiving care.

Severe harm: Any patient safety incident that appears to have resulted in permanent harm to one or more persons receiving care.

Death: Any patient safety incident that directly resulted in the catastrophic death of one or more persons receiving care.

(National Patient Safety Agency (2004) *Seven Steps to Patient Safety*. London: NPSA)

Duty to give an explanation and apology

Once a notifiable patient safety incident has arisen with a patient the nurse must give that patient a full explanation of what is currently known and details of any further inquiry to be carried out. The patient must also receive an apology. Both the explanation and apology must be made in person. The duty to explain and apologise includes a requirement to support the patient during this process. This might include the provision of an interpreter to ensure the patient understands the explanation and is able to ask questions of the nurse. It also includes the need to give emotional support to the patient.

Once the patient has received an explanation and apology the nurse is required to provide the patient with a written note of the discussion and must ensure that a written notice of the incident and copies of correspondence are kept for later inspection by the CQC.

Activity 3.6 *Reflection*

A woman experiencing pain and swelling in her left lower leg went to her scheduled outpatient appointment with a nurse practitioner to review her chronic care needs. Although the woman mentioned her leg pain to the nurse practitioner, the detailed discussion of her other problems meant the possibility that the pain was due to a deep vein thrombosis was overlooked by the nurse.

Over the next four days the woman experienced increased pain, swelling and difficulty walking. When she attended the emergency department a deep vein thrombosis was diagnosed, requiring three days of inpatient treatment.

In groups consider:

Does this situation meet the definition of a notifiable safety incident?

If it does what action should be taken by the nurse practitioner?

An answer is provided at the end of the chapter.

Statutory duties in Wales, Northern Ireland and Scotland

There is currently no equivalent statutory organisational duty of candour with the legal force of the one imposed in England in place in the other devolved health services but there are general duties for those services to be open and raise concerns.

In Wales the National Health Service (Concerns, Complaints and Redress Arrangements) (Wales) Regulations 2011 place a duty on the health boards providing NHS care to be open when harm may have occurred:

> *[W]here a concern is notified by a member of the staff of the responsible body, the responsible body must, where its initial investigation determines that there has been moderate or severe harm or death, advise the patient to whom the concern relates, or his or her representative, of the notification of the concern and involve the patient, or his or her representative, in the investigation of the concern.*
> (National Health Service (Concerns, Complaints and Redress Arrangements) (Wales) Regulations 2011 regulation 12(7))

The Scottish and Northern Ireland governments are committed to imposing a statutory duty of candour in their devolved health services but the legislation has yet to be implemented (The Health (Tobacco, Nicotine etc. and Care) (Scotland) Bill and Department of Health Social Services and Public Safety 2015).

Professional duty of candour

In its response to the Francis report (House of Commons, 2013) the government made clear that a statutory organisational duty of candour alone was not enough to promote openness and honesty in the NHS. In the government's view it was critical to ensure that registered health professionals also had an individual duty of candour imposed on them.

Imposing a professional duty of candour on all registered health professionals, and this includes nurses, ensures a consistent approach to candour and the reporting of errors. A professional duty also ensures that those who seek to obstruct others in raising concerns will be in breach of their professional code and guilty of professional misconduct.

The Professional Standards Authority (PSA) oversees the regulation of health and social care professionals by regulating the professional regulators including the NMC. The PSA were charged by the government to ensure clear and consistent guidance and standards for the duty of candour by the professional regulators. Currently only two regulators, the General Medical Council (GMC) and the NMC, have explicit standards requiring their registrants to be open and candid with patients in their professional Codes.

The statutory regulators of health and social care professionals have issued a joint statement on the professional duty of candour that establishes a common professional duty on registered health professionals even though it may be expressed in different ways in their statutory codes. The statutory regulators must promote the professional duty of candour expressed in the joint statement and hold registered professionals accountable against it.

The jointly agreed professional duty of candour requires that

> *[e]very healthcare professional must be open and honest with patients when something goes wrong with their treatment or care which causes, or has the potential to cause, harm or distress.* (General Chiropractic Council et al., 2014)

Nurse's professional duty of candour

The NMC has implemented this joint statement on the requirements of a professional duty of candour as standard 14 of the revised *Code*. The standard requires that nurses must be open and candid with all service users about all aspects of care and treatment, including when any mistakes or harm have taken place.

To achieve the standard registered nurses must:

- act immediately to put right the situation if someone has suffered actual harm for any reason or an incident has happened which had the potential for harm;
- explain fully and promptly what has happened, including the likely effects, and apologise to the person affected and, where appropriate, their advocate, family or carers; and
- document all these events formally and take further action (escalate) if appropriate so they can be dealt with quickly.

Guidance on the duty of candour

The NMC and the GMC (2015) have issued joint guidance on the implementation of their professional duty of candour. The guidance makes clear that:

- Openness and honesty begins before care and treatment and patients must be fully informed about their care and this includes the risks as well as the benefits of the options available.
- The professional duty of candour is not intended for circumstances where a patient's condition gets worse due to the natural progression of their illness. It applies when something goes wrong with a patient's care, and they suffer harm or distress as a result.
- When a nurse realises that something has gone wrong, and after doing what they can to put matters right, the district nurse or someone from the healthcare team must speak to the patient. The most appropriate team member will usually be the lead or accountable clinician.
- Nurses must speak to the patient as soon as possible after they realise something has gone wrong with their care. There is no need to wait until the outcome of an investigation to speak to the patient, but you should be clear about what has and has not yet been established.
- Nurses should apologise to the patient who will expect to be told three things as part of that apology: what happened, what can be done to deal with any harm caused and what will be done to prevent someone else being harmed.
- Nurses must embrace a learning culture by reporting errors so that lessons can be learnt quickly and patients can be protected from harm in the future.

Activity 3.7 *Research*

Download and read the nursing case studies on the duty of candour from **www.nmc.org.uk/globalassets/sitedocuments/nmc-publications/case-studies.pdf**

The aim of the statutory and professional duty of candour is to promote openness in healthcare that will protect patients and improve public confidence in nursing. Nurses must ensure they discharge their duty of candour to protect their patients. Nurses who fail to be open and honest with patients can be called to account by the NMC.

Fitness to practise

The NMC admits that it would be impossible to compile a definitive list of the type of breaches of *The Code* it investigates (NMC, 2015a). However, the cases regularly considered include:

- physical, sexual or verbal abuse;
- theft;
- failure to provide adequate care (for registrants who are employers and managers this can include failing to maintain an acceptable environment of care);
- failure to keep proper records;
- failure to administer medicines safely;
- deliberately concealing unsafe practice;
- committing criminal offences;
- continued lack of competence despite opportunities to improve.

As the NMC is concerned with public safety, the degree of misconduct must initially reach a level that gives rise to concern for public safety. This often means that a nurse called to account by the NMC for professional misconduct faces several different charges, which taken together give rise to a concern for public safety. The NMC expects the nurse's employer to take appropriate disciplinary action where lesser matters of misconduct, such as arriving late for work, are concerned.

Case study 3.9: Protecting public safety

A care home manager was struck off the nursing register over a catalogue of uncaring treatment suffered by residents (Kirby, 2004). She was found guilty of seven counts of professional misconduct, including failing to take reasonable steps to maintain patients' dignity.

The Conduct and Competence Committee was told that she:

- *caused up to five sets of patients' unlabelled false teeth to be kept in a box;*
- *failed to ensure patients were dressed in their own underwear and clothing;*
- *failed to ensure there were adequate stocks of incontinence pads and toilet paper;*
- *failed to ensure adequate care was provided for a patient with a painful sore;*
- *failed to ensure adequate records were kept for another patient's weight.*

A fifth area of accountability in England

Registered nurses in England are subject to a fifth sphere of accountability that sits between the employer and profession. In response to concerns over the safety and quality of health services the Health and Social Care Act 2008 was enacted, and created:

- a new healthcare regulator, the Care Quality Commission (CQC);
- new regulations for organisations providing health and adult social care services;
- new regulations for the health and social care workforce.

At the heart of the regulations is the requirement for service providers, including nursing services, to be registered with the CQC, which has the authority to impose fundamental standards on service providers that are enshrined in law (CQC, 2014). Everyone working in health and social care, including nurses, is expected to contribute to the achievement of these standards. Where there is a risk of failing to meet the standards it must be raised to the appropriate person so that remedial action can be taken. The CQC has far-reaching powers to take action against those who do not meet these standards (CQC, 2014).

Care Quality Commission (CQC)

The CQC is the independent regulator of health and social care in England. The commission regulates health and adult social care services provided by the NHS, local authorities, private companies and voluntary organisations. Its main statutory duty is to protect and promote the health, safety and welfare of those who use health and adult social care services in England. To meet that duty, the CQC has the power to formulate policies and standards with which health and adult social care services have to comply. These include the following:

- Registration of health services to ensure that required standards of safety and quality are being met.
- Monitoring of health providers to check that they are meeting essential standards of safety and quality.
- Using enforcement powers to take speedy and effective action where services are not to the required standard.
- Carrying out periodic reviews of services to assess how well those providing and arranging services are performing.
- Offering advice and making recommendations to help improve services.

(CQC, 2009)

Registration with the CQC

Under the Health and Social Care Act 2008 all providers of health services, including NHS trusts providing maternity services in England, have to register with the CQC if they are undertaking regulated activities as defined in the Health and Social Care Act 2008 (Regulated Activities) Regulations 2014.

All service providers must submit evidence, including evidence from people who use the services, confirming that each standard and outcome imposed for the regulated activity is complied with (Health and Social Care Act 2008 (Regulated Activities) Regulations 2014). Where a service provider does not meet the required standard it must be declared and an action plan submitted with the reasons for non-compliance and how they will be achieved.

Fundamental standards under the Health and Social Care Act 2008 (Regulated Activities) Regulations 2014 came fully into force on 1 April 2015 and are listed in Table 3.1.

Table 3.1: Fundamental standards imposed by the Health and Social Care Act 2008 (Regulated Activities) Regulations 2014

- Care and treatment must be appropriate and reflect service users' needs and preferences.
- Service users must be treated with dignity and respect.
- Care and treatment must only be provided with consent.
- Care and treatment must be provided in a safe way.
- Service users must be protected from abuse and improper treatment.
- Service users' nutritional and hydration needs must be met.
- All premises and equipment used must be clean, secure, suitable and used properly.
- Complaints must be appropriately investigated and appropriate action taken in response.
- Systems and processes must be established to ensure compliance with the fundamental standards.
- Sufficient numbers of suitably qualified, competent, skilled and experienced staff must be deployed.
- Persons employed must be of good character, have the necessary qualifications, skills and experience, and be able to perform the work for which they are employed (fit and proper persons requirement).
- Registered persons must be open and transparent with service users about their care and treatment (the duty of candour).

Activity 3.8 *Group work*

Fundamental Standards

Download a copy of the CQC Fundamental Standards from **www.cqc.org.uk/sites/default/files/20150324_guidance_providers_meeting_regulations_01.pdf**

In groups choose three standards and compare the requirements to achieve the standard against the practice you observed on your last clinical placement.

Highlight which standards were achieved and which standards require an improvement in practice.

As this activity is based on your own experience and reflections, there is no outline answer at the end of the chapter.

CQC and healthcare regulators

The roles of the CQC and healthcare regulators are likely to clash given the nature of their function. The CQC is the regulator of healthcare in England whereas the NMC regulates nursing and midwifery. To ensure that the regulatory systems do not come into conflict, both bodies signed a memorandum of understanding in September 2010 outlining areas of cooperation. Where the NMC or CQC encounters concerns which it believes may fall within the remit of the other, they will convey the concerns with supporting information to a named officer with relevant responsibility at the other organisation. For example, the CQC can convey its concerns about a nurse's fitness to practise to the NMC. Similarly, the NMC can convey any concerns about nursing services which may call into question their registration with the CQC.

Case study 3.10: CQC demands improvement in nursing care

The CQC demanded that an NHS trust in England make improvements after inspectors visited the hospital three times and found concerns with some services. There was evidence of nine poor discharges in the previous six months and 10 cases of poor care involving discharges.

This included a patient discharged without being properly dressed and without equipment needed to keep them safe at home. In another case a patient was sent to a care home with no medication and no information about what drugs had been given before they were discharged.

Two patients with dementia were moved to the discharge lounge during the night to make space for new patients. There was minimal staffing at night, and this was raised with the hospital which put plans in place to prevent it happening again.

During one of the days the CQC visited the trust, only four of the 21 wards were fully staffed.

(Health Service Journal, *2012)*

Strengthening public confidence in the NMC

The NMC is itself regulated by the Professional Standards Authority (previously called the Council for Healthcare Regulatory Excellence), which oversees the disciplinary decisions of the main bodies of the healthcare professions. It has the power under section 29 of the National Health Service Reform and Health Care Professions Act 2002 to seek a judicial review of a disciplinary decision of a healthcare regulatory body where it considers that decision to be unduly lenient.

Case study 3.11: Unduly lenient decision

In Professional Standards Authority for Health and Social Care v Nursing and Midwifery Council *[2016] EWHC 754 (Admin) the nurse had been acting manager of a care home when complaints were brought to his attention regarding the treatment of several elderly residents by a member of staff. The nurse failed to refer those allegations to a safeguarding team, but he also made an offensive remark that dementia patients did not know what they were talking about; told other members of staff to stop making enquiries into the allegations; and used a written note from staff concerning the abuse of a resident as notepaper. At a hearing before the NMC panel only the failure to submit referrals to safeguarding and conducting an inappropriate investigation were put in the charges. The offensive remark and obstruction of the investigation were not considered. Although the panel found the nurse guilty of professional misconduct they decided that his fitness to practise was not impaired.*

The Professional Standards Authority argued that the panel's decision was not based on a full account of the incident and its finding was unduly lenient.

The court allowed the PSA appeal and held that it was important for a disciplinary body to have regard to the need for protection of the public. The importance of the omitted allegations was obvious and would provide valuable assistance to the NMC panel in determining whether the nurse had a serious underlying attitudinal problem which could affect his ability to care for the elderly. Those allegations should have been in the charges. The panel's failure to consider the allegations rendered its decision unduly lenient. The case was remitted to a differently NMC panel for rehearing.

It can be seen that you are accountable to the profession through the provisions of the Nursing and Midwifery Order 2001. This empowers the NMC to maintain a professional register of practitioners and to determine the standards of education and training necessary to enter the register and to establish standards for practice in order to remain on the register. The standards expected of a registered practitioner are set out in *The Code* (NMC, 2015a).

The role of accountability is to hold nurses answerable for their acts or omissions to a range of higher authorities with whom there is a legal relationship that binds the nurse to their rules and regulations.

Four areas of law are drawn together to provide maximum protection to the public from the harmful acts or omissions of registered nurses. By making you accountable, the law regulates your practice and deters you from conduct that might pose a threat to the public.

It is essential that, to practise safely and avoid being held to account for your actions, you must inform your practice with the requirements of the criminal, civil and contract law, and ensure that your conduct at all times meets the provisions of the NMC's *Code.*

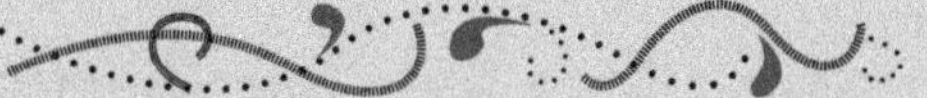

Chapter summary

- The concepts of professionalism and accountability are frequently misunderstood.
- To be accountable is to be answerable for your acts and omissions.
- You are personally accountable for your practice.
- You are answerable for your acts and omissions regardless of advice or directions from another professional.
- You do not have control or authority over who holds you to account or what you are accountable for.
- The purpose of accountability is to ensure that the public and patients are not harmed and to provide redress to those who have been harmed.
- To provide maximum protection to the public and patients four areas of law are drawn together and can individually or collectively hold you to account.
- A nurse will not generally be able to argue that they are unaccountable because of a lack of experience.
- The regulatory body for the profession is the Nursing and Midwifery Council (NMC), and it is concerned with protecting the public.
- Fitness to practise may be impaired by misconduct, lack of competence, a conviction or caution, physical or mental ill health, a finding by any other health or social care regulator or licensing body that a registrant's fitness to practise is impaired or a fraudulent or incorrect entry in the NMC's register.
- The NMC is itself regulated by the Professional Standards Authority, which oversees the disciplinary decisions of the main regulatory bodies of the healthcare professions.

Activities: Brief outline answers

Activity 3.4: Evidence-based practice and research (page 47)

1. Society through the public law: the nurse is likely to face a criminal charge of attempting to murder these patients. If found guilty, a term of imprisonment is the most likely punishment rather than a fine or community order.

2. The profession through the Nursing and Midwifery Order 2001: the nurse will be asked to justify her actions by a Conduct and Competence Committee of the NMC. If guilty of professional misconduct, the most likely sanction will be a striking-off order given the seriousness of the allegations.

3. The employer through the law of contract: the employer can hold the nurse accountable through reasonable disciplinary measures. An investigation of the incident will be conducted and if his or her employer reasonably believes that s/he is guilty of misconduct, s/he can be dismissed by her employer for breach of contract.

4. The patient through the civil law: the patients have been left with irreversible brain damage and will argue that the trust caring for them breached their duty of care, causing harm. They will sue for compensation in the civil courts.

Activity 3.6: Reflection (page 55)

A notifiable patient safety incident that triggers the statutory duty of candour is defined under paragraph 8 of the Health and Social Care 2008 (Regulated Activities) Regulations 2014, regulation 20. This states that:

> *In relation to a health service body, 'notifiable safety incident' means any unintended or unexpected incident that occurred in respect of a service user during the provision of a regulated activity that, in the reasonable opinion of a health care professional, could result in, or appears to have resulted in –*
>
> *the death of the service user, where the death relates directly to the incident rather than to the natural course of the service user's illness or underlying condition, or*
>
> *severe harm, moderate harm or prolonged psychological harm to the service user.*

Harm is defined by the National Patient Safety Agency (2004) as:

> ***Low Harm:*** *Any patient safety incident that required extra observation or minor treatment and caused minimal harm, to one or more persons receiving care.*
>
> ***Moderate Harm:*** *Any patient safety incident that resulted in a moderate increase in treatment and which caused significant but not permanent harm, to one or more persons receiving care.*
>
> ***Severe Harm:*** *Any patient safety incident that appears to have resulted in permanent harm to one or more persons receiving care.*

In your group discussion, you will have considered whether the nurse practitioner should have diagnosed a DVT during her assessment and examination of the patient and the nature of the harm to the woman as a result of missing the DVT at the outpatient appointment. If you conclude that the nurse practitioner did miss the chance to provide early treatment for the patient's DVT then you are also likely to conclude that it did not result in permanent harm and so is not classed as severe harm. You might have concluded that the harm was more that minimal and could not be classed as low harm. If you consider that four days of pain, swelling and limited mobility requiring a further three days of inpatient treatment was a moderate increase in treatment causing significant but not permanent harm, then the nurse's failure to diagnose the DVT resulted in moderate harm that triggers the statutory duty of candour. The nurse practitioner is now required, on behalf of the NHS trust, to give that patient a full explanation of what is currently known and details of any further inquiry to be carried out. The patient must also receive an apology. Both the explanation and apology must be made in person. The duty to explain and apologise includes a requirement to support the patient during this process. This might include the provision of an interpreter to ensure the patient understands the explanation and can ask questions of the nurse. It also includes the need to give emotional support to the patient. Once the patient has received an explanation and apology the NHS trust is required to provide the patient with a written note of the discussion and must ensure that a written notice of the incident and copies of correspondence are kept for later inspection by the CQC.

Further reading

Information on the types of claims made against the NHS in England can be found in this document:

National Health Service Litigation Authority (2009) *Report and Accounts 2008–2009.* London: The Stationery Office.

To give you an insight into how the NMC protects the public by encouraging them to report concerns about nurses it is well worth reading:

Nursing and Midwifery Council (NMC) (2004) *Complaints about Unfitness to Practise: A guide for members of the public.* London: NMC.

It is vital that as a student nurse you understand in practical terms the number and types of cases the NMC deals with in a typical year so we recommend you read:

Nursing and Midwifery Council (NMC) (2015) *Annual Fitness to Practise Report 2014–15.* London: NMC.

Useful website

The Nursing and Midwifery Council website is essential reading for student nurses. Here you will find additional guidance, news, consultations for you to contribute to and dates of fitness to practise hearings that you should make every effort to attend at least once during your training to experience accountability at work first hand: **www.nmc-uk.org**.

Chapter 4
Equality and human rights

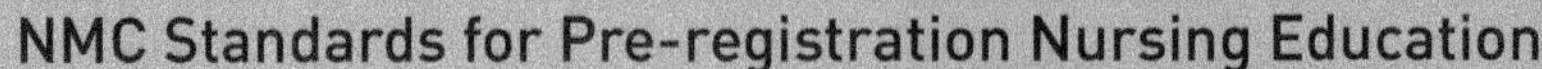

NMC Standards for Pre-registration Nursing Education

This chapter will address the following competencies:

Domain 1: Professional values

2. All nurses must practise in a holistic, non-judgemental, caring and sensitive manner that avoids assumptions, supports social inclusion; recognises and respects individual choice; and acknowledges diversity. Where necessary, they must challenge inequality, discrimination or exclusion from access to healthcare.

Domain 2: Communication and interpersonal skills

1. All nurses must build partnerships and therapeutic relationships through safe, effective and non-discriminatory communication. They must take account of individual differences, capabilities and needs.
3. All nurses must be aware of their own values and beliefs and the impact this may have on their communication with others. They must take account of the many different ways in which people communicate and how these may be influenced by ill health, disability and other factors, and be able to recognise and respond effectively when a person finds it hard to communicate.

Chapter aims

By the end of this chapter you will be able to:

- explain what is meant by a 'right';
- describe the purpose of the Human Rights Act 1998;
- discuss how the Human Rights Act 1998 affects the delivery of healthcare;
- outline how disabled people are protected from discrimination;
- illustrate the measures enacted to outlaw discrimination on the grounds of race;
- state the role of the Equality and Human Rights Commission.

Introduction

This chapter explores the notion of rights as they apply to nursing and will focus in particular on human rights. The provisions and key concepts of the Human Rights Act 1998 are introduced and explored with the emphasis on how a rights-based legal system affects nursing practice. Leading on from this, the chapter highlights how the state's obligations under the Human Rights Act 1998 have resulted in stronger laws protecting people from discrimination. Disability discrimination and race discrimination are explored in the context of healthcare.

A right is an interest recognised and protected in law. The traditional method of bestowing rights in the legal systems of the UK was to place obligations on others to act or refrain from acting in a particular way. For example, patients have a right not to be harmed when in your care. You have an obligation – a legal duty – to be careful when nursing patients. Where you fail in that duty and cause harm to the patient you will be liable in the law of negligence. In the UK, Parliament is able to create, remove and change the law and the obligations imposed by them.

Following the atrocities of the Second World War, the European Convention on Fundamental Rights and Freedoms (Council of Europe, 1950) (the Convention) was created by the Council of Europe to formalise the relationship between individuals and the government of the country in which they live. The main purpose of the Convention is to limit a state's interference with the rights of the citizens, because some rights are considered so fundamental that they must be respected in every individual's case.

Activity 4.1 *Reflection*

Defining a human right

Before reading on, write down what you understand by the term 'human rights'.

An outline answer is given at the end of the chapter.

The rights enshrined in the European Convention on Human Rights underpin all the domestic laws of the United Kingdom. The European Convention is based on the Universal Declaration on Human Rights from the United Nations (1948). They require each individual to be treated with respect, dignity and compassion. Registered nurses have a duty to respect and uphold people's human rights under the provisions of the NMC *Code* (2015a), standard 1.5.

Dignity and human rights

Dignity is a vitally important concept in nursing and it is essential that you understand its scope and your duty to uphold the dignity of the patients in your care.

The right to be treated with dignity is proclaimed in article 1 of the Universal Declaration of Human Rights (1948):

> *All human beings are born free and equal in dignity and rights. They are endowed with reason and conscience and should act towards one another in a spirit of brotherhood.*

Article 1 of the Charter of Fundamental Rights of the European Union 2000 also asserts that *Human dignity is inviolable. It must be respected and protected.*

The term 'dignity' is not specifically set out in the European Convention but it clearly underpins the fundamental rights and freedoms it set out. The European Court of Human Rights has emphasised that

> *[t]he very essence of the Convention is respect for human dignity and human freedom.* (*Pretty v United Kingdom* [2002])

Respecting and protecting dignity is a fundamental element of nursing those who are vulnerable to ill health or disability.

> *Human dignity is all the more important for people whose freedom of action and choice is curtailed, whether by law or by circumstances such as disability. We need to be able to use [the European Convention on Human Rights] to promote respect for the inherent dignity of all human beings but especially those who are most vulnerable to having that dignity ignored.* (Baroness Hale of Richmond, 2004)

To avoid discrimination it is necessary to treat the sick and disabled differently, because their situation is significantly different from that of the able-bodied. The state and its organisations, such as the NHS, have a duty to take reasonable and appropriate measures to uphold the human rights of those who are vulnerable due to ill health or disability. For nurses this means upholding dignity by showing empathy and humane concern for their patients that ensures nursing care ameliorates and compensates for their disabilities.

In all your dealings with vulnerable or disabled patients you must show your respect for the patient as a unique individual, through understanding, empathy and compassion. As a registered nurse you will be called on daily to discharge your professional duty to ensure that you deliver the fundamentals of care by caring for, feeding and toileting those who need assistance with these most intimate and sensitive activities. Dignity has an obvious role to play in these fundamental elements of nursing care. Sadly, it is during these intimate and sensitive interventions that the dignity of the vulnerable is too often ignored.

Case study 4.1: Failing to treat a patient with dignity

A hospital staff nurse was struck off the professional register by the NMC who found her fitness to practise was impaired by misconduct because she failed to maintain the privacy and dignity of a patient. Whilst helping the patient to use a bedpan, the nurse left the room blinds up and left the door of the room open.

(NMC, 2016)

Activity 4.2 encourages you to download and read the findings of the Francis report into care provided by the Mid Staffordshire NHS Foundation Trust that will shock the conscience of all decent-minded student nurses. Remember your patients are not simply numbers – they are husbands, wives, sons, daughters, fathers, mothers, grandparents. They are people who rightly expect to be well cared for and treated with kindness, respect and compassion.

Activity 4.2 | *Research*

Independent Inquiry into Care Provided by Mid Staffordshire NHS Foundation Trust

Download Volume 1 of the Francis report from **www.midstaffsinquiry.com/assets/docs/Inquiry_Report-Vol1.pdf**

Read Section A of the report, detailing the experience of patients, then identify what you consider to be breaches of dignity and human rights in the care of patients that are set out in the report.

We have seen that article 1 of the Universal Declaration of Human Rights (United Nations, 1948) calls upon us to *act towards one another in a spirit of brotherhood.* The principle is not a new one and the challenge for you is to ensure that it is observed. Your compassion as a nurse is a vital aspect of your humanity and respect for the dignity and human rights of the patients in your care.

Although the UK was an early signatory to the European Convention on Human Rights (Council of Europe, 1950), enforcing human rights was a difficult and protracted process as Parliament had never incorporated the Convention into domestic law. This was changed by the Human Rights Act 1998, making the main provisions of the Convention enforceable in UK law (see the box below).

Main rights incorporated into the Human Rights Act 1998

Schedule 1, part I, the Convention: Rights and Freedoms

Article 2	Right to Life
Article 3	Prohibition of Torture
Article 4	Prohibition of Slavery and Forced Labour
Article 5	Right to Liberty and Security
Article 6	Right to a Fair Trial
Article 7	No Punishment Without Law
Article 8	Right to Respect for Private and Family Life
Article 9	Freedom of Thought, Conscience and Religion

Article 10	Freedom of Expression
Article 11	Freedom of Assembly and Association
Article 12	Right to Marry
Article 14	Prohibition of Discrimination
Article 16	Restrictions on Political Activity of Aliens
Article 17	Prohibition of Abuse of Rights
Article 18	Limitation on Use of Restrictions on Rights

The Human Rights Act 1998 works by unlocking Convention rights, making them enforceable before UK courts and tribunals. It is unlawful for public authorities, including the NHS, to act in a way that is incompatible with these rights (Human Rights Act 1998, section 6).

The box below shows that public authorities are those that have or carry out a public function.

Main public authorities in healthcare

- Courts and tribunals
- NHS trusts
- Private and voluntary sector contractors when undertaking public functions under contract to the NHS
- Local authorities, including social services
- General practitioners (GPs), dentists, opticians and pharmacists when undertaking NHS work
- Clinical commissioning groups, foundation trusts and local health boards
- Bodies that have functions of a public nature (e.g. a professional regulatory body), even if they also have private functions

How the Human Rights Act 1998 works

The laws of the UK continue to apply in the same way. The duties imposed on a nurse when caring for a patient through the laws of negligence, consent and confidentiality continue to be applied. However, where a person, such as a patient, believes that a law or the way a law is enforced breaches a fundamental right of the Convention, they can challenge that law in court. The courts supervise the decisions of public authorities when human rights are in question (*R (Mahmood) v Secretary of State for the Home Department* [2001]).

The Human Rights Act 1998 requires that all legislation is interpreted and given effect so as to comply with Convention rights, regardless of when the Act in question came into force (Human Rights Act 1998, section 3). The courts will do their best to apply this principle to avoid the need to change the law.

Case study 4.2: Who can be a nearest relative?

In R (on the application of SSG) v Liverpool City Council (1), Secretary of State for Health (2) and LS (Interested Party) *[2002], a woman argued that her human rights were breached by a requirement of the Mental Health Act 1983 that stipulated that in a same sex relationship the partner could not be recognised as the nearest relative unless they had lived together for five years. For heterosexual cohabitees this period was six months.*

The court held that to comply with the Human Rights Act 1998 the Mental Health Act 1983 had to be read so as to permit same sex partners the same rights as heterosexual partners. This could be done without the need to amend the law.

Where the law is in breach of a fundamental human right, then the courts will declare that it is incompatible with the Human Rights Act 1998 and leave it to Parliament to amend the offending Act (Human Rights Act 1998, section 4). This is achieved by Parliament making a remedial order to amend the legislation to bring it into line with Convention rights.

Case study 4.3: Remedial order amending the Mental Health Act 1983

In R (H) v Mental Health Review Tribunal for North East London Region *[2001], the Court of Appeal declared sections 72 and 73 of the Mental Health Act 1983 incompatible with the Human Rights Act 1998, as they failed to put the burden of proof for the continued detention of patients on to the health service. The Minister for Health issued a remedial order amending the sections and requiring the Mental Health Review Tribunal to discharge a patient where the hospital failed to show that the criteria for detention were met.*

Obligations created by the Human Rights Act 1998

Positive obligations

Article 1 of the European Convention on Human Rights requires that steps are taken to secure fundamental rights and freedoms for citizens. This creates a positive obligation to ensure that appropriate laws and policies are in place to protect citizens and allow them to enjoy the rights and freedoms contained in the Convention.

Case study 4.4: The law failed to protect a child from a beating

In A v United Kingdom *[1998], an unruly nine-year-old boy was beaten by his stepfather, who was subsequently charged with assault occasioning actual bodily harm. At trial the stepfather was acquitted after the jury accepted the defence of reasonable chastisement.*

continued . . .

The boy then took the UK government to the European Court of Human Rights, alleging a breach of their positive obligation to protect him from inhuman and degrading treatment and punishment under article 3 of the Convention. The court held that English law failed to protect children as it allowed the defence of reasonable chastisement and so breached article 3. The government gave an undertaking to the court that English law would be amended to increase protection.

Negative obligations

A negative obligation requires that a state and its public authorities respect human rights in their day-to-day dealings with individuals. For example, state schools are forbidden to use corporal punishment to control unruly children.

In addition to the duties imposed by law and *The Code,* nurses also have a negative obligation not to breach the human rights of patients in their care.

Case study 4.5: Giving treatment to a sick child against the wishes of the mother

In Glass v United Kingdom *[2004], a severely physically and mentally disabled child (G) complained that the UK had violated his right to physical integrity under the European Convention on Human Rights 1950, article 8. On his readmission with respiratory failure, the hospital insisted that he was dying and that diamorphine should be given to relieve his obvious distress. His mother disagreed and objected to the proposed treatment in the belief that it would harm G's chances of recovery. Diamorphine was administered but the child's condition improved and he returned home.*

The court upheld the complaint that his treatment was contrary to his mother's wishes and the hospital had breached its negative obligation to respect his right to physical integrity under article 8 of the Convention.

Absolute, limited and qualified rights

Absolute rights

Not all rights within the Convention carry the same weight in law. Absolute rights such as the right to life (article 2), protection from torture, inhuman and degrading treatment and punishment (article 3), and the prohibition on slavery and enforced labour (article 4) may not be deviated from in any circumstances.

Case study 4.6: No-lift policies and human rights

In R (on the application of A and Others) v East Sussex County Council and Another *[2003], the High Court held that a no-lift policy, which completely banned manual handling or only allowed it where a person's life was in danger, would breach the absolute right to life (article 2) or the right to freedom from torture, inhuman and degrading treatment and punishment (article 3). The court held that, in some circumstances, such as a fire endangering a patient's life or where a patient might be left for too long in their own excrement or might develop pressure sores if not moved, then manual handling might be the only way to protect the patient from a breach of these fundamental human rights.*

Limited rights

Limited rights such as the right to liberty (article 5) have limited exceptions under explicit and finite circumstances set out in the Convention itself.

For example, if the right to liberty was absolute, then the state would not be able to imprison criminals or detain patients with mental disorders or diseases that were a danger to public health. Therefore article 5(1)(a) of the Convention allows for the lawful detention of a person after conviction by a competent court, while article 5(1)(e) provides for the lawful detention of persons for the prevention of the spreading of infectious diseases, and of persons of unsound mind.

Qualified rights

The third class of rights in the Convention are qualified rights. Qualified rights include the right to respect for private and family life (article 8), religion and belief (article 9), freedom of expression (article 10) and assembly and association (article 11).

Qualified rights have general exceptions and derogation; that is, relaxation of the legal rule is allowed where it:

- has its basis in law; and
- is done to secure a permissible aim set out in the relevant article; and
- is necessary in a democratic society to fulfil a pressing social need, pursue a legitimate aim and be proportionate to the aims being pursued.

Proportionality is a principle that requires any interference with a Convention right to be carefully designed to meet the objective in question and must not be arbitrary or unfair.

Case study 4.7: Disproportionate use of a care order

In C and B (Children) (Care Order: Future Harm) *[2000], the Court of Appeal held that the granting of a care order in respect of two children on the grounds that their mother might cause them significant harm in the future if her mental health deteriorated was a disproportionate response to the assessed risk. The court revoked the care orders and imposed supervision orders in their place.*

Human rights and nursing practice

The right to life (article 2)

The European Court of Human Rights has stated that this right

> *ranks as one of the most fundamental provisions in the Convention ... Together with Article 3 ... it ... enshrines one of the basic values of the democratic societies making up the Council of Europe.*
> (*NHS Trust A v M* [2001])

Article 2 imposes on the state and its authorities a positive obligation to protect the right to life. The state must take appropriate steps to preserve life and this has been recognised in the health-care context. In *Association X v United Kingdom (7154/75)* (1978), the European Commission on Human Rights stated that the concept that everyone's life shall be protected by law requires the state not only to refrain from taking life intentionally, but to take appropriate steps to safeguard life. This would suggest that article 2 covers both the intentional deprivation and careless endangering of life.

The purpose of article 2 is to emphasise the principle of the sanctity of life and, in *Pretty v DPP* [2001], a woman in the latter stages of motor neurone disease wanted a pardon for her husband if he assisted her to take her own life. The House of Lords held that article 2 gave rise to a right to life, not a right to die, and that the sanctity of life demanded by article 2 could not allow the state to sanction the intentional human intervention to end life.

The only inroad into the sanctity of human life allowed by article 2 has been the withholding of life-sustaining treatment. In *NHS Trust A v M* [2001], the High Court declared that, where the continuation of treatment was no longer in the best interests of a patient, action to discontinue that treatment would not constitute an intentional deprivation of life. The court held that the withdrawal of treatment would not breach the positive obligation to take adequate and appropriate steps to safeguard life if that treatment was futile.

The remit of article 2 is extremely narrow. It is only engaged when there is intentional or careless human intervention to end life. Active euthanasia would be a breach of article 2. Withholding life-sustaining treatment, such as artificial hydration and nutrition, is not a breach of article 2 if continued treatment is futile or the patient chooses not to continue with such treatment.

Prohibition of torture, inhuman or degrading treatment or punishment (article 3)

Although an absolute right, article 3 contains three different thresholds, namely torture, inhuman treatment and degrading treatment. For article 3 to be engaged one of the three thresholds must be breached.

Activity 4.3 ***Reflection***

Inhuman or degrading treatment

Reflect back on your clinical practice placement and briefly highlight some instances where you believe an intervention might amount to inhuman or degrading treatment. Please do not identify the placement or the patients, but just general examples. For instance, you could write that a delay in attending to a patient who was doubly incontinent amounts to inhuman and degrading treatment.

An outline answer is given at the end of the chapter.

Torture consists of deliberate inhuman treatment, causing very serious and cruel suffering. The threshold for torture was reduced in *Selmouni v France* [1998], when the European Court of Human Rights held for the first time that a sustained beating amounted to torture not inhuman treatment. The effect of lowering the threshold for torture is to lower the threshold for inhuman and degrading treatment and, while few patients would claim to have been tortured, they will find it easier to argue that treatment was inhuman or degrading in nature.

Indeed, in *Tanko v Finland* [1994], the European Commission on Human Rights refused to exclude the possibility that a lack of proper medical care, in a case where someone is suffering from a serious illness, could amount to treatment contrary to article 3.

Inhuman treatment or punishment

Inhuman treatment or punishment is less severe than torture. It includes less serious physical assaults, inhuman detention conditions and a lack of proper medical care.

Case study 4.8: Lack of proper treatment

In D v United Kingdom *[1997], the European Court of Human Rights held that to deport a man in the advanced stages of AIDS would be a breach of article 3. Withdrawal of the care, support and treatment he was currently receiving in the UK would have serious consequences and would expose him to a real risk that he would die in distressing circumstances, which would amount to inhuman treatment contrary to article 3.*

Degrading treatment or punishment

Treatment is degrading if it is ill-treatment that is also grossly humiliating. Treatment is capable of being degrading within the meaning of article 3, whether or not it arouses feelings of fear, anguish or inferiority in the victim. It is enough if judged by the standard of right-thinking bystanders that it would be viewed as humiliating or debasing the victim, showing a lack of respect for, or diminishing, their human dignity (*R (Burke) v GMC and Others* [2004]).

If a nurse witnessed the degrading treatment of a patient, then that would engage the patient's rights under article 3 even if the patient was too ill or incapable to be aware of the degrading treatment themselves.

The healthcare exception

A key exception to the principle of inhuman or degrading treatment applies to the provision of healthcare. In *Herczegfalvy v Austria* (1993), the European Court of Human Rights recognised that it is for medical authorities to decide on the therapeutic methods to be used, if necessary by force, to preserve the physical and mental health of patients.

A measure that is a therapeutic necessity cannot be regarded as inhuman or degrading. The court must be satisfied that the medical necessity of the treatment is convincingly shown to exist. The interpretation of the term 'convincingly shown' by the Court of Appeal in *R (on the application of N) v M* [2002] required that:

- the decision to proceed with treatment had to be in accordance with a respected body of professional opinion as set out in *Bolam v Friern HMC* [1957]; and
- be in the best interests of the patient.

Both parts of the definition have to be complied with in order to satisfy the burden of proof that the care or treatment is medically necessary.

Therefore, inhuman or degrading treatment must attain a minimum level of severity if it is to fall within the scope of article 3. This level depends on all the circumstances of the case, such as the nature and context of the treatment, the manner and method of its execution, its duration, its physical or mental effects and, in some instances, the sex, age and state of health of the patient (*T and V v United Kingdom* [1999]).

Article 3 concerns fundamental issues of respect, dignity and humanity and can apply to healthcare.

Case study 4.9: Detention without appropriate psychiatric treatment was inhuman and degrading

A man was arrested and detained by the police under the Mental Health Act 1983. He was held in a cell for more than 72 hours while an appropriate placement was found. During this time he repeatedly banged his head on the wall, drank from the toilet and smeared himself with faeces. He was eventually transferred to a clinic for treatment.

The European Court of Human Rights took into account his vulnerability throughout his detention and the fact that he had been in real need of psychiatric treatment. They held that his initial care in police custody had diminished his dignity and breached his right under article 3.

(MS v UK, *[2012]*)

Although article 3 has a broader remit than article 2, nevertheless it still requires a high threshold to be crossed before its provisions are engaged. Only where patients are subject to the severest forms of unnecessary distress will their rights under article 3 be engaged.

Respect for private and family life, home and correspondence (article 8)

Article 8 concerns the everyday right of individuals to respect for their private and family life, home and correspondence. However, as a qualified right article 8(2) allows scope for intrusion into this right on a variety of grounds, including the protection of health.

To be justified, any intrusion must be in accordance with the law and be proportionate to the aim being achieved.

The Convention interprets the concept of private life very broadly. In *Pretty v United Kingdom* [2002], the European Court of Human Rights held that

> *the concept of 'private life' is a broad term not susceptible to exhaustive definition. It covers the physical and psychological integrity of a person. It can sometimes embrace aspects of an individual's physical and social identity ... Article 8 also protects a right to personal development, and the right to establish and develop relationships with other human beings and the outside world. The Court considers that the notion of personal autonomy is an important principle underlying the interpretation of its guarantees. The very essence of the Convention is respect for human dignity and human freedom.*
> (*Pretty v United Kingdom* [2002] at 61)

As a qualified right the threshold for engagement is relatively low. Any interference with your patient or the way they live their lives needs to be justified and proportionate. For example, in *R v Bigwood* [2000], a woman was stabbed by her husband and received medical treatment and documentation of her wounds. Evidence including photographs was compiled by the police who charged the husband with wounding. The wife later retracted the complaint but the prosecution wished to proceed with the evidence they had collected. The wife argued that to do so without her permission was a breach of her right to respect for her private life. The judge agreed and the indictment was stayed.

The personal autonomy protected by article 8 means that it is for a competent patient, not the nurse or doctor, to decide what treatment they should be given in order to meet their need for dignity and avoid what the patient would find distressing. A competent patient's article 8 rights to physical and psychological integrity, to autonomy and dignity will therefore prevail over any rights or obligations located in articles 2 and 3 of the Human Rights Act 1988, schedule 1, part 1. Any positive obligations of the state under article 2 or article 3 necessarily cease at the point at which they would otherwise come into conflict with, or intrude into, the competent patient's rights of autonomy and self-determination under article 8 (*R (Burke) v GMC and Others* [2004]).

In order to show that their practice is in accordance with the law, nurses would need to demonstrate that they had followed the specific legal requirements for the care they have undertaken. For example, nurses would need to demonstrate that patients had exercised their right to self-determination by obtaining an effective consent before treatment and that they had carried out that treatment in a manner that reflected the extent of their duty of care towards the patient.

Article 8 is the most influential of the Convention articles that directly affect the provision of healthcare. It adds statutory force to the capable adult's right to self-determination – a right that can be exercised in defiance of the right to life (article 2) and right to freedom from inhuman and degrading treatment (article 3) of the Human Rights Act 1998, schedule 1, part 1.

To promote equality of rights and prevent discrimination, Parliament has enacted a range of statutes to supplement the Human Rights Act 1998. In particular, the law prohibits discrimination on the grounds of disability or race and the health service as a public body has a duty to promote equality in the provision of services. It is essential that nurses are aware of the legal and policy issues that are in place to prevent discrimination.

Equality Act 2010

To simplify and strengthen anti-discrimination law the Equality Act 2010 drew together and consolidated provisions relating to disability, race and sex discrimination.

Key provisions of the Equality Act 2010

- Places a duty on public bodies to consider reducing social and economic inequalities when taking strategic decisions.
- Extends definitions of discrimination to include discrimination by association or false perception.
- Allows employers to take positive actions in terms of under-represented groups.
- Extends the circumstances in which a person is protected against discrimination because of a protected characteristic.
- Allows people to make a claim if they are directly discriminated against because of a combination of two protected characteristics.
- Makes it unlawful to discriminate against adults because of their age when providing goods, facilities and services.
- Introduces new measures to address pay inequality in the workplace.
- Makes discrimination relating to the use of pre-employment health questionnaires unlawful.
- Introduces new power of employment tribunals to make recommendations.

Protection under the Equality Act 2010

Protection from unlawful discrimination is provided by the Equality Act 2010 in relation to the following protected characteristics:

- disability
- gender reassignment
- pregnancy and maternity (including breastfeeding)

- race
- religion and belief
- sex
- sexual orientation.

Discrimination

The purpose of the Equality Act 2010 is to prohibit discrimination against people because of a protected characteristic.

Activity 4.4 — *Group work*

In a group, discuss your understanding of the word discrimination.

Then discuss how an NHS hospital might discriminate against a person.

As this activity is based on your own ideas and experience, there is no outline answer at the end of the chapter.

The word discrimination comes from the Latin *discriminare*, meaning to distinguish between. Discrimination is now taken to be more than distinction; it is an action based on prejudice resulting in unfair treatment of people.

Under the Equality Act 2010 it is unlawful to discriminate against a person because of one or more protected characteristics. Discrimination arises when for a reason that relates to a protected characteristic they are treated less favourably than others to whom that reason does not apply and it cannot be shown that this treatment was objectively justified.

Different forms of discrimination are recognised under the Equality Act 2010.

Direct discrimination

Direct discrimination occurs where a health service treats someone less favourably because of one or more protected characteristics.

Case study 4.10: Lesbian couple's legal battle to get fertility treatment on the NHS

A lesbian couple were eventually allowed free fertility treatment on the NHS when their local health authority accepted that to continue to deny them access to the service was direct discrimination on the grounds of sexual orientation.

The couple were initially refused access to a specialised conception service as they were not classified as an infertile couple biologically incapable of conceiving. On this basis, it was claimed that they did not meet the necessary criteria to receive NHS-funded treatment.

Indirect discrimination

Indirect discrimination occurs when a health service's rules, policies and procedures have a worse impact on people who share a particular protected characteristic than on people who do not share that characteristic.

Case study 4.11: Optician's unfair payment scheme

An optician had a rule that said glasses could be paid for in instalments by anyone who was in work.

This rule particularly disadvantaged people who were retired as they could not take up the offer. The rule was held to be an example of indirect discrimination on the grounds of age.

Discrimination arising from disability

Health service providers and their staff must not treat disabled people unfavourably because of something connected to their disability where they cannot show that what they are doing is objectively justified. This only applies if they knew, or could reasonably have been expected to know, that the person was disabled.

Activity 4.5 *Research*

Discrimination arising from disability

Download and read *74 deaths and counting* from **www.mencap.org.uk/74deaths**

It highlights how discriminatory decision-making in healthcare results in the early death of those with disability.

Discrimination by association

Nurses must not treat someone worse than someone else because they are associated with a person who has a protected characteristic.

Case study 4.12: Mother discriminated against at work because of disability of her child

Discrimination by association is a codification (see Chapter 1) of a judgment of the European Court of Justice in Coleman v Attridge Law *[2008] where a mother argued that she was discriminated against and harassed at work because of the disability of her child. She said she was refused the same flexibility of working hours as colleagues who were parents of non-disabled children. She also said that abusive and insulting comments were made about both her and her child, whereas no such comments*

continued . . .

were made when other employees had to ask for time off, or a degree of flexibility, in order to look after non-disabled children. Her employer countered by saying the claims were not true and, even if they were, discrimination only applied to a person with a disability.

The European Court of Justice ruled that the prohibition of direct discrimination is not limited to people who are themselves disabled. It also includes less favourable treatment of an employee based on the disability of his child, whose care is provided primarily by the employee.

Discrimination arising from an incorrect perception

A nurse or other healthcare worker must not treat someone worse than someone else because they incorrectly think that person has a protected characteristic.

Case study 4.13: A case of mistaken gender

A GP's receptionist tells a woman that the practice will not take her on their patient list because they believe she is a transsexual person. This is not in fact the case but the woman is still the victim of discrimination.

Combined discrimination: dual characteristics

The Equality Act 2010 allows a claim for direct discrimination because of the combination of two protected characteristics, also known as dual discrimination.

A person might be discriminated against based on a combination of two characteristics such as age and race. The person must show that the alleged discrimination was because of the combination of two characteristics. A comparison has to be made to the treatment of a person who does not share either of the characteristics in the combination.

Case study 4.14: Combined discrimination

A BBC presenter lost her job when the programme she worked on moved to a prime time slot. She claimed this was due to her being an older woman and that a younger woman or an older man would not have been treated in the same way. The employment tribunal agreed that she had been the victim of discrimination.

Victimisation due to a complaint about discrimination

A service provider must not treat someone badly or victimise them because they have complained about discrimination or helped someone else complain, or done anything to uphold their own or someone else's equality law rights.

The provisions relating to association, perception and victimisation can apply to anyone, even if they do not have one of the protected characteristics themselves.

Case study 4.15: Victimisation because of a complaint about discrimination

A customer, a registered nurse, complains that a member of staff in a hospital café told the woman she was with that she was not allowed to breastfeed her baby except in the toilets. As a result of the complaint the café tells the nurse she is barred altogether. This is victimisation and unlawful under the Equality Act 2010 even though the nurse was not the person breastfeeding.

Age discrimination in the provision of goods and services

The Equality Act 2010 extended protection from discrimination on the grounds of age to include the provision of goods and services. Since 2012 it has been unlawful to discriminate against adults aged over 18 because of their age when providing goods, facilities and services, and carrying out public functions. Therefore an NHS body will not be able to refuse to provide a service to those over 60 years old unless it is lawfully or medically justified. Similarly, a nurse will not be able to refuse to provide a service based on age without such lawful or medical justification. The provision of products or services for people of different ages will not be affected where this is justified, such as providing heating allowance for those over 60 years of age. Age discrimination includes people in an age group who are being treated less favourably. For example, if an older people's nursing service refuses to provide care to people under 60 who, for example, have suffered a stroke, then that would be age discrimination. The extension of protection against age discrimination to include goods and services has been hailed by critics of the health services as a vital tool to combat ageism in the NHS.

In their review of age equality in health and social care, Carruthers and Ormondroyd (2009) found that:

- age discrimination remains an issue for health and social care;
- most examples of age discrimination are of indirect discrimination but these have just as detrimental an impact;
- the extension of age discrimination to the provision of health and social care should come into force at the same time as for other sectors (2012);
- negative attitudes and narrow assumptions about age, but particularly about older people, are an important cause of age discrimination;
- discriminatory behaviour often contributes to poor quality care – tackling age discrimination is necessary to achieving high quality care;
- the distribution of resources within the health and social care system will need to conform to the new legislative requirements, and in some situations will require a redistribution of resources so that needs are met more fairly.

Such is the extent of age discrimination in the health service that it was feared the government would either have to delay the application of this provision to the health service for several years in order to give the NHS time to change its systems and services, or exclude the NHS altogether. However, health services have been bound by the provision since 2012 (Williams, 2009).

Chapter summary

- The Human Rights Act 1998 incorporates the main provisions of the European Convention on Human Rights into British law.
- Human rights are fundamental freedoms that require everyone to be treated with dignity and compassion.
- The Human Rights Act 1998 requires public authorities including the NHS to comply with Convention rights.
- Convention rights give rise to positive and negative obligations.
- Convention rights may be absolute, limited or qualified.
- The right to life prohibits intentional deprivation of life, but allows the withholding of life-sustaining treatment.
- The right to freedom from torture, inhuman or degrading treatment prohibits interventions causing unnecessary distress or loss of dignity.
- The right to respect for private and family life requires respect for a patient's autonomy and dignity.
- Some 20 per cent of adults of working age are considered to have a disability.
- The Equality Act 2010 simplifies and strengthens anti-discrimination law.
- The Equality Act 2010 protects people from unlawful discrimination in protected characteristics.
- Direct discrimination occurs where a health service treats someone less favourably because of one or more protected characteristics.
- The Equality Act 2010 allows a claim for direct discrimination because of the combination of two protected characteristics, also known as dual discrimination.
- A health service provider must not victimise a person because they have complained about discrimination.

Activities: Brief outline answers

Activity 4.1: Reflection (page 67)

Human rights refer to the basic rights and freedoms to which all humans are entitled. Such rights include civil, social, economic and political rights.

Activity 4.3: Reflection (page 75)

The examples you give may at first appear to be inhuman or degrading but the threshold set out in law says that treatment cannot be inhuman or degrading if it is a therapeutic necessity – that is, it is in the best interests of the patient and accords with a practice accepted by a responsible body of professionals.

Look again at your list and consider if the situations you raise meet the therapeutic necessity criteria.

Further reading

For a broader discussion on health and human rights we would recommend one of the following titles:

Annas, G, Marks, S, Gruskin, S and Grodin, M (2004) *Perspectives on Health and Human Rights.* London: Routledge.

McHale, J and Gallagher, A (2004) *Nursing and Human Rights.* London: Butterworths.

For a more focused discussion of human rights and disability, consider reading:

Clements, L and Read, J (2007) *Disabled People and the Right to Life: The protection and violation of disabled people's most basic human rights.* London: Routledge.

Shakespeare, T (2006) *Disability Rights and Wrongs.* London: Routledge.

For a broader discussion on diversity in healthcare we recommend:

Spector, R (2008) *Cultural Diversity in Health and Illness,* 6th edn. London: Prentice Hall.

Useful websites

A full copy of the Human Rights Act 1998 can be found at: **www.opsi.gov.uk**

Recent judgments and other information from the European Court of Human Rights are published here: **www.echr.coe.int/ECHR/EN/Header/Case-Law/HUDOC/HUDOC+database/**

The National Health Service Litigation Authority maintains a human rights information service with newsletters and case sheets here: **www.nhsla.com/Pages/Home.aspx**

The government's guidance on equality, diversity and human rights pages (**www.dh.gov.uk/en/Managingyourorganisation/Equalityandhumanrights/index.htm**) has now been archived and can be accessed via **webarchivenationalarchives.gov.uk**

For more general cases of discrimination advice and support, look at the Equality and Human Rights Commission website: **www.equalityhumanrights.com/**

www.statisticsauthority.gov.uk UK Statistics Authority

Chapter 5
Consent to treatment

NMC Standards for Pre-registration Nursing Education

This chapter will address the following competencies:

Domain 1: Professional values

4. All nurses must work in partnership with service users, carers, families, groups, communities and organisations. They must manage risk, and promote health and well being while aiming to empower choices that promote self-care and safety.

Domain 2: Communication and interpersonal skills

8. All nurses must respect individual rights to confidentiality and keep information secure and confidential in accordance with the law and relevant ethical and regulatory frameworks, taking account of local protocols. They must also actively share personal information with others when the interests of safety and protection override the need for confidentiality.

Domain 3: Nursing practice and decision-making

9. All nurses must be able to recognise when a person is at risk and in need of extra support and protection and take reasonable steps to protect them from abuse.

Chapter aims

By the end of this chapter you will be able to:

- discuss the relationship between the ethical principle of autonomy and the law of trespass to the person;
- outline the role of consent in healthcare;
- describe the elements of a valid consent;
- define decision-making capacity;
- discuss the provisions for providing care and treatment to a person who lacks decision-making capacity.

Introduction

We saw in Chapter 2 that respect for the moral principle of autonomy is essential when making decisions about the care and treatment of a patient. Chapter 4 showed that respect for autonomy is further enhanced by the provisions of the Human Rights Act 1998 through the right to life, right to be free from torture, inhuman or degrading treatment, and the right to respect for a private life. This chapter examines the legal expression of those rights and principles through the law relating to consent. It begins with an exploration of the role of autonomy and consent in healthcare and moves on to consider the elements of a valid consent in law. Leading on from this the chapter takes you through the process of obtaining consent before introducing the key concept of decision-making capacity and how the provisions of the Mental Capacity Act 2005 set out the requirements for assessing capacity and making decisions for those who are unable to make care and treatment decisions for themselves. The chapter concludes by considering the limits to consent and its role in end of life care.

Nursing is very much a hands-on, interpersonal profession and nurses regularly need to touch their patients in order to examine them or provide care and treatment (*F v West Berkshire HA* [1990]). The right to touch an individual is limited in law and there is an initial presumption that it must not occur without permission.

The right to self-determination

The law recognises that adults have a right to determine what will be done to their bodies (*Schloendroff v Society of New York Hospitals* [1914]). Touching a person without consent is generally unlawful and will amount to a trespass to the person or, more rarely, a criminal assault. Bodily integrity is held in very high regard by the law. Unlike other civil wrongs, such as negligence, which requires harm, any unlawful touching is actionable even if done with the best of motives. As Dame Elizabeth Butler-Sloss stated in *Re MB (Caesarean Section)* [1997]:

> *The right to determine what shall be done with one's own body is a fundamental right in our society.*
>
> *The concepts inherent in this right are the bedrock upon which the principles of self-determination and individual autonomy are based. Free individual choice in matters affecting this right should, in my opinion, be accorded very high priority.*

Case study 5.1: Saving a patient's life without permission?

In Williamson v East London and City HA *[1998], a woman returned to hospital to have a breast implant replaced. The surgeon saw her before the operation to examine her and obtain consent for the replacement of the implant. During the examination the surgeon felt lumps under the woman's armpit, but did not say anything at this time. When in theatre the surgeon decided to look more closely at the area of concern and went on to surgically remove the lumps.*

continued . . .

The woman sued the surgeon for trespass to the person. The court held that the surgeon should have obtained consent for the removal of the lumps during the pre-operation examination. He had proceeded without permission and this was a trespass. Some £32,000 was awarded in damages.

The situation described in Case Study 5.1 highlights the high regard in which the law holds the right to self-determination by protecting individuals from violations of bodily integrity. Arguably, the surgeon had saved the woman's life, but he had done so without permission. The damages awarded reflect the seriousness of touching a patient without permission by acting in a paternalistic way and not respecting the patient's autonomy and right to decide.

The propriety of treatment

Permission to touch a patient through obtaining consent is an important defence to a claim of unlawful touching or trespass to the person. Consent, however, provides more than a defence to a claim of trespass to the person – it goes to the very heart of the propriety of treatment.

In *Airedale NHS Trust v Bland* [1993], Lord Mustill considered:

> *[a]ny invasion of the body of one person by another is potentially both a crime and a tort. How is it that nurses can with immunity perform on a consenting patient an act which would be a very serious crime if done by someone else?*
>
> *The answer must be that bodily invasions in the course of proper medical treatment stand completely outside the criminal law. The reason why the consent of the patient is so important is not that it furnishes a defence in itself, but because it is usually essential to the propriety of medical treatment.*
>
> *Thus, if the consent is absent, and is not dispensed with in special circumstances by operation of law, the acts of the nurse lose their immunity.*
> (*Airedale NHS Trust v Bland* [1993], Lord Mustill at 797)

Lord Mustill suggests that the very rightness of an examination or treatment is underpinned by the patient's consent. Where the action of the nurse falls outside what is considered proper treatment, those acts will lose their immunity.

Case study 5.2: Inappropriate treatment

In R v Nicholson *[2012] a nurse was employed in the surgical recovery room of a hospital looking after patients who were coming round after general anaesthetic. On several occasions he sexually assaulted women under his care, some of whom were recovering from anaesthesia. The allegations included the inappropriate touching of breasts and of the pubic area of female patients under the guise of providing care and treatment. He was sentenced to 13 years imprisonment that was upheld on appeal.*

Proper treatment

The Court of Appeal gave guidance on what constitutes proper treatment when it considered an intervention that might otherwise be inhuman or degrading treatment under article 3 of the European Convention on Human Rights 1950. As mentioned in Chapter 4, in *R (on the application of N) v M* [2002] the court held that treatment that was a medical necessity could not be inhuman or degrading as long as the medical necessity was convincingly shown to exist; that is, the treatment:

- was in accordance with a standard accepted by a responsible professional opinion – known as the *Bolam* test after *Bolam v Friern HMC* [1957]; and
- was in the patient's best interests.

If either strand is not met, the medical necessity of the treatment is not satisfied and the actions of the nurse will lose their immunity.

Quality of consent

As well as requiring nurses to restrict their touching of patients to that required in the course of proper treatment, the law also demands that the quality of consent reflects the sensitive nature of an intimate procedure.

When giving consent for such a procedure patients are entitled to expect that the nurse is qualified to carry it out.

Case study 5.3: Breast examination by a computer technician

In R v Tabassum *[2000], a man examined the breasts of three women after they consented to participate in a survey he said he was doing in relation to breast cancer. All the women assumed the man was medically qualified in some way as he wore a white coat, but he was not. When the women discovered this they complained to the police. The man argued that he had only touched the women in the way to which they had consented and that he had no sexual motive. The Court of Appeal held that sexual motive was irrelevant. For intimate examinations patients were entitled to a person who was qualified to carry out the procedure. As Tabassum was not medically qualified in any way, the necessary quality of the consent was absent and so the consent was not valid. Tabassum was sentenced to two years' imprisonment for indecent assault.*

The principle that intimate examinations and treatments must be carried out by suitably qualified people was highlighted in the case of the deputy manager of a care home who was convicted of assaulting one of her residents. In *R v Williams* [2004], the deputy manager of a care home attempted to carry out a manual evacuation of faeces on a resident in her care. Although she had ten years' experience in the care sector, she was not qualified to carry out the procedure.

The resident was left screaming in pain with Williams refusing to call a doctor as it would reflect badly on the home. The deputy manager was convicted of assault and sentenced to three months in prison.

Intimate examinations and treatment, therefore, require that:

- a suitably qualified or supervised person undertakes the procedure;
- the consent of the patient is obtained before the procedure; and
- the procedure is deemed to be proper medical treatment.

Where any of those conditions are not met, the actions of the nurse lose their immunity and both criminal and civil liability might arise.

Chaperones

Further protection for the nurse and patient against allegations of wrongdoing may be provided by the use of a chaperone.

Activity 5.1 **Reflection**

It is not uncommon for a nurse to be asked to act as a chaperone for a patient.

- Write down what you consider to be the role of the chaperone.
- Who do you think should fulfil that role in healthcare?

Now read below for further information.

The role of chaperones for intimate examinations and treatments was considered by the *Independent Investigation into How the NHS Handled Allegations About the Conduct of Clifford Ayling* (DH, 2004), where a doctor was convicted of 12 counts of indecent assault on his female patients.

The inquiry found no common definition of the role of a chaperone. Four differing definitions were used (DH, 2004: para. 2.51):

- a chaperone provides a safeguard for a patient against humiliation, pain or distress during an examination and protects against verbal, physical, sexual or other abuse;
- a chaperone provides physical and emotional comfort and reassurance to a patient during sensitive and intimate examinations or treatment;
- an experienced chaperone will identify unusual or unacceptable behaviour on the part of the healthcare professional;
- a chaperone may also provide protection for the healthcare professional against potentially abusive patients.

It can be seen from these definitions that a chaperone's role may be passive, as a simple witness to the examination, or active, as someone who participates in the procedure by providing comfort and reassurance, and is skilled in identifying unacceptable behaviour.

The Ayling Inquiry (DH, 2004: paras 2.58–2.60) recommended that:

- each NHS trust has a chaperoning policy and makes this explicit to patients and resources it accordingly;
- there must be accredited training for the role and an identified managerial lead with responsibility for the implementation of the policy;
- any reported breaches of the chaperoning policy must be formally investigated and treated, if deliberate, as a disciplinary matter;
- best practice demands that the chaperone policy must ensure that:
    - no family member or friend of a patient should be expected to undertake any formal chaperoning role;
    - the presence of a chaperone during a clinical examination and treatment must be the clearly expressed choice of a patient;
    - the patient must have the right to decline any chaperone offered if they so wish;
    - chaperoning should not be undertaken by other than trained staff: the use of untrained administrative staff as chaperones is not acceptable.

Elements of a valid consent

To be a valid defence to a claim of trespass, consent needs to satisfy three key elements. It must be:

- full;
- freely given; and
- reasonably informed.

Full consent

When obtaining consent, you must ensure that the patient agrees to all the treatment you intend to carry out. Proceeding with treatment that the patient is unaware of, or has refused to agree to, will be a trespass to the person and actionable in law (*Williamson v East London and City HA* [1998]).

Nurses must, therefore, take care to explain all the treatment or touching that will occur when obtaining consent from a patient and ensure that additional treatment or touching is subject to further consent.

Case study 5.4: Lack of full consent

In Devi v West Midlands RHA *[1981], a Sikh woman, aged 29 with four children, was sterilised without her consent and knowledge while undergoing an abdominal operation to repair a perforation of her uterus, because doctors felt that if she became pregnant again the womb might rupture.*

The court held that the surgery had been performed without a full consent. It was clear from the evidence that the woman's religious beliefs forbade sterilisation or contraception. As a result of the sterilisation she developed a serious mental health problem and lost all libido, so that her marriage was put under strain. Having regard to her religious beliefs and cultural background, the sterilisation was a real substantial loss that had been performed without consent.

Freely given consent

Consent is an expression of autonomy and must be the free choice of the individual. It cannot be obtained by undue influence. This does not mean that a nurse cannot influence a patient's decision. Indeed, part of the nurse's role is to explain the benefits of treatment to patients in order to obtain consent. Even suggesting that, by refusing to take medicine or other treatment, the patient will get the nurse rebuked is not considered to be undue influence. In law, to be undue the influence must erode the free will of the patient. It must be so forceful that the patient excludes all other considerations when making their choice, such as in situations where a threat of force or harm forces a patient to accept treatment.

Case study 5.5: No undue influence

In Centre for Reproductive Medicine v U *[2002], a widow appealed against a decision permitting the destruction by a reproductive centre of her late husband's sperm, which they had surgically removed and stored. Prior to the sperm being removed, he had signed a consent form in which he had agreed that the sperm could be used after his death. He later withdrew this aspect of his consent at the request of a specialist nursing sister, when it was explained that use after death caused ethical problems.*

Mrs U contended that her husband had withdrawn his consent reluctantly and only because he believed that, if he did not, treatment would cease or be postponed. She argued he had been unduly influenced by the nurse.

The court found that Mr U's withdrawal of his consent to the posthumous storage and use of his sperm had not been due to undue influence. The nurse had influenced his decision by explaining the difficulty of allowing the posthumous use of sperm, but she had not unduly influenced him. Mr U had listened to the nurse, asked questions, weighed his options and arrived at a freely given decision. Without an effective consent the continued storage and later use of his sperm had been rendered unlawful.

Undue influence may also be brought to bear by family members. Nurses must be certain that the choice being made is that of the patient and is not due to the outside influence of family members. In *Re T (Adult: Refusal of Treatment)* [1992], a woman who initially consented to an operation changed her mind following a visit from her mother, a person with strong views on the use of blood, and would only proceed without blood products. When Miss T later required a blood transfusion, the court held that her refusal of treatment had been negatived by the undue influence of her mother, that her refusal of treatment was not freely given and that the transfusion could proceed.

Reasonably informed consent

The law is clear that part of a nurse's duty of care is to give advice and information to a patient, so that the patient understands the nature of the treatment proposed and can make a rational choice (*Hills v Potter* [1983]). The courts do not distinguish between advice given in a therapeutic and non-therapeutic context (*Gold v Haringey HA* [1987]).

The basis of the duty to give information is derived from two areas of law: the law of trespass and the law of negligence.

Trespass to the person

In trespass a real or effective consent requires that the nurse explains in broad terms the nature of the treatment to the patient. As long as the broad nature of the touching has been explained, no cause of action in trespass will arise. In *Potts v NWRHA* (1983), a patient successfully sued for battery when she was led to believe that she was having a routine post-natal vaccination. In fact, she was given the long-acting contraceptive Depo-Provera. If a nurse gives misinformation or false information to a patient, consent will be negatived and liability in trespass will arise.

Negligence

The second type of information required to be given to a patient concerns the risks inherent in any treatment. Here the courts have been quick to point out that a failure to disclose risks does not vitiate a real consent and no action is possible in trespass (*Hills v Potter* [1983]). The proper cause of action in disclosure of risks cases falls in negligence.

Breach in the standard of care

Nurses owe a duty to their patients to take reasonable care not to cause harm. Advising patients about the risks associated with treatment and about less risky available options for treatment forms part of that duty of care (*Sidaway v Bethlem Royal Hospital* [1985]).

Activity 5.2 — *Critical thinking*

Knowledge of risks

- How much information do you think a patient should be given about their treatment?
- Should they be told every last detail or just what you consider important?

An outline answer is provided at the end of the chapter.

The issue of how much information a patient should receive about risks was initially considered by the House of Lords in *Sidaway v Bethlem Royal Hospital* [1985]. In this case a woman underwent surgery for persistent pain, which carried a less than 1 per cent risk of damage to the spine even if performed properly. This risk occurred and the woman suffered severe injuries. She claimed she had not been warned of the risk and would not have consented to the surgery had she been told. Their Lordships held that the surgeon had acted in accordance with an accepted body of practice at the time and there was no negligence.

Move from Bolam to a prudent patient approach

It has been seen that a nurse's duty of care to a patient includes giving advice and information about the inherent risks of the proposed treatment (*Sidaway v Bethlem Royal Hospital* [1985]). Failure to warn of material risks that then caused harm would result in an action for negligence (*Chatterton v Gerson* [1981]).

For the last thirty years the amount of information about the risks inherent in treatment to be disclosed to a patient when obtaining consent was generally left to the nurse or other health professional to decide based on the *Bolam test* (*Bolam v Friern HMC* [1957]). That is, nurses were required to disclose information that a respected body of their professional peers would disclose to the same patient in the same circumstances.

The United Kingdom Supreme Court has now ruled that this paternalistic approach to the duty to warn of risks is no longer acceptable in twenty-first-century Britain as the relationship between nurses and their patients is now very different from 1985. Patients are now active partners in decisions about their healthcare and should have the right to sufficient information about the treatment and any alternatives to enable them to make an informed choice (*Montgomery v Lanarkshire Health Board* [2015]).

Case study 5.6: Prudent patient test

In Montgomery v Lanarkshire Health Board *[2015] a woman of short stature with diabetes was under the care of an obstetrician as she was expected to have a large baby. Although the risk to her baby of shoulder dystocia, where the baby's shoulders would be unable to pass through the pelvis, was some 9 to 10 per cent this risk was not disclosed to the mother nor was the alternative possibility of delivering the baby by caesarean section. Shoulder dystocia did occur and the baby suffered severe disability from the resulting occlusion of the umbilical cord.*

In their judgment the Supreme Court held that nurses and other health professionals could no longer rely on the paternalistic Bolam test *as the standard for disclosing information about risks inherent in treatment. The court found that greater importance was now attached to personal autonomy and, when asked to make a decision about treatment that might have an effect on their health and well being, patients were entitled to information about risks and about alternative treatment that might be available.*

Since the introduction of the Human Rights Act 1998 the courts have increasingly reflected the fundamental values of the European Convention on Human Rights (1950) including the value of self-determination set out in the right to respect for a private and family life (Human Rights Act 1998, schedule 1, part 1, article 8).

The duty to advise patients of the risks of proposed treatment no longer falls within the scope of the Bolam test. An adult person of sound mind is entitled to decide which, if any, of the available forms of treatment to undergo, and their consent has to be obtained before treatment interfering with bodily integrity is undertaken (*Tracey v Cambridge Uni Hospital NHS Foundation Trust and others* [2014]).

Nurses are now under a duty to take reasonable care to ensure that a patient is aware of any material risks involved in any recommended treatment, and of any reasonable alternative or variant treatments. Nurses can no longer selectively choose what information to disclose (*Montgomery v Lanarkshire Health Board* [2015]).

Material risks

What constitutes a material risk has also been changed by the Supreme Court judgment in *Montgomery*. In *Sidaway* the materiality of a risk was largely based upon the percentage chance of it occurring. A risk with less than a 10 per cent chance of occurring was not generally disclosed.

In *Pearce v United Bristol Healthcare NHS Trust* [1999] the court confirmed that significant risks, again regarded as those with around a 10 per cent chance of occurring, should be disclosed. Lord Woolf held that

> *[i]n a case where it is being alleged that a plaintiff has been deprived of the opportunity to make a proper decision as to what course he or she should take in relation to treatment, it seems to me to be the law, … that if there is a significant risk which would affect the judgment of a reasonable patient, then in the normal course it is the responsibility of a [health professional] to inform the patient of that significant risk, if the information is needed so that the patient can determine for him or herself as to what course he or she should adopt.*
> (at paragraph 21)

In *Montgomery v Lanarkshire Health Board* [2015] the Supreme Court now requires nurses to judge the materiality of a risk by considering

> *whether, in the circumstances, a reasonable person in the patient's position would be likely to attach significance to the risk, or the [nurse] was or should reasonably be aware that the particular patient would be likely to attach significance to it.*
> (at paragraph 87)

This prudent patient approach to the duty to disclose risks brings the law in the United Kingdom into line with the law in other common law jurisdictions including the United States (*Canterbury v Spence* [1972]), Canada (*Reibl v Hughes* [1980]) and Australia (*Rogers v Whitaker* [1992]).

Impact on nursing practice

In *Montgomery v Lanarkshire Health Board* [2015] the Supreme Court made clear that whilst the case concerned the duty of a consultant obstetrician to disclose risks the principles established in the judgment are relevant to other health professionals including nurses.

Nurses must therefore ensure that they provide patients with information about treatment that a prudent patient would want to know. This change in the law is also reflected in the revised NMC *Code* (2015a) at standard 2 that requires nurses to listen to people and respond to their preferences and concerns. This includes respecting a person's right to be involved in decisions about their health, well being and care.

The nurse–patient partnership

The Supreme Court decision in *Montgomery v Lanarkshire Health Board* [2015] together with changes to the regulatory standards for nurses and the health service signal a fundamental shift away from a paternalistic nurse–patient relationship to a patient-centred nurse–patient partnership, with the emphasis placed on the patient's wishes and views on their care. This shift in emphasis can be traced back to the Francis report (House of Commons, 2013) into the Mid Staffordshire NHS Foundation Trust and the government's response to that report (DH, 2014) which resulted in:

- the introduction of fundamental standards under the Health and Social Care Act 2008 (Regulated Activities) Regulations 2014 that came fully into force on 1 April 2015 and form the basis of inspections by the Care Quality Commission (CQC);
- a revised code of professional standards and behaviour from the Nursing and Midwifery Council (NMC, 2015a) that came into force on 31 March 2015; and
- a decision of the UK Supreme Court in *Montgomery v Lanarkshire Health Board* [2015] that acknowledged that the general approach to a health professional–patient relationship now had to be based on partnership rather than paternalism.

Health and Social Care Act 2008 (Regulated Activities) Regulations 2014 (see Chapter 3)

The regulations contain new fundamental standards relating to safety and quality that all providers of regulated healthcare must meet and this includes nursing services. The fundamental standards set in law a clear baseline below which care must not fall and the CQC will be able to take enforcement action against providers that do not meet those standards. Some of these standards have criminal offences attached, and the CQC can bring prosecutions if these are breached and the breach causes avoidable harm or risk of such harm.

Regulations 9, 10 and 11 of the 2014 regulations require that nurses ensure that their care is person centred and that service users are respected, involved and informed of their options at each stage of their care. This includes:

- Collaborating with the service user to assess need and preferences for care and treatment.
- Designing care and treatment to meet the service user's preferences.
- Enabling and supporting service users to understand the care or treatment choices available and the balance of risks and benefits involved in any particular course of treatment.
- Providing relevant persons with the information they would reasonably need.
- Making reasonable adjustments to enable the service user to receive their care or treatment.

(Health and Social Care Act 2008 (Regulated Activities) Regulations 2014, regulations 9, 10 and 11)

The fundamental standards set out in the 2014 regulations require partnership with patients with their wishes and preferences at the centre of care and treatment.

NMC *Code* of standards of professional practice and behaviour (see Chapter 3)

The revised NMC *Code* (2015a) came into force on 31 March 2015 and the influence of the Francis report (House of Commons, 2013) is clear. A key theme underpinning the *Code* is prioritising people and this includes working in partnership with patients. This is spelt out in standard 2 of the revised *Code* that requires nurses to listen to people and respond to their preferences and concerns. This includes working in partnership with people to make sure care is delivered effectively.

Nurses must also:

- recognise and respect the contribution that people can make to their own health and well being;
- encourage and empower people to share decisions about their treatment and care;
- respect the level to which people receiving care want to be involved in decisions about their own health, well being and care;
- respect, support and document a person's right to accept or refuse care and treatment; and
- recognise when people are anxious or in distress and respond compassionately and politely.

(NMC, 2015a at standard 2)

Decision of the Supreme Court in *Montgomery v Lanarkshire Health Board* [2015]

The limited right to self-determination allowed by the law of trespass ran contrary to policy developments in the NHS and a nurse's obligation under the revised *Code* (2015a) that emphasises a partnership with patients and a restated desire to ensure that patients are involved in decisions about their health service provider, place of treatment and crucially the form of treatment (DH, 2012a).

The Supreme Court decision gives legal force to the professional requirement on nurses to listen to people and respond to their preferences and concerns. It also underpins the requirement for a patient-centred partnership set out in the Health and Social Care Act 2008 (Regulated Activities) Regulations 2014 that are the basis of inspections by the CQC.

The judgment recognises the changing relationship between nurses and their patients which is now based on partnership and the recognition of personal autonomy rather than the paternalistic nurse knows best approach of last century.

Obtaining consent

Activity 5.3 *Reflection*

- Note down the methods you have used to obtain consent from patients when on a clinical placement.
- What is the most common form of obtaining consent used by you?

Now read below for further information.

Nurses may obtain consent in two ways. A patient may express their consent – that is, a patient makes known their willingness to be touched. Express consent can be written or oral. Written consent is usually obtained where a procedure is invasive, such as surgery, or perceived as carrying a material risk, such as an immunisation, and is often taken by means of a consent form.

A consent form provides a degree of evidential certainty to the nurse that the patient agrees to treatment. It should not be relied on too heavily, however. Lord Donaldson, in *Re T (Adult: Refusal of Treatment)* [1982], pointed out that a consent form was only as useful as the understanding of the person signing it. When obtaining consent, whether in writing or orally, it is essential that an explanation of treatment and other material facts must be recorded in the patient's file to corroborate the consent.

The second form of consent is an implied consent. This is permission implied through the actions of the patient to a request to provide treatment. An obvious example would be a patient holding out an arm and rolling up a sleeve when asked for permission to take their blood pressure.

Case study 5.7: Implied consent

In O'Brien v Cunard SS Co *[1891], a woman was vaccinated against smallpox on a boat bound for Boston. Told by the doctor she should be vaccinated, she held out her arm and rolled up her sleeve to accept the injection. When she later sued for trespass the court held that consent had been implied by her actions.*

It can be seen from *O'Brien* that consent is implied from the action of the patient in response to a request to give treatment. It does not mean that agreeing to come to hospital or allowing a nurse into their home implies that a patient agrees to treatment. Every episode of care or treatment must be subject to a valid consent.

Case study 5.8: Every episode of care requires a valid consent

In Mohr v Williams *[1905], a patient agreed to a repair on a defect to their right ear. While the patient was under anaesthetic the surgeon decided to examine the left ear and, on finding the same defect, continued the operation and repaired it. The patient sued for trespass, arguing that the surgeon did not have consent for the left ear repair. The surgeon argued that, by expressly consenting to the right ear repair, the patient had implied consent for the left ear as well.*

The court disagreed with the surgeon. There was no consent and it could not be implied. Every episode of care or treatment had to have its own distinct consent. The surgeon had committed a trespass to the person.

Evidential certainty

As a matter of law each form of consent, whether it be given verbally, in writing or implied, is equally effective and it does not matter which method you use. From an evidential perspective, it is clear that a written consent provides evidence that consent was obtained. Whatever method you use to obtain consent, it is essential that your contemporaneous entry in the patient's record corroborates that consent was given and that the patient was happy to proceed with treatment. As most examinations and treatments are conducted on a one-to-one basis, a contemporaneous note of the procedure is vital to rebut any allegation of wrongdoing (*McLennan v Newcastle HA* [1992]).

Withdrawing consent

Consent is a continuous process and may be withdrawn at any time. A withdrawal of consent is indistinguishable from an initial refusal to consent. Nurses must accept that, if a patient changes their mind and refuses to continue with treatment, it must cease or trespass to the person will occur.

Where the patient then decides to continue with the treatment, it is not necessary to explain the risks inherent in the procedure all over again.

Case study 5.9: Withdrawing consent

In Ciarlariello v Schacter *[1991], a patient underwent a cerebral angiogram before which the doctor explained the effect and risks of the procedure. During the course of a second angiogram the patient became agitated and insisted that the procedure be stopped.*

Later the patient consented to the continuation of the procedure, during which she suffered a stroke and was paralysed. The patient sued, arguing that she would not have agreed to carry on if she had been reminded of the risks.

The court held that it was impracticable to apply the same stringent requirements of informing a patient of the risks of treatment, particularly a patient under sedation, once the procedure had commenced, and that the doctor had not been negligent.

The right to decide on treatment

In *Re T (Adult: Refusal of Treatment)* [1992], the Court of Appeal held that the right to decide presupposes an ability or a capacity to do so. Decision-making capacity is the key to autonomy. If a patient has capacity, their decisions are binding on you. An adult patient with decision-making capacity has the right to accept or refuse treatment even if doing so will lead to their death. This reflects the fundamental respect for autonomy in healthcare. It is not for you to judge a capable patient's decision on treatment against your values (*Re MB* (*Caesarean Section*) [1997]).

Case study 5.10: Refusal of life-sustaining blood transfusion

A 22-year-old mother died just hours after giving birth to twins, because doctors were forbidden from giving her a blood transfusion as she was a Jehovah's Witness (Attewill, 2007).

Complications set in after the birth that required an immediate emergency transfusion. Although the care team explained the consequences of not having treatment, the patient refused the blood because of her religious beliefs.

As a capable adult patient she was entitled to refuse the blood and the care team were required in law to accept her decision, even though the consequences were that the patient died.

Limits to autonomy and consent

Although the law holds respect for autonomy in high regard, the right to consent is limited by both common law and statute.

A person cannot consent to an action that would lead to their death, and a nurse who killed a patient even where the patient requested it would face a charge of murder.

Case study 5.11: Killing a patient

In R v Cox *[1992], a consultant gave a patient a lethal injection when she reminded him that he had promised not to let her suffer.*

She was cremated before the details of the incident became known and so the doctor was only convicted of attempted murder.

Decision-making capacity

Decision-making capacity is the ability to make a decision and it is the key to autonomy *(Re T (Adult: Refusal of Treatment)* [1992]). It is based on the person understanding and using information about treatment when making a decision.

Decision-making capacity can vary over time and can vary depending on the decision to be made. A patient might have the requisite capacity to make a simple decision but not the requisite capacity to make a complex decision.

Case study 5.12: Capacity to marry and make a will

An 84-year-old man chose to marry his 24-year-old maid when he was very ill and frail. Once married, his will became void and he made a new one bequeathing his considerable estate equally between his new wife and his adult children.

When he died a short while after, his wife knew that she would inherit considerably more of his estate if he had died without making a valid will. She argued that he did not have the capacity to make a will. His children countered by saying that, if that was the case, he did not have the capacity to marry his maid.

In the case of In the Estate of Park *[1953], the court held that the complexity and level of understanding required when making a will was far greater than the capacity required to agree to marry someone. The court decided that the man was capable of agreeing to marry and marrying his wife, but lacked the capacity to make a new will.*

Capacity is based on a test of understanding and is not a professional or status test. You cannot assume lack of capacity because of a person's age, physical appearance, condition or an aspect of their behaviour.

Patients who lack decision-making capacity

Patients aged 16 and over are assumed in law to have the ability to make decisions about their healthcare and their consent to treatment is required before it can proceed.

Where the patient lacks decision-making capacity, the Mental Capacity Act 2005 and its guiding principles ensure that their rights and interests are at the centre of the decision-making process (see the box below).

Box 5.1: The principles of the Mental Capacity Act 2005

- A person must be assumed to have capacity unless it is established that he or she lacks capacity.
- A person is not to be treated as unable to make a decision unless all practicable steps to help him or her to do so have been taken without success.
- A person is not to be treated as unable to make a decision merely because he or she makes an unwise decision.
- An act done, or decision made, under this Act for or on behalf of a person who lacks capacity must be done, or made, in his or her best interests.
- Before the act is done, or the decision is made, regard must be had to whether the purpose for which it is needed can be as effectively achieved in a way that is less restrictive of the person's rights and freedom of action.

The Mental Capacity Act 2005 requires you to assume that a person aged 16 or older has the capacity to make decisions, even unwise decisions, for themselves. You are able to act on a patient's decision to accept or refuse treatment without the need to assess decision-making capacity. The need to assess capacity only arises where the behaviour or circumstances of the person triggers a doubt in your mind about their ability to make a decision. The principle stresses a person's right to autonomy and is further supported by requiring steps be taken to maximise decision-making capacity.

Activity 5.4 — *Critical thinking*

Practical steps to help a person make decisions

The law recognises that some people require support to make decisions. What practicable steps could you take to help a person make a decision about care and treatment?

Now read below for further information.

The Code of Practice of the Mental Capacity Act 2005 (Department for Constitutional Affairs, 2007) suggests that practical steps to help a person make a decision might include:

- using simple language and, where appropriate, pictures and objects rather than words;
- arranging for the person to have the information in their preferred language;
- consulting whoever knows the person well on the best methods of communication;
- choosing the best time and location where the person feels at ease;
- waiting until the person's capacity improves before requiring a decision.

Where a person is considered to lack decision-making capacity, any action or decision taken must be in their best interests (see pages 105–6).

The final guiding principle of the Mental Capacity Act 2005 requires you to act in the least restrictive way possible. This important requirement will ensure that any interference with a person's rights and freedom to make decisions will be limited to that required to meet the immediate needs of the individual.

Assessing decision-making capacity

A person lacks capacity where an impairment or disturbance of the mind or brain affects their ability to make a particular decision. It does not matter whether the lack of capacity is permanent or temporary.

Case study 5.13: Temporary lack of capacity

In Re MB (Caesarean Section) *[1997], the Court of Appeal held that the panic instilled by a needle phobia drove so forcibly into the mind of the patient that she was unable to weigh the consequences of refusing treatment and was temporarily incapable.*

The test for decision-making capacity is a two-stage functional test based on the decision to be made at that time rather than a general ability to make decisions; that is:

1. Is there a permanent or temporary impairment or disturbance to the functioning of a patient's mind or brain?
2. If there is, how far does it affect the person's ability to make a decision?

A person will not be capable of making a decision if, due to an impairment or disturbance to the mind or brain, they are unable to:

- understand the treatment information relevant to the decision; or
- retain the information long enough to make a decision; or

- use or weigh the information as part of the process of arriving at a decision; or
- communicate that decision by any means.

Case study 5.14: Does the patient have decision-making capacity?

In Re C (Adult: Refusal of Treatment) *[1994], a man detained in Broadmoor special hospital and suffering from paranoid schizophrenia, with a false belief that he was a doctor, developed gangrene in his right foot. He refused consent for an amputation and took the hospital to court to ensure that no treatment would proceed without his express consent.*

The judge decided that Mr C had decision-making capacity, because, despite his profound mental health problem, he understood the surgeon's advice about the dangers of refusing treatment. He retained that treatment advice and repeated it back to the judge. Then he showed that he had used the treatment information when weighing up his options by telling the judge that he might die without the amputation but he was prepared to trust in God.

It will generally be for the person providing treatment to determine whether a patient has decision-making capacity. Where the issue is more serious, with many people involved in the care and treatment, the person in charge, usually the senior doctor, will determine if the patient has decision-making capacity. If a dispute over capacity remains unresolved, the courts will determine decision-making capacity.

Stages of the assessment process

The trigger phase

You must assume that a patient 16 years or older has capacity to consent to care or treatment unless a concern triggers a doubt about the person's decision-making capacity.

The practical support phase

You cannot say a person lacks decision-making capacity unless you have taken practical steps to help them to make a decision.

The diagnostic threshold

Are you able to discern an impairment or disturbance to the functioning of the person's mind or brain? It does not matter if this is permanent or temporary. If you cannot determine such an impairment or disturbance, no further action can be taken under the Mental Capacity Act 2005.

The assessment phase

How far does the impairment or disturbance to the person's mind or brain affect their ability to make a decision? Where a person cannot:

- understand treatment information; or
- retain treatment information; or
- use or weigh treatment information when making a decision; or
- communicate their decision in some way;

then you can reasonably conclude that they lack capacity for that particular decision.

Designated decision-makers

The Mental Capacity Act 2005 has two formal powers that allow a third party to make decisions on behalf of a person who lacks decision-making capacity These powers can give the designated decision-maker the right to consent to or refuse medical treatment. Where a designated decision-maker with authority is in place for a patient, their consent must be obtained before care and treatment can lawfully be given.

Personal welfare lasting power of attorney

A power allowing another to consent on behalf of a person who lacks capacity to make decisions can be created through a personal welfare lasting power of attorney. The power must be created by the person (the donor) when they are capable and can only come into force when the person lacks capacity and the power of attorney has been registered with the Office of the Public Guardian.

A person can also create a lasting power of attorney that allows another to manage their property and affairs.

Court of Protection deputy

When continuing decisions need to be made on behalf of a person who lacks capacity and there is no lasting power of attorney in place, the Court of Protection may appoint a person, called a deputy, to make personal welfare decisions on behalf of the incapable patient that can include the right to consent to or refuse treatment.

The court must be satisfied that the deputy is willing and able to fulfil the role and that appointing a deputy is a proportionate response to the needs of the patient.

Advance decisions refusing treatment

As well as having designated decision-makers able to make consent to treatment decisions, a person can make an advance refusal of treatment. Where a valid applicable advance refusal is in place, the wishes of the patient must be respected and treatment withheld. Compulsory treatment for mental disorder under the Mental Health Act 1983, other than electroconvulsive therapy (ECT), can override a valid and applicable advance decision refusing healthcare.

Case study 5.15: Advance decision refusing treatment

In Re AK (Adult Patient) (Medical Treatment: Consent) *[2001], a man with motor neurone disease had a long-established advance decision refusing treatment that stated that, two weeks after he lost the ability to communicate, his care team were to withhold his artificial nutrition and hydration. The court confirmed that the conditions expressed by the patient when an adult with capacity had now come into effect and it was lawful to withhold the treatment.*

Although advance decisions can be made orally, where they are to apply to life-sustaining treatment, the Mental Capacity Act 2005, section 25, requires that they are:

- made in writing;
- signed by the person or signed on their behalf in their presence;
- witnessed in writing in the presence of the person;
- verified by a statement made by the maker that expressly and specifically states that the advance decision is to apply even if life is at risk.

Best interests

The Mental Capacity Act 2005 provides a checklist of factors that must be considered when determining whether care and treatment is in the best interests of a patient who lacks capacity.

This holistic approach to best interests ensures that the wishes of the patient and views of those caring for the patient are taken into account.

When determining whether care and treatment is in an incapable patient's best interests you must:

- consider all the relevant circumstances;
- consider whether the decision can wait until the person regains capacity;
- as far as reasonably practicable, permit and encourage the person to participate in their care and treatment;
- not be motivated by a desire to bring about the death of the patient;
- consider, as far as is reasonably ascertainable:
  - the person's past and present wishes and feelings (and, in particular, any relevant written statement made when they had capacity);
  - the beliefs and values that would be likely to influence their decision if they had capacity;
  - other factors that they would be likely to consider if they were able to do so;

- take into account, if it is practicable and appropriate to consult them, the views of the following, as to what would be in the person's best interests:
  - anyone named by the person as someone to be consulted on the matter in question or on matters of that kind;
  - anyone engaged in caring for the person or interested in his or her welfare;
  - any donee of a lasting power of attorney granted by the person;
  - any deputy appointed for the person by the court.

Independent mental capacity advocate

Where no suitable person is available to be consulted on what would be in the best interests of the patient, there may be a duty to instruct an independent mental capacity advocate (IMCA).

The IMCA will make representations about the person's wishes, feelings and beliefs, and call the decision-maker's attention to the factors relevant to their decision.

IMCAs will only be involved where the decision concerns:

- serious medical treatment; that is, treatment that involves providing, withdrawing or withholding treatment in circumstances where:
  - in a case where a single treatment is being proposed, there is a fine balance between its benefits to the patient, and the burdens and risks it is likely to entail for him or her;
  - in a case where there is a choice of treatments, a decision as to which one to use is finely balanced; or
  - what is proposed would be likely to involve serious consequences for the patient;
- a change in the person's accommodation, where it is provided by the NHS or local authority; or
- authorised detention under the deprivation of liberty safeguards.

Protection from liability

Where care and treatment for an incapable adult proceeds following an assessment of capacity and determination of best interests, the caregiver is protected from liability in the law relating to consent.

Restraint

Restraint is defined as

> *the use or threat of force where the person is resisting and any restriction of liberty of movement whether or not the person resists.*

This wide definition includes even mild forms of restraint, such as holding an incapable person's hand to prevent them wandering away and holding an arm to keep it still when taking a blood sample. Restraint is permitted but only when the person using it reasonably believes it is necessary to prevent harm to the incapable person.

The restraint used must be proportionate to both the likelihood of the harm and the seriousness of the harm.

Court of Protection

The Court of Protection is a specialist court that hears cases and settles matters concerning people who lack capacity. The court can also appoint deputies (see page 104) and give them powers to make ongoing decisions for capable adults.

Office of the Public Guardian

The Office of the Public Guardian is responsible for the supervision of deputies appointed by the court and for supporting deputies in their role.

It also has a role in protecting people subject to the court's powers from abuse or exploitation by:

- keeping a register of lasting powers of attorney;
- keeping a register of orders appointing deputies;
- supervising deputies appointed by the court;
- receiving reports from attorneys;
- dealing with enquiries and complaints about deputies and attorneys.

Mental capacity law in Scotland

Scotland has had a legal framework for the management of the financial and welfare needs of incapable adults since 2001. The first major piece of legislation enacted by the Scottish parliament after devolution was the Adults with Incapacity (Scotland) Act 2000, the main provisions of which are set out in Box 5.2.

Box 5.2: Key provisions of the Adults with Incapacity (Scotland) Act 2000

A continuing power of attorney appointed by an individual, while capable, to manage property and/or financial affairs.

A welfare attorney appointed by an individual, while capable, to manage welfare matters after loss of capacity.

A person authorised by the Public Guardian to use the funds of an incapable adult for the benefit of that adult.

A guardian appointed by a sheriff who may have financial and/or welfare powers.

A person authorised to make welfare and financial decisions under an intervention order by the sheriff to deal with a specific issue.

Power for managers in authorised establishments to manage a resident's finances where no one else is available to act.

Provision for doctors to treat an incapable adult without consent.

Guiding principles

The 2000 Act provides various powers for making decisions and taking action on behalf of an incapable adult. An adult is defined by the Act as a person aged 16 years or over. Incapable is also statutorily defined as

> *incapable of acting or making decisions or communicating decisions or understanding decisions or retaining the memory of decisions in relation to any particular matter, by reason of mental disorder or of inability to communicate due to physical disability.*
> (Adults with Incapacity (Scotland) Act 2000, section 1(6))

The powers can cover property and financial affairs or personal welfare matters that include decisions about healthcare. To ensure a consistent approach when deciding whether to intervene on behalf of an incapable adult the Act requires that the general principles in part 1 are always applied (see Box 5.3).

Box 5.3: Adults with Incapacity (Scotland) Act 2000, part 1, section 1

General principles

Principle 1 Benefit

Any person intervening in the life of the incapable adult must be satisfied that there is a benefit to the adult and that such benefit cannot be achieved without the intervention.

Principle 2 Minimum intervention

The intervention must be the least restrictive option in relation to the freedom of the incapable adult. (This means that the method of intervention to be selected must be the least restrictive option and that the person who is authorised to intervene must act in the least restrictive way.)

Principle 3 Take account of the wishes of the adult

The views of the incapable adult must be sought, by any means possible. (If the adult can communicate by any means, it is a legal requirement to obtain the views of that adult, even if that means using an interpreter.)

Principle 4 Consultation with relevant others

The views of the nearest relative, the primary carer, any person already appointed to act for the adult and any other person who appears to be relevant must be sought.

Principle 5 Encourage the adult to exercise whatever skills he or she has

The adult must be encouraged to exercise whatever skills he or she has concerning property, financial affairs or personal welfare, and to develop new such skills.

Medical treatment

Where arrangements have been made for another to make decisions regarding the welfare of an incapable adult that includes consent to treatment, then the Act requires nurses, along with other health professionals, to obtain consent from that person before proceeding with treatment of the incapable adult. The power to consent to treatment may be bestowed by a welfare power of attorney, a welfare guardianship order or by an intervention order issued by the court.

Where no such arrangements are in place, then part 5 of the Adults with Incapacity (Scotland) Act 2000 makes separate provision for the medical treatment of incapable adults. This allows the medical practitioner primarily responsible for the treatment of the person to issue a certificate stating that the adult is incapable of deciding about the medical treatment in question. The certificate of incapacity has to be in a prescribed form and must specify the period during which the authority remains valid. This period is determined by what the medical practitioner primarily responsible for the medical treatment of the adult considers appropriate to the condition or circumstances of the adult. The Act, however, places a maximum limit of one year from the date of the examination on which the certificate is based.

The completion of an incapacity certificate triggers a general authority to do what is reasonable in relation to medical treatment to safeguard or promote the physical or mental health of the adult.

As the certificate can only be signed by medical practitioners, nurses cannot instigate treatment with an incapable adult unless it is an emergency.

End of life decisions

The NMC's *Code* imposes on registered nurses a duty to *recognise and respond compassionately to the needs of those who are in the last few days and hours of life* (at standard 3.2).

Withdrawing treatment

We saw in Chapter 2 that nurses and doctors sometimes have to exercise clinical judgement and come to the conclusion that to continue with treatment is futile and it should be withdrawn. Where the decision to withdraw treatment concerns life-sustaining treatment, some patients worry they will be unreasonably denied treatment towards the end of their life (GMC, 2010).

Case study 5.16: Fear of inappropriate withdrawal of treatment

A man moving into the latter stages of cerebral ataxia that would leave him aware of his surrounds but unable to move or communicate in any way was concerned that the artificial nutrition and hydration needed to keep him alive would be prematurely withdrawn by his care team. He wanted the court to confirm that he had the right to demand that the treatment should continue until he died.

The Court of Appeal held that nurses and doctors could only withdraw treatment needed to sustain life when it was futile to continue with that treatment. Any nurse who withdrew life-sustaining treatment before this time would not merely be in breach of duty but would be guilty of murder. Patients do not have the right to demand treatment as it is a matter for the clinical judgement of the health professionals involved but where there is a dispute over the lawfulness of withdrawing or withholding treatment then those health professionals might need a declaration from the court as a matter of good practice.

*(*R (On The Application Of Oliver Leslie Burke) (Respondent) v General Medical Council (Appellant) and The Disability Rights Commission and 8 Others (Interveners) *[2005])*

It can be seen from the Court of Appeal decision in *Burke* that whilst there is initially a very strong presumption in favour of taking steps that would prolong life the obligation is not absolute (*R (Burke) v GMC and Others* [2004]). Nurses are not required to continue treatment or to intervene when to do so would be futile for as important as the sanctity of life is it may have to take second place to human dignity (*Airedale NHS Trust v Bland* [1993]).

While it is never acceptable to deny a person treatment with the intention of ending their life, there may be circumstances where it would not be in their best interests to continue with or to receive treatment that would keep them alive (*Airedale NHS Trust v Bland* [1993]).

It is essential therefore that nurses apply the law in relation to futile treatment and use it to inform their practice when considering the withdrawal of treatment. In doing so the nurse will avoid an allegation of wilful neglect, gross negligence or even murder (*R (Burke) v GMC* [2005]) (see Chapter 7 for more on this).

The nurse's duty of care

Exercising clinical judgement forms part of a nurse's duty of care to their patients. The duty is a

> *single comprehensive duty covering all the ways in which you are called on to exercise skill and judgement in the improvement of the physical and mental condition of the patient.*
> (*Sidaway v Bethlem Royal Hospital* [1985] (Lord Diplock at 894))

It is an enduring duty that cannot be easily shed because once a patient has been seen that duty of care arises, a duty to provide and go on providing treatment whether the patient is competent or incompetent, conscious or unconscious. Nurses are under a continuing obligation that cannot lawfully be withdrawn unless arrangements are made for the responsibility to be taken over by someone else or a capable patient refuses treatment (*R (Burke) v GMC* [2005]).

Refusal of treatment

Adults with capacity have the right to decide whether or not to accept treatment and where such a voluntary informed decision is made it must be respected by the nurse (DH, 2009).

Consent is a continuous process and may be withdrawn at any time. A withdrawal of consent is as indistinguishable as an initial refusal to consent (*Ciarlariello v Schacter* [1993]). The House of Lords in *Airedale NHS Trust v Bland* [1993] held that

> *the principle of self-determination requires that respect must be given to the wishes of the patient so that if an adult patient of sound mind refuses, however unreasonably, to consent to treatment or care by which his life would or might be prolonged, the doctors responsible for his care must give effect to his wishes, even though they do not consider it to be in his best interests to do so. … To this extent the principle of the sanctity of human life must yield to the principle of self-determination …*
> (Lord Goff of Chieveley at 864)

Case study 5.17: The right to refuse life-sustaining treatment

As a result of a blood vessel in her neck rupturing, a woman had been left tetraplegic and in need of artificial respiration in order to sustain her life. She said that she did not wish to continue her life in this way and withdrew her consent for artificial ventilation to continue. The NHS trust refused her request to turn off the ventilator.

continued . . .

The court held that a patient with serious physical disability had the same right to personal autonomy and to make decisions as any other person with mental capacity. The woman possessed the mental capacity to make decisions regarding her treatment and so the administration of artificial respiration by the trust against her wishes amounted to an unlawful trespass and had to be withdrawn.

(Re B (Consent to Treatment: Capacity) *[2002]*)

The law and regulatory guidance is clear: a valid refusal of treatment must be respected even if serious consequences or even death results.

Where the patient lacks decision-making capacity then any decision to withdraw life-sustaining treatment must be shown to be in the patient's best interests (*Aintree University Hospitals Foundation Trust v James* [2013]).

Human rights and withdrawing treatment

It was seen in Chapter 4 that nurses have a duty to ensure that they respect the human rights of their patients.

Activity 5.5 *Reflection*

Before reading on, note which articles of the European Convention of Human Rights are, in your view, likely to be engaged by a decision to withdraw life-sustaining treatment.

Turn to Chapter 4 for further information on the rights contained in the Convention.

Now read on.

In deciding whether or not to continue with treatment for an incapable adult a nurse would have to have regard to the patient's right to life, right to be free from torture inhuman and degrading treatment and their right to respect for a private and family life that includes respect for autonomy and dignity (Human Rights Act 1998, schedule 1, part 1, articles 2, 3 & 8).

Although the right to life is held in high regard by the Convention the European Court of Human Rights recognises that the right does not extend to giving treatment which would be futile (*NHS Trust A v M* [2001]).

Case study 5.18: Futile treatment does not engage article 2, the right to life

In perhaps the first case to come before the courts following the commencement of the Human Rights Act on 2 October 2000, a hospital trust sought a declaration that it was lawful to discontinue the administration of artificial hydration and nutrition to a patient diagnosed as being in a permanent vegetative state in 1997 after having suffered anoxic brain damage. The trust submitted that it would not be in her best interests to continue the treatment but were concerned that withdrawing treatment might now be contrary to her right to life under article 2 of the Human Rights Convention.

The court held there was no obligation on the state to prolong the woman's life and the withdrawal of treatment would not breach the requirement contained in article 2 to take adequate and appropriate steps to safeguard life as the positive obligation upon a state to protect life was not an absolute obligation to treat a patient if that treatment would be futile.

(NHS Trust A v M *[2001])*

Similarly the right to life would not be engaged where providing treatment would preserve life at the expense of a person's dignity or right to self-determination in breach of their rights under articles 3 and 8 of the Convention (*R (Burke) v GMC* [2005]).

The law does allow for the withholding or withdrawing of treatment necessary to sustain life where it is futile and it is no longer in the patient's best interests to receive it (*An NHS Trust v Mr and Mrs H* [2012]). The key question for nurses is under what circumstances does life-sustaining treatment become futile?

Activity 5.6 — *Reflection*

Write down the circumstances that would lead you to conclude that continued treatment is futile and could be withdrawn.

Now read on.

When does continued treatment become futile?

The lower courts have applied a number of different tests over the last 15 years to determine if a patient's treatment is futile.

An early test adopted by the House of Lords, then our most senior court, in *Airedale NHS Trust v Bland* [1993] set a high threshold for futility and required treatment to have no therapeutic purpose of any kind before it could be regarded as futile. In *R (On The Application Of Oliver Leslie Burke) (Respondent) v General Medical Council (Appellant) & The Disability Rights Commission & 8 Others (Interveners)* [2005], the Court of Appeal reminded nurses of that high threshold whilst acknowledging that where that threshold was met treatment could be withdrawn:

> *There is a very strong presumption in favour of taking all steps which will prolong life, and save in exceptional circumstances, or where the patient is dying, the best interests of the patient will normally require such steps to be taken. In case of doubt it falls to be resolved in favour of the preservation of life. But the obligation is not absolute. Important as the sanctity of life is, it may have to take second place to human dignity.*
> (Lord Phillips at 304)

The general presumption in law is that a patient's best interests requires the continuation of treatment to preserve life but this presumption is rebuttable.

The case of *Aintree University Hospitals NHS Foundation Trust v David James* [2013] began a more recent debate when treatment should be regarded as futile.

Activity 5.7 — *Group work*

In groups, read the case summary below and discuss whether continued treatment and CPR are futile, giving reasons for your answer.

Mr James was admitted to hospital due to a complication with his stoma but then developed multi-organ failure, with respiratory failure, cardiovascular failure and renal failure and remained in hospital on ventilator support in the critical care unit. His condition continued to deteriorate and the hospital wished to place a Do Not Attempt Resuscitation instruction on his medical records but his family disagreed. His medical team gave evidence to the Court of Protection that attempts at CPR and invasive support would be painful and would put the patient at risk of further complications.

His family argued that treatment was not futile because CPR had been successful in the past and it would therefore not be in the patient's best interests to withhold treatment. They argued that treatment should be given unless it was unlikely to prevent death or manage a crisis.

Now read on.

When the Court of Protection considered Mr James's case the judge agreed with the family that as CPR had been successful previously it would not be in the patient's best interests to impose a Do Not Attempt Resuscitation order now. In the view of the judge the high threshold for considering treatment as futile had not been met.

The Court of Appeal took a different view and sought to introduce a much lower threshold for futility. In their view treatment was futile if

> *[i]t did not secure a therapeutic benefit for the patient, that is to say the treatment must, standing alone or with other medical care, have the real prospect of curing or at least palliating the life threatening disease or illness from which the patient is suffering.*

To consider futility based on the past success of an intervention or its ability to cope with a crisis situation without having regard to the lack of improvement it would bring to the patient's health generally was too narrow a view (*Aintree University Hospitals NHS Foundation Trust v David James* [2013] (Rt Hon Sir Alan Ward at 33 to 39)).

Concerns over the need for a therapeutic benefit for a treatment not to be considered futile led to the case being brought before the United Kingdom Supreme Court.

Supreme Court appeal

The Supreme Court set out the correct approach to making decisions about whether to give life-sustaining treatment in the case of persons lacking the capacity to make such decisions for themselves.

Their Lordships held that the focus when making decisions in such cases must be whether it was in the patient's best interests to give the treatment, rather than whether it was in the patient's best interests to withhold or withdraw treatment.

If continued treatment is not in the patient's best interests, then it would be lawful for a nurse to withhold or withdraw that treatment. The Supreme Court further held that it would in fact be unlawful to continue with the treatment and nurses who acted reasonably and without negligence in these circumstances would not be in breach of their duty towards the patient by withholding or withdrawing treatment.

Activity 5.8 *Group work*

In *Aintree University Hospitals Foundation Trust v James* [2013] Lady Hale stressed the duty on health professionals, including nurses, to have regard to the Mental Capacity Act 2005 Code of Practice (2007) when making decisions for or on behalf of those who lack decision-making capacity (Mental Capacity Act 2005, section 42).

The Supreme Court held that paragraphs 5.31 to 5.33 of the Code of Practice, that set out how best interests should be worked out when making decisions about life-sustaining treatment, were an accurate statement of the law and nurses must inform their decision-making by reference to this part of the Code of Practice.

In groups read paragraphs 5.31 to 5.33 of the Code of Practice and highlight in bullet form the key requirements for determining best interests for life-sustaining treatment.

When you have done that, read on.

When considering the best interests of patients receiving continued life-sustaining treatment nurses adopt a holistic approach and they are required to:

- consider the patient's welfare in the widest sense to include not just medical but social and psychological issues as well;
- consider the nature of the medical treatment in question, what it involves and its prospects of success;
- consider what the outcome of that treatment is likely to be;
- try to put themselves in the place of the patient and ask what the patient's attitude to the treatment would be;
- consult others who are looking after the patient or interested in his welfare, for their view of what his attitude would be.

When considering the nature of the treatment nurses must decide whether treatment would be futile in the sense of being ineffective or of no benefit to the patient. In this context nurses must accept that recovery does not mean a return to full health, but the resumption of a quality of life which the patient would regard as worthwhile. Even where a nurse considers that continued treatment is a burden on the patient that burden must be weighed against the benefits of a continued life. That weighing process will require a nurse to consider wider issues than the therapeutic value of the treatment. They must also have regard to the patient's welfare and give great weight to the right to family life.

Activity 5.9 — **Research**

The Supreme Court confirmed that health professionals, including nurses, who required further guidance on withdrawing life-sustaining treatment should follow what they called the sensible advice of the GMC in its guidance on *Treatment and care towards the end of life: good practice in decision-making* (2010).

*Download and read the guidance recommended by the Supreme Court that is available from **www.gmc-uk.org/End_of_life.pdf_32486688.pdf***

Do Not Attempt Resuscitation orders

The lawfulness of the decision to withhold cardiopulmonary resuscitation (CPR) from the patient in *Aintree University Hospitals Foundation Trust v James* [2013] lay at the centre of the Supreme Court's judgment. CPR is used by nurses and other health professionals in response to patients whose cardiac or respiratory function ceases. In the case of many patients, however, the likelihood of resuscitation being successful is very small. Where a decision is taken that any attempt at resuscitation would be futile then a notice is placed on the patient's file that CPR should not be attempted. In hospital and care home settings some 80 per cent of patients who die do so with a Do Not Attempt Resuscitation notice (DNAR) in place. In the view of the Court of Appeal more than 50 per cent of the population will be the subject of a decision, taken in advance of their deaths, that they will not receive cardiopulmonary resuscitation if they have an arrest (*Tracey v Cambridge Uni Hospital NHS Foundation Trust and others* [2014]).

Lawfulness of DNAR notice

Case study 5.19: Lawfulness of a DNAR notice

In Re R (adult: medical treatment) *[1996] a 23-year-old man born with a malformation of the brain and cerebral palsy had been admitted to hospital on five occasions, and after the last of these admissions his consultant psychiatrist concluded that in her opinion it would be in his best interests to allow nature to take its course the next time he experienced a life-threatening crisis and allow him to die with dignity and comfort. His parents agreed and a Do Not Attempt Resuscitation, DNAR, notice was signed to this effect.*

The court held that a do not resuscitate policy was lawful where CPR was unlikely to be successful.

In *R (adult: medical treatment)* [1996] the court recognised that two areas of law had to be considered and carefully weighed before arriving at a decision not to resuscitate a patient. That is the duty of care to the patient that includes a duty to provide treatment has to be weighed against the principle that there is no duty to provide treatment where doing so would be futile (*Airedale NHS Trust v Bland* [1993]).

In *Aintree University Hospitals Foundation Trust v James* [2013] the United Kingdom Supreme Court held that it would be lawful to consider treatment futile if it was not in the patient's best interests to receive it. The ruling confirms the approach adopted in *R (adult: medical treatment)* [1996] that a DNAR notice would be lawful where it was decided that it would not be in the patient's best interests to provide treatment.

The value of DNAR notices to nurses

In addition to allowing a patient to die with dignity, free from unnecessary, futile treatment, DNAR notices also protect nurses from an allegation of wilful neglect towards a patient in their care as the initial presumption in favour of providing CPR is lawfully rebutted.

Case study 5.20: Conviction for wilful neglect for refusing to perform CPR on a patient

A registered nurse was in charge of a nursing home for elderly patients who were mentally ill when a healthcare assistant told her that a patient's breathing was shallow and his pulse was faint. The nurse said she panicked and did not perform cardiac pulmonary resuscitation (CPR) and, although she called for an ambulance, the patient had died by the time it arrived. She was charged and convicted with wilful neglect and appealed.

continued . . .

The Court of Appeal held that she had been properly convicted as the offence was complete if a nurse deliberately neglected to do that which ought to have been done in the treatment of the patient. She could not escape liability on the basis that the treatment would have made no difference to the patient and panic was not a defence to the charge.

*(*R v Patel *[2013])*

Requirement to consult the patient

The decision to place a DNAR notice on a patient's record is generally taken by the doctor in charge of the patient's care in consultation with nurses involved in the patients care.

Controversy over the decision to issue a DNAR notice often arises from patients and their families who were not consulted about the notice and were unaware that it had been issued (*R (On The Application Of Oliver Leslie Burke) (Respondent) v General Medical Council (Appellant) & The Disability Rights Commission & 8 Others (Interveners)* [2005]). The Court of Appeal has now directed that a patient with capacity or the family of a patient who lacks capacity should be consulted before a decision about issuing a DNAR notice is made (*Tracey v Cambridge Uni Hospital NHS Foundation Trust and others* [2014]).

Case study 5.21: Consultation before issuing a DNAR notice

In Tracey v Cambridge Uni Hospital NHS Foundation Trust and others *[2014] a man sought judicial review of the decisions of an NHS trust concerning the treatment of his wife who had terminal lung cancer and had been admitted to hospital following a road traffic accident. The trust had placed a Do Not Attempt Resuscitation notice on her medical file that was cancelled after three days when the family expressed concern about it. Three days later, her condition deteriorated and another notice was imposed after consultation with her family and she died two days later.*

The Court of Appeal held that article 8 of the European Convention of Human Rights, the right to respect for a private and family life, home and correspondence, was engaged by a DNAR decision because it concerns how an individual chooses to pass the closing days and moments of their life and how they manage their death.

The Court of Appeal ruled that:

- Clinicians had to involve the patient in a DNAR decision.
- NHS trusts and health boards should have a clear and accessible DNAR policy that should be given to the patient as part of the DNAR decision.
- A DNAR decision engaged article 8 of the European Convention on Human Rights 1950 and this required the provisos discussed below.

Article 8: Respect for private and family life, home and correspondence

Chapter 4 highlighted that article 8 concerns the everyday right of individuals to respect for their private and family life, home and correspondence. However, as a qualified right article 8(2) gives scope for intrusion into this right on a variety of grounds including the denial of futile treatment.

The Convention interprets the concept of private life very broadly. It includes the right to autonomy and self-determination and to psychological and physical integrity that includes personal dignity.

Case study 5.22: The European Court of Human Rights view of private life

In Pretty v United Kingdom *[2002] the European Court of Human Rights held that:*

> *The concept of 'private life' is a broad term not susceptible to exhaustive definition. It covers the physical and psychological integrity of a person. It can sometimes embrace aspects of an individual's physical and social identity.*
>
> *Article 8 also protects a right to personal development, and the right to establish and develop relationships with other human beings and the outside world. The Court considers that the notion of personal autonomy is an important principle underlying the interpretation of its guarantees. The very essence of the Convention is respect for human dignity and human freedom.*

*(*Pretty v United Kingdom *[2002] 35 EHRR 1 at 61)*

To be justified, any intrusion with an article 8 right must be in accordance with the law and be proportionate to the aim being achieved. This implies an obligation to have procedures in place to ensure the effective respect for the rights. The Convention guarantees rights that are practical and effective not theoretical or illusory. Since a DNAR decision is one that potentially deprives a patient of life-saving treatment there must be a presumption in favour of patient involvement. That is nurses must involve the patient in the DNAR decision and there would need to be convincing reasons not to involve the patient (*Tracey v Cambridge Uni Hospital NHS Foundation Trust and others* [2014]).

The Court of Appeal in *Tracey* held while a nurse would be correct to consider it inappropriate and therefore not a requirement of article 8 to involve the patient in the process if they consider that to do so is likely to cause the patient to suffer physical or psychological harm, nurses must be wary of being too ready to exclude patients from the process on the grounds that their involvement is likely to be distressful. The Court of Appeal acknowledged that it was very likely that many patients would find it distressing to discuss the question whether CPR should be withheld from them in the event of a cardiorespiratory arrest. Nurses who form the view that the patient will not suffer harm if consulted would not be justified in excluding the patient from the decision because they may find the topic distressing.

Consulting the patient's family

Although the Court of Appeal ruling in the *Tracey* case concerned the need to consult with an adult who had decision-making capacity before issuing a DNAR notice, the High Court has now confirmed that where the patient lacks decision-making capacity then the family must be consulted instead (*Winspear v City Hospitals Sunderland NHSFT* [2015]).

Case study 5.23: Consultation with the family about the appropriateness of a DNAR notice

In Winspear v City Hospitals Sunderland NHSFT *[2015] a mother claimed that an NHS trust had breached her son's rights under European Convention on Human Rights, article 8, by placing a Do Not Attempt Resuscitation notice on his clinical record without consulting her.*

The son was 28, lacked decision-making capacity and suffered from various health conditions including cerebral palsy, epilepsy and spinal deformities and had been admitted to hospital with a chest infection. A specialist registrar placed the notice on the son's record without consulting the mother because he considered that CPR would be futile in the event of a cardiac arrest.

The High Court held that the principles in R (on the application of Tracey) v Cambridge University Hospitals NHS Foundation Trust *[2014] applied to adult patients who lacked capacity. Before making a decision not to attempt cardiopulmonary resuscitation, it was necessary to consult a person in accordance with the Mental Capacity Act 2005 if practicable and appropriate. A failure to consult without good reason would violate the patient's rights under ECHR article 8.*

Accessible and clear DNAR policy

Any interference with an individual's right to a private life has to be in accordance with the law (European Convention on Human Rights, article 8(2)). The Court of Appeal in *Tracey* held that this requires a DNAR policy that describes the circumstances in which nurses would be entitled to interfere with a patient's article 8 rights by coming to a DNAR decision. Their Lordships further held that the DNAR policy must be accessible and clear to be compatible with the Human Rights Convention. That is, any interference with the right to a private life, as in the case of a DNAR decision, must be:

- sufficiently accessible to the individual who is affected; and
- sufficiently precise to enable him to understand its scope and foresee the consequences of his action.

A DNAR decision would not satisfy these criteria if it was not made in accordance with a clear and accessible policy. The right to be consulted and notified about DNAR decisions would be undermined if the patient was not aware of the criteria by which the GP reached the decision to complete a DNAR notice.

Assisted dying

The debate over whether the considered and deliberate ending of the life of a terminally or incurably ill patient should be lawful has now been considered by both the Houses of Parliament and our highest domestic court, the United Kingdom Supreme Court.

Sanctity of life continues to be a principle protected by the law. Any action calculated to endanger or recklessly threaten life is a crime severely punished by the law. However, from a moral stance in the United Kingdom and from a legal stance in other countries, such as the Netherlands, Belgium and Switzerland, the notion that death must be avoided at all costs is being replaced. There is an increasing consensus that for some death is preferable to the intractable pain and suffering that results from their incurable or terminal illness.

Euthanasia

The term euthanasia is derived from the Greek meaning 'easy death' or 'dying well'. This broad definition adds to the confusion over the contemporary meaning of the word. It is difficult to argue that a person should not be entitled to an 'easy death' and this is the basis of palliative care in the United Kingdom. Nurses who deliver palliative care to their patients would rightly argue that this does not equate to euthanasia. A more realistic definition of the concept would be the process whereby life is ended by another to avoid the distressing effects of an illness (Kennedy and Grubb, 1998).

Active euthanasia

Active euthanasia is a process where the death of a person results from a specific act directed at causing their death. The intention of the person carrying out the act must be that the person will die (Kennedy and Grubb, 1998). An intention to relieve suffering by giving sedation and analgesia whose secondary effects are to shorten life is not considered active euthanasia and is lawful under the principle of double effect (*Airedale NHS Trust v Bland* [1993]).

The principle of double effect

Any care or treatment given to a patient that is motivated by a desire to bring about a patient's death is unlawful (Mental Capacity Act 2005, section 4) and could result in prosecution for murder.

Case study 5.24: Doctor guilty of attempted murder

In R v Cox *(1992) a consultant rheumatologist was convicted of attempted murder after he admitted injecting a patient with potassium chloride to end her pain and suffering. The woman had been a patient of the doctor for some 13 years, and was terminally ill with what was described in court as the worst case of rheumatoid arthritis they had encountered. In the 18 years before her death, she had been admitted to hospital 20 times. Her pain was agonising. Any movement caused intense discomfort and she screamed at the slightest touch.*

continued . . .

The charge of attempted murder was brought because it could not be proved conclusively that the injection had killed her. Despite the verdict, the consultant was given a suspended sentence and was only reprimanded by the GMC; he was allowed to continue practising medicine.

Murder in common with most criminal offences requires two elements to be present in order to prove the offence has been committed. These elements are a blameworthy act – or the *actus reus* – and the state of mind of the accused – the *mens rea*. Both must be present at the time of committing the offence. With murder the prosecution would need to prove that the accused intended to cause death or serious harm to the victim and did so through a blameworthy act.

Case study 5.25: A case of murder

In R v O *[2005] a man was convicted of murder when he killed the victim by striking him over the head with a wooden plank in a racially motivated attack. In this case the defendant directly intended to seriously harm or kill the victim.*

The necessary intention for murder can also be made out through the less direct actions of a person, often referred to as oblique intention.

Case study 5.26: Oblique intention for murder

In R v Woollin *[1999] a man was charged with murder when he killed his child by throwing it across a room towards a soft play pen. The child struck its head on the wooden arm of a chair and died. Woollin argued that he had not intended to kill or do serious harm to the child. The House of Lords considered how a judge should direct a jury in circumstances in which a defendant did an act which caused death without the purpose of killing or causing serious harm.*

*The House of Lords held that where a person foresees with virtual certainty that their actions will result in death or serious harm, the inference may be irresistible that they intended that result, however little they may have desired or wished it to happen (*R v Woollin *[1999] (Lord Steyn)).*

The decision in Woollin would seem to suggest that if a nurse or any other health professional administered a controlled drug to a patient to relieve pain but foresaw serious harm or death as virtually certain, even though they did not wish it, because of the size of the dose being given, then it is possible a jury would conclude that the necessary intention for murder was made out.

However, it appears the courts do differentiate between an intention to murder and an intention to relieve pain. Ever since the case of *R v Bodkin Adams* [1957] the courts have recognised that increased doses of sedation and analgesia may be given to relieve pain even though the unwanted effect of such treatment is to shorten life under the principle of double effect. The courts accept that nobody should die in pain and effective palliative care can require what seems like very high doses of analgesia and sedation in the form of controlled drugs (*Airedale NHS Trust v Bland* [1993]). In *Pretty v DPP* [2001] Lord Steyn seemed to play down his ruling in *Woollin* in the context of healthcare when he held that, 'under the double effect principle medical treatment may be administered to a terminally ill person to alleviate pain although it may hasten death. This principle entails a distinction between foreseeing an outcome and intending it' (*Pretty v DPP* [2001] (per Lord Steyn at 65)).

This distinction can be illustrated by comparing the cases of Harold Shipman and David Moor.

Case study 5.27: Intention to kill

Harold Shipman, a GP, was convicted of 15 counts of murder after a jury accepted that his intention, when administering high doses of analgesia in the form of controlled drugs to his patients, was to kill not relieve pain. A subsequent inquiry following his conviction found that he had killed at least 218 patients.

(The Shipman Inquiry, 2004)

Case study 5.28: Intention to relieve pain

In R v Moor *[2000] a well-respected GP was charged with murder after a journalist published an article quoting him as saying that he had used high doses of controlled drug analgesia and sedation to help patients to a pain-free death. At his trial the jury accepted that Dr Moor had used high doses of controlled drugs to relieve pain under the principle of double effect and that he was not motivated by a desire to kill his patients. He was found not guilty of murder.*

Another doctor, a Dr Martin, was charged with murder and accused of giving his patients six times the normal dose of controlled drug. He was also acquitted of murder by a jury who accepted that he was administering the drugs under the principle of double effect and his intention was to relieve pain even though it did hasten the patients' deaths (Strokes, 2005).

It can be seen that where there is any suggestion that the action of the nurse or other health professional is motivated by bringing about the patient's death and not solely to relieve pain then a charge of murder or attempted murder may result. It is essential that nurses carefully and accurately record their use of controlled drugs in palliative care and also record the extent of pain experienced by the patient. It is essential that the nurse's philosophy towards palliative care is underpinned by a desire to keep the patient pain free and that this is reflected in both words and deeds.

Case study 5.29: Ward sister convicted of attempted murder

In R v Salisbury *[2005] a ward sister was convicted of the attempted murder of two of her patients after the jury heard evidence that she had administered high doses of diamorphine and was overheard telling a patient to 'give in, it is time to go'. The Court of Appeal agreed with the jury and accepted that the ward sister had administered controlled drugs to her patients with the intention of killing them and had been motivated by a desire to free up beds.*

While the principle of double effect is endorsed and applied by the courts, active euthanasia is not currently tolerated and the position of the law has changed little since Justice Devlin's summing up in the case of *R v Bodkin Adams* [1957] at 366:

> *If the acts done are intended to kill and do kill it does not matter if a life is cut short by weeks or months, it is just as much murder as if it were cut short by years.*

Passive euthanasia

Passive euthanasia is distinguished from active euthanasia, as the means of ending life is not by the use of a direct action such as a lethal injection of drugs, but by withholding treatment and care necessary to keep the person alive. Steinbock (1980) argues that active and passive euthanasia are indistinguishable as omitting to treat is as potent as actively killing a person. In his view there is no difference between giving a lethal injection and omitting antibiotics for an infection if the intention is that the person should die as a result.

In law, however, there is a real distinction in culpability where a death occurs as a result of an action by a third person compared to a death resulting from a person omitting to act. We are all protected in law from harmful acts, but criminal liability for harm that results from a failure to act is reserved for circumstances where a duty to act arises.

Case study 5.30: Note the impact of a duty to act in the following cases

In R v Stone & Dobinson *[1977] a couple were convicted of manslaughter for failing to get medical attention for Stone's frail anorexic sister who they had taken in and agreed to look after. The woman was found dead in her bed, emaciated, covered in pressure sores, urine and faeces, some six months after moving in.*

In R v Smith *[1979] a woman who had a dread of doctors and hospitals died when she refused to allow her husband to call for assistance when complications occurred during labour at home. Although initially charged with manslaughter Smith was directed to be found not guilty as his wife had given a valid refusal of treatment and so absolved him of his duty to seek assistance.*

In *Burke v GMC & others* [2005] a man was concerned that the artificial nutrition required to keep him alive would be withdrawn when it was still of benefit to him and he would suffer as the result of slowly dying from thirst and starvation. He challenged the lawfulness of the GMC's guidance on withholding treatment and made it clear in an advanced statement that he wanted to be kept alive by artificial means. The Court of Appeal held that:

> *It seems to us that for a doctor deliberately to interrupt life-prolonging treatment in the face of a patient's expressed wish to be kept alive, with the intention of thereby terminating the patient's life, would leave the doctor with no answer to a charge of murder.*
> (*Burke v GMC & others* [2005], Lord Phillips at paragraph 34)

It is clear from the judgment in *Burke* that to terminate a person's life by passive means, such as withholding life-sustaining treatment or denying the person treatment for an infection, when there continues to be a positive duty to care for the patient is unlawful. Nurses cannot make a determination of a patient's best interests on the basis that they are better off dead (*Aintree University Hospitals Foundation Trust v James* [2013]). Any withholding or withdrawing of treatment must be on the grounds that such treatment is futile and of no benefit to the patient (*Aintree University Hospitals Foundation Trust v James* [2013], *Airedale NHS Trust v Bland* [1993]). Arguably such an intervention cannot be considered a form of euthanasia. Dying slowly from an untreated infection or lack of hydration is not the release from suffering envisaged by the proponents of euthanasia.

Assisted dying

Assisted dying or assisted suicide is now being advanced an acceptable way of lawfully ending the lives of those in intolerable pain or suffering. Rather than a person being killed by another to end their suffering, they are given the means to end their own lives when they feel they can no longer go on living with their condition. Currently this form of intervention is prohibited under the Suicide Act 1961. Although it is no longer an offence to take one's own life (Suicide Act 1961, section 1) it remains an offence to

> *assist or encourage a suicide.*
> (Suicide Act 1961, section 2(1) as amended by the Coroners and Justice Act 2009, section 59)

Assisted suicide is prohibited whether performed by a relative, friend or a nurse and a person who does so would be liable on conviction to fourteen years in prison.

The aim of the prohibition is to protect vulnerable people from being pressured into killing themselves by unscrupulous family or friends.

Case study 5.31: Pressured into attempting suicide

In R v McShane *[1977] a daughter was found guilty of trying to persuade her 89-year-old mother, who was residing in a nursing home, to kill herself so that she could inherit her mother's estate. The police obtained incriminating evidence of the daughter by using a hidden camera at the nursing home that showed the daughter handing her mother drugs, hidden in a packet of sweets, with a pinned note on her mother's dress telling her not to 'bungle it!'*

Whilst such protection is laudable, the same provisions have prevented people who cannot take their own lives because of a debilitating condition from being helped to do so by a friend, relative or health professional.

In *Pretty v DPP* [2001] the House of Lords refused to grant Diane Pretty's application for a judicial review challenging the decision of the Director of Public Prosecutions (DPP), who had refused to give an undertaking that he would not prosecute her husband if he assisted in her suicide at some time in the future.

The European Court of Human Rights subsequently confirmed that the Suicide Act 1961 did not violate the European Convention on Human Rights as:

- The right to life protected under article 2 did not include a right to die at a chosen time.
- It was not the government subjecting Mrs Pretty to inhuman or degrading treatment under article 3 but the motor neurone disease from which she suffered.
- Mrs Pretty's right to respect for her private life under article 8 was not absolute. The right could be restricted by the government passing legislation which had the legitimate aim of protecting vulnerable individuals from being forced into agreeing to be assisted to die.
- Banning assisted suicide therefore was not a disproportionate or unlawful action by the government.

However a softening of this stance was signalled in *R (on the application of Purdy) v Director of Public Prosecutions* [2009], where the House of Lords ruled that the DPP should issue guidelines for prosecutors setting out when it would be in the public interest to bring charges under the Suicide Act 1961, section 2.

Currently the Crown Prosecution Service is unlikely to prosecute relatives and friends of a person who makes a clear and consistent request to be helped to die if they act out of compassion.

A woman who bought a lethal drug on the internet and mixed it into a form that could be taken by her parents who had entered a suicide pact was not prosecuted as the CPS decided that it would not be in the public interest to do so. The woman had acted out of compassion in response to a direct request from her parents (Marsden, 2014).

Those who force the person into killing themselves or seek to profit from their death still face prosecution (Director of Public Prosecutions, 2010).

The guidelines also state that public interest factors that tend to favour prosecution include circumstances where

> *the suspect was acting in his or her capacity as a medical doctor, nurse, other healthcare professional, a professional carer [whether for payment or not], or as a person in authority, such as a prison officer, and the victim was in his or her care.*
> (Director of Public Prosecutions, 2010, p6)

This clause in the guideline is seen as forbidding nurses and health professionals from participating in action that would assist the death of patients in their care.

After four failed attempts at introducing legislation through private members' bills in the House of Lords campaigners tried to change the law on euthanasia in the United Kingdom by bringing cases to the Supreme Court. The appeals were from three people who had severe physical disabilities and wanted the right to ask health professionals to assist them to end their lives (*R (on the application of Nicklinson) v Ministry of Justice* [2014]).

Supreme Court ruling

In *R (on the application of Nicklinson) v Ministry of Justice* [2014] nine Supreme Court Justices delivered a multi-layered and divided judgment on two appeals. In the first appeal a man suffered a catastrophic stroke leaving him paralysed except that he could move his head and his eyes. He wanted to end his life, but needed assistance to do this. A second man who joined the appeal was unable to move any part of his body except his right hand. His condition was irreversible and he wished to end his life. Both men sought the same declarations from the Supreme Court that:

- It would be lawful for a health professional to kill him or to assist him to end his life; and
- The current state of the law relating to assisted dying is incompatible with the right to a private life under article 8 of the Convention.

The second appeal before the Supreme Court concerned a third man who suffered a brainstem stroke in 2008 leaving him unable to move. He wished to end his life by travelling to make use of the Dignitas service in Switzerland.

On the question of whether the current law on assisted suicide is incompatible with article 8 of the European Convention on Human Rights, the Supreme Court held that it was a matter for the United Kingdom to decide. Under human rights law there is a margin of appreciation applied to how broad Convention rights are interpreted among different member states of the Council of Europe. It takes account of the cultural and historical differences between countries. In the case of assisted dying what is right for the Netherlands may not be right for the United Kingdom. Whether the current law is incompatible with article 8 is, therefore, a domestic question for the United Kingdom to decide under the Human Rights Act 1998.

A majority of the Supreme Court held that it has the constitutional authority to make that decision but decided not to do so at that time. However, the Supreme Court made it clear that while the sensitive and controversial nature of assisted dying did not justify the court ruling out the possibility that it could make a declaration of incompatibility, it would be inappropriate for a court to make that decision before giving Parliament the opportunity to consider the position. Parliament rejected the latest attempt to introduce an assisted dying law in September 2015 when the Commons rejected the assisted dying bill introduced by Rob Marris, a Labour MP who had argued that it was about ensuring peaceful deaths rather than euthanasia, by voting it down by 330 votes to 118.

On the second appeal, the Supreme Court unanimously ruled that while it was appropriate to ask the DPP to publish guidance on decisions about prosecutions under section 2 of the Suicide Act 1961, it would be inappropriate to tell the DPP what to put in that guidance. The exercise of judgement by the DPP needed a degree of flexibility in the guidelines so that the variety of relevant factors, and the need to vary the weight to be attached to them according to the circumstances of each individual case, are all able to be considered.

Chapter summary

- The moral principle of autonomy is given its legal expression in the law relating to consent.
- Consent imposes on nurses a legal obligation to respect an individual's autonomy and self-determination.
- Consent is essential to the propriety of care and treatment.
- A legally valid consent will protect the practitioner from the tort of trespass to the person and the criminal offence of assault and battery.
- A valid consent must be full, free from duress and reasonably informed.
- An adult with decision-making capacity is able to refuse treatment even if such refusal might lead to his or her death.
- Where there is doubt about the capacity of a person aged 16 or older to make a treatment decision, their capacity must be assessed in accordance with the guiding principles of the Mental Capacity Act 2005.
- Treatment for a person who lacks capacity can only proceed if it is in their best interests.
- Best interests must be determined in accordance with the checklist of factors set out under the Mental Capacity Act 2005.
- The Mental Capacity Act 2005 allows for designated decision-makers to consent to treatment for people who lack capacity.
- Changes to the regulatory framework and law require a shift away from paternalism to partnership in the nurse–patient relationship.
- The fundamental standards set out in the Health and Social Care Act 2008 (Regulated Activities) Regulations 2014 now require partnership with patients with their wishes and preferences at the centre of care and treatment.
- Standard 2 of the revised NMC *Code* also places a professional obligation on nurses to listen to people and respond to their preferences and concerns by working in partnership with patients.
- The Supreme Court has also ruled that the amount and type of information about care and alternative treatment, their benefits and risks must be based on what a prudent patient would want to know to help them make an informed decision.
- Nurses must work in partnership with their patients and respect their right to be involved in decisions about their care and treatment.
- The courts have long recognised that continued life-sustaining care and treatment for very sick and critically ill patients can be futile.

continued . . .

- The general presumption in law is that a patient's best interests requires the continuation of treatment to preserve life, but this presumption is rebuttable.
- Treatment that is futile can be lawfully withheld or withdrawn.
- The courts require all decisions about the withholding of treatment to be based on a best interests approach.
- Futility is now based on a broader view of the best interests of the patient and requires a consideration of wider welfare issues such as the right to family life.
- DNAR notices are routinely used by community health services and GPs who decide that providing CPR to a patient would be futile and not in their best interests.
- The Court of Appeal has found that a DNAR notice engages the right to a private life under article 8 of the European Convention on Human Rights (1950).
- GPs and nurses are now required to involve the patient in the DNAR decision.
- A clear and accessible DNAR policy must set out the criteria used to reach the decision to complete a DNAR notice.
- The principle of double effect allows for increased doses of analgesia and sedation to be given to a patient to relieve pain even if it does hasten death. This is lawful as long as there is no suggestion that the nurse is motivated by bringing about the death of the patient.
- Euthanasia is a process whereby life is ended by another to avoid the distressing effects of an illness. It is unlawful in the United Kingdom.
- Assisted dying is a process where a person is given the means to end their own life.
- Currently assisting or encouraging a suicide is unlawful, but those with emotional ties to a person will not face prosecution if they acted from compassion.
- Assisted dying is a process where a person is given the means to end their own life. It is unlawful to aid, abet, procure or counsel a suicide under section 2 of the Suicide Act 1961.
- Arguments for a change in the law centre on patient autonomy and beneficence.
- Assisted dying is lawful in Belgium, Luxembourg, Switzerland and the Netherlands.
- The Supreme Court has held that it was a matter for the United Kingdom to decide if its law on assisted dying was incompatible with the European Convention on Human Rights.
- The Supreme Court has the constitutional authority to make that decision, but decided not to do so at this time, preferring to allow Parliament to consider the issue first.

Activities: Brief outline answers

Activity 5.2: Critical thinking (page 92)

The degree of information to be given to a patient about risks is based on the standard of care in *Bolam*.

Sufficient information must be given to enable the patient to make a choice. There is a two-edged duty:

- to disclose material risks;
- to withhold information where a patient would be frightened if told all risks where the likelihood of occurrence was very small.

The issue of how much information a nurse should give in response to a general enquiry about risks was considered by the Court of Appeal in *Blyth v Bloomsbury HA* [1993]. The answer depends on:

- the circumstances;
- the nature of the enquiry;
- the nature of the information which is available;
- its reliability and relevance;
- the condition of the patient.

A different test applies to patients who ask specific questions about risks inherent in treatment. When a specific question is asked about risks, patients are entitled to full and honest answers.

Further reading

For a detailed consideration of consent in healthcare consider reading:

McLean, S (2009) *Autonomy, Consent and the Law.* London: Routledge-Cavendish.

For a more general guide to consent in healthcare read:

Department of Health (2001) *Good Practice in Consent* (HSC 2001/023). London: The Stationery Office.

An essential companion to student nurses working with people who lack decision-making capacity in England and Wales is:

Department for Constitutional Affairs & Welsh Assembly Government (2007) *Mental Capacity Act 2005 Code of Practice.* London: The Stationery Office.

For students working with persons who are deprived of their liberty, the DoLs Code of Practice is an essential read:

Ministry of Justice (2008) *Deprivation of Liberty: Code of Practice to supplement the main Mental Capacity Act 2005 Code of Practice.* London: The Stationery Office.

Useful websites

The Department of Health website offers current information on consent to examination and treatment and model consent forms at: **www.gov.uk/government/publications/reference-guide-to-consent-for-examination-or-treatment-second-edition**

Reference Guide for Consent to Examination or Treatment, from the Welsh Assembly Government (WHC (2006) Consent to Examination or Treatment): **http://wales.gov.uk/topics/health/publications/health/** and search for 'consent'.

Current guidance on the operation of the Mental Capacity Act in England can be obtained from **www.justice.gov.uk** by searching on 'Mental Capacity Act'.

Scottish government website on the Adults with Incapacity (Scotland) Act 2000 with information and guidance on the operation of the Act: **www.scotland.gov.uk/Topics/Justice/law/awi**

The Scottish government offers advice on the operation of the Adults with Incapacity (Scotland) Act 2000 at **www.scotland.gov.uk/Topics/Justice/law/awi**

Chapter 6
Mental health

NMC Standards for Pre-registration Nursing Education

This chapter will address the following competencies:

Domain 1: Professional values

1. All nurses must practise with confidence according to *The Code: Professional standards of practice and behaviour for nurses and midwives* (NMC, 2015a), and within other recognised ethical and legal frameworks.
6. All nurses must understand the roles and responsibilities of other health and social care professionals and seek to work with them collaboratively for the benefit of all who need care.

Domain 2: Communication and interpersonal skills

4. All nurses must recognise when people are anxious or in distress and respond effectively, using therapeutic principles, to promote their well-being, manage personal safety and resolve conflict ... They must know when to consult a third party and how to make referrals for advocacy, mediation or arbitration.

Domain 3: Nursing practice and decision-making

7. All nurses must be able to recognise and interpret signs of normal and deteriorating mental and physical health and respond promptly to maintain or improve the health and comfort of the service user, acting to keep them and others safe.

Chapter aims

By the end of this chapter you will be able to:

- state the principles of the Mental Health Act 1983;
- describe the requirements for compulsory admission;
- outline the key detention provisions of the Mental Health Act 1983;
- evaluate the safeguards designed to protect patients undergoing treatment for a mental disorder;
- discuss the arrangements for the rehabilitation and aftercare of patients detained for treatment.

Introduction

This chapter examines how the law seeks to protect, manage and enable treatment for people who suffer from mental health problems. The discussion focuses on the principles and provisions of the Mental Health Act 1983 and the nurse's role when providing care and treatment within that legal framework. The discussion moves on to consider the principles of compulsory detention and consent to treatment for mental disorder. The chapter ends by summarising the provisions of the Mental Health Act 1983 that relate to the aftercare of patients who have received hospital treatment for their mental disorder.

The position of the patient with mental health problems is now more legalised than ever before (Unsworth, 1987). In addition to the provisions of the Mental Health Act 1983, a strong body of case law has developed that deals with fundamental issues of liberty, autonomy and respect.

The Mental Health Act 1983

In England and Wales, mental healthcare is regulated through the provisions of the Mental Health Act 1983 as amended by the Mental Health Act 2007.

Despite a long-standing policy of community-focused service delivery and support, the legislation continues to centre on:

- entry into;
- care in; and
- discharge from institutions.

The fundamental aim of the 1983 Act is to strengthen the rights of patients made subject to its compulsory powers. This is achieved through five key principles that all have a liberal thrust.

- Increased recourse to review of detention.
- Enhanced civil and social status.
- Ideology of entitlement.
- Least restrictive alternative.
- Multidisciplinary review of medical decisions.

Increased recourse to review of detention

Detention in hospital has been limited by time since the Lunacy Act 1890. Detained patients have a right to appeal against detention through the Mental Health Review Tribunal (MHRT), which considers whether the criteria for detention continue to be met.

A right of appeal for those detained for assessment was introduced for the first time by the Mental Health Act 1983.

Case study 6.1: Discharge by a Mental Health Review Tribunal

In R (on the application of C) v Secretary of State for the Home Department *[2002], the Court of Appeal dismissed an application by the Home Secretary calling for a decision to discharge a patient by the MHRT to be quashed.*

The Court of Appeal held that the MHRT had heard evidence that the patient no longer met the detention conditions of the Mental Health Act 1983 and would therefore be discharged.

To ensure that all detained patients have their case independently reviewed, hospital managers now have a duty to refer a case to the MHRT where the patient has not appealed and remains detained in hospital for six months following their admission (Mental Health Act 1983, section 68).

Hospital managers are also empowered to conduct their own reviews of detention and order discharge where three or more agree that the detention conditions are not met (Mental Health Act 1983, section 23).

Case study 6.2: Discharge can only be ordered where three or more managers agree

In R (Tagoe-Thompson) v Central and North West London Mental Health NHS Trust *[2002], a man suffering from paranoid schizophrenia appealed to the hospital managers against his detention for treatment under section 3 of the Mental Health Act 1983.*

Three managers met to review the detention and two agreed that the patient should be discharged. However, as one of the panel objected, the court agreed that the patient could not be discharged as the requirement of section 23 of the Mental Health Act 1983, giving the power of discharge to the hospital managers, required it to be exercised by three or more people.

Enhanced civil and social status

This principle was advocated mainly on therapeutic rather than legal grounds. One way the law was able to implement this principle was through the right to vote. Informal in-patients were given the right to vote by allowing them to register their entitlement using a previous address (Representation of the People Act 1983).

Detained patients did not gain the right to vote until an amendment to the House of Lords Reform Act 2001 granted it subject to the patient's capacity to decide.

Ideology of entitlement

This principle promoted the concept of access to services as a legal right. Patients who have been detained for treatment are entitled to aftercare services as a right.

There is a duty on the health and social services to continue to provide aftercare until it appears to them that the patient is no longer in need of that service (Mental Health Act 1983, section 117). The duty is owed to individual patients who cannot be charged for the aftercare services.

Case study 6.3: Aftercare is a duty owed to individual patients

In R (on the application of Stennett) v Manchester City Council *[2002], patients who had been discharged from hospital after detention for treatment for a mental disorder complained to the court that they were required to pay for their stay in a care home. The House of Lords held that the provision of aftercare was a right owed to patients detained for treatment under the Mental Health Act 1983, section 117. The local authority and the health service were not entitled to ask patients to pay for that aftercare and so their care home fees would have to be reimbursed.*

Least restrictive alternative

Any use of formal powers under the 1983 Act must be the least restrictive means of meeting the needs of the patient. The approved mental health professional (AMHP) (see pages 136–7) has a duty to ensure that the person is actively resisting admission to hospital and that compulsory admission is the most appropriate method of dealing with the case.

The AMHP must also certify that the detention order used is the least restrictive method of meeting the needs of the patient.

Multidisciplinary review of medical decisions

When formal admission under the Mental Health Act 1983 is considered, this falls to the AMHP whose role is to ensure that the person appears to be suffering from a mental disorder that warrants compulsory confinement. This initial safeguard ensures that people who do not have a mental disorder or those who do not actively resist admission are not improperly detained.

Further multidisciplinary reviews of medical decisions occur under part 4 of the 1983 Act, which provides safeguards concerning consent to treatment in certain cases. For example, patients who are subject to the consent to treatment provisions have a legal right to be supported through the treatment process by an independent mental capacity advocate (Mental Health Act 1983, section 130A).

The Mental Health Act Commission is an independent watchdog that oversees the implementation of the 1983 Act, and safeguards and promotes the rights of patients subject to the Act's compulsory powers. They make both announced visits and unannounced inspections of every mental health facility in order to:

- keep under review the operation of the Mental Health Act 1983 in respect of patients detained or liable to be detained under that Act;
- visit and interview, in private, patients detained under the Mental Health Act in hospitals and mental nursing homes;

- consider the investigation of complaints where these fall within the Commission's remit;
- appoint registered medical practitioners and others to give second opinions in cases where this is required by the Mental Health Act;
- publish and lay before Parliament a report every two years;
- monitor the implementation of the Code of Practice and propose amendments to ministers.

Scope of the Mental Health Act 1983

Part 1, section 1 of the Mental Health Act 1983 makes it clear that the Act shall have effect with respect to *the reception, care and treatment of mentally disordered patients, the management of their property and other related matters.* From the outset it is clear that the 1983 Act only applies to people who suffer from a mental disorder.

Definition of mental disorder

Mental disorder is the legal term used by the 1983 Act to establish who can be made subject to its provisions. It is defined as

> *[a]ny disorder or disability of the mind.*
> (Mental Health Act 1983, section 1(2))

As the definition is very broad, two safeguards are included to narrow the scope of the 1983 Act. A person with a learning disability cannot be compulsorily admitted for treatment or guardianship unless their disability is associated with abnormally aggressive or seriously irresponsible conduct (Mental Health Act 1983, section 1(2A)). Furthermore, dependence alone on alcohol or drugs cannot be considered a mental disorder for the purpose of the Act (Mental Health Act 1983, section 1(3)).

Case study 6.4: The Mental Health Act 1983 only applies to the care and treatment of a person's mental disorder

In St George's Healthcare NHS Trust v S *[1998], a pregnant woman with pre-eclampsia was detained under section 2 of the Mental Health Act 1983 when she refused hospital treatment for this life-threatening physical condition. The court held that her detention was unlawful because she did not have a mental disorder and the 1983 Act cannot be used to detain someone just because their thinking seemed unusual, irrational or contrary to public opinion. The Mental Health Act 1983 can only be used to justify detention for mental disorder.*

Principles of compulsory detention

The process of detention aims to ensure that the only people made subject to the compulsory provisions of the 1983 Act are those who:

- are or appear to be suffering from a mental disorder; and
- are actively resisting admission to hospital.

In all other cases, informal admission under the provisions of section 131 of the Mental Health Act 1983 is more appropriate.

Deprivation of liberty

Compulsory detention means that a person is deprived of their liberty. Detention on the grounds that a person is suffering from a mental health problem is not in itself unlawful. As long as it is in accordance with the law, it will comply with the European Convention on Human Rights (Council of Europe, 1950). As specified in *Winterwerp v The Netherlands* [1979], the law must show that:

- unless it is an emergency;
- the person is reliably shown by objective medical evidence to be suffering from a mental disorder; and
- the disorder is of a nature or degree that warrants continued compulsory confinement.

Activity 6.1 *Evidence-based practice and research*

Detention conditions

Look at the requirements for detention for each of the powers detailed in Appendix 6.1 (see pages 153–5). Do these requirements meet the conditions specified by the European Court of Human Rights in *Winterwerp v The Netherlands* [1979]?

An outline answer is given at the end of the chapter.

Compulsory admission

The detention process is a division of responsibility between three key people:

- the approved mental health professional;
- a registered medical practitioner; and
- the patient's nearest relative.

Approved mental health professionals

Approved mental health professionals (AMHPs) include nurses and social workers who have been approved by the local authority as having appropriate competence in dealing with people who have a mental disorder (Mental Health Act 1983, section 114).

The AMHP generally makes the application for detention once they are satisfied that the person is suffering from a mental disorder and is actively resisting admission to hospital and has a duty to conduct a suitable interview with the person before making the application. The AMHP provides a safeguard against the misuse of detention powers and cannot be directed by their local authority or employer to apply for a person's detention.

Registered medical practitioners

Reliable, objective medical evidence is a fundamental requirement of lawful detention and an application for detention must be founded upon two medical recommendations (one in an emergency). One doctor must also be an approved clinician recognised by the primary care trust as being competent in the diagnosis of mental disorder. This requirement meets the need for objective medical evidence under human rights law (MHA 1983, section 12).

The medical recommendation must also indicate that the person is suffering from a mental disorder of a nature or degree that warrants continued compulsory confinement.

The degree of the disorder is its current severity. The nature of the disorder is its prognosis and the person's past history, including previous admissions and compliance with treatment. Only one of these criteria needs to be satisfied to meet the requirements for detention.

Case study 6.5: Nature or degree of the disorder warrants compulsory confinement

In R v Mental Health Review Tribunal for South Thames Region Ex p. Smith *[1998], a patient appealed against his detention when he was returned to hospital having been absent without leave for a year with no medical intervention. While the court agreed that the* ***degree*** *of his disorder did not warrant detention, the* ***nature*** *of his disorder, which had been shown to have deteriorated rapidly and because of which he became a danger to the public by making explosive devices, did warrant his continued confinement.*

The nearest relative

The nearest relative is a statutory friend allocated to a detained patient. The person is drawn from a hierarchy of relatives set out under section 26 of the 1983 Act, with the person in the highest category becoming the nearest relative unless someone lower down the list:

- ordinarily resides with the patient; or
- cares for the patient.

Where there are two or more people in the same category, the older person will be the nearest relative.

Case study 6.6: A person who ordinarily resides with or cares for the patient

In Dewen v Barnet Healthcare Trust and Barnet London Borough Council *[2000], a man detained for treatment under the Mental Health Act 1983 argued that his son, not his daughter, should be his nearest relative as he was older than his sister. He also argued that his detention was unlawful as his son would have objected to his detention.*

The court held that, although the son would normally be regarded as the nearest relative, being the older of two people in the same category, his sister took precedence as nearest relative because she provided care on a regular basis for her father. She had agreed to his detention for treatment of his paranoid schizophrenia and so the detention was lawful.

The hierarchy of nearest relative means:

- husband, wife or civil partner;
- son or daughter;
- mother or father;
- brother or sister;
- grandparent;
- grandchild;
- uncle or aunt;
- nephew or niece;
- a person who is not a relative, but with whom the patient has been living for not less than five years.

The purpose of the nearest relative is to provide a statutory friend for the detained patient, and that person has the power to:

- make applications to admit a person under compulsion; where the AMHPs make the application they have to take reasonable steps to inform the nearest relative about an application, and are required to have regard to any wishes expressed by the nearest relative;
- veto an application for treatment (section 3) and guardianship (section 7);
- be given information by the hospital managers about the patient's detention and discharge unless the patient objects;
- discharge their relative from detention by giving 72 hours' notice to an authorised person at the hospital; the discharge can be barred by the responsible clinician and a further application cannot be made for six months; the nearest relative then has 28 days to make an application to a Mental Health Review Tribunal for discharge;

- apply to the tribunal for discharge in respect of a patient detained by a criminal court under section 37 of the Act;
- have the right to be involved in any consideration as to the aftercare needs of a patient unless the patient objects;
- make a formal complaint to the hospital managers and the Mental Health Act Commission.

A nearest relative may be removed by the county court if they act unreasonably or are otherwise unsuitable. The patient, another relative, a person living with the patient or an AMHP can apply to have a nearest relative removed and replaced by the court (Mental Health Act 1983, section 29(2)).

Detention

The properly completed Mental Health Act forms are sufficient authority to detain the patient and convey them to the named hospital. Once in hospital the managers have a duty, usually delegated to a registered nurse, to inform the patient of the conditions of detention and their right to appeal or complain (Mental Health Act 1983, section 132).

Under the civil detention provisions a person can be detained either for assessment or for treatment. Where a person is detained for treatment, appropriate medical treatment must be available. This is defined as medical treatment appropriate to the patient's case, taking into account the nature and degree of the mental disorder and other circumstances of his or her case.

Case study 6.7: Treatment to include control and supervision

In Reid v United Kingdom *(2003) a patient argued that he was unlawfully detained as he was not having medical treatment. The court held that treatment could include control and supervision to prevent harm to himself or others because of his abnormally aggressive behaviour.*

Informal admission

A person can enter hospital for assessment and treatment of their mental disorder without the need to be detained. Since 1959, formal admission to hospital has been reserved for those who actively resist admission. Informal admission is used for those who consent, those who are incapable of deciding on admission and those who come into hospital informally rather than be detained (Mental Health Act 1983, section 131).

A 16- or 17-year-old child must consent themselves to admission on an informal basis. Where the child lacks the capacity to make the decision or refuses admission on an informal basis, the decision cannot be made by a person with parental responsibility.

Holding powers

Informal patients who wish to leave hospital against medical advice can be made subject to the holding powers under section 5 of the 1983 Act (see Appendix 6.1, pages 153–5). The approved clinician or their nominated deputy may hold a patient for up to 72 hours to allow for an assessment to be made with a view to their detention under section 2 or section 3. Where the immediate attendance of an approved clinician cannot be secured, a nurse of the prescribed class may hold the person for up to six hours or until the clinician arrives on the ward (see Appendix 6.1).

For the purposes of the power to detain a patient in hospital for a maximum of six hours under section 5(4) of the Mental Health Act 1983, a nurse of the prescribed class is a first- or second-level registered nurse whose registration includes an entry indicating that the nurse's field of practice is either mental health or learning disabilities nursing (Mental Health (Nurses) (England) Order 2008 (SI 2008/1207)).

Mentally disordered people who commit offences

Where a person commits an offence when suffering from a mental disorder, the Crown Prosecution Service and police must wherever possible divert the person away from the criminal justice system and arrange for the person's care and treatment (Crown Prosecution Service, 2004).

Even where prosecution is in the public interest, because of the seriousness of the crime, the courts have a range of options under the Mental Health Act 1983 to enable the person to be assessed and to receive care and treatment. Similarly, prison inmates who are in need of care and treatment can be transferred to hospital. These provisions are summarised in Appendix 6.2 (pages 156–7).

Consent to treatment

Compulsory admission and treatment under the Mental Health Act 1983 are dealt with separately. Detention under the Act does not necessarily mean compulsory treatment. Section 56 of the Act specifically excludes most of the emergency provisions and holding powers from the consent to treatment provisions, including patients detained by virtue of:

- an emergency application (section 4);
- holding powers under sections 5(2) or (4);
- remand to hospital for a report on their mental condition (section 35);
- a detention by the police (sections 135 or 136);
- a detention in a place of safety (sections 37(4) or 45A(5)).

They also do not apply to a patient who is:

- conditionally discharged and not recalled to hospital (sections 42, 73 or 74);
- a community patient and not recalled to hospital (section 17A); or
- subject to guardianship (section 7).

The approved clinician

The care of a detained mental health patient is supervised by an approved clinician who is called the patient's responsible clinician. This person is not necessarily a consultant psychiatrist. Amendments introduced by the Mental Health Act 2007 have extended the professionals who can be appointed as approved clinicians to include consultant clinical psychologists, consultant nurses and occupational therapists.

The approved clinician will supervise the patient's treatment, grant leave and, where necessary, renew a detention order or discharge the patient from hospital (Mental Health Act 1983, sections 20 and 145).

Even though the provisions of the Mental Health Act 1983 allow for compulsory treatment without consent, it is essential that care and treatment are given in a climate of consent with respect for the rights and dignity of the patient. The European Convention on Human Rights places a negative obligation – a duty not to breach a patient's human rights – on mental health nurses. Treatment for mental disorder can engage rights under article 3: the right to be free from torture, inhuman and degrading treatment, and article 8: the right to respect for private and family life, which includes respect for personal autonomy and dignity.

Case study 6.8: Treatment that is medically necessary is not inhuman or degrading

In Herczegfalvy v Austria *[1993], the European Court of Human Rights held that mental healthcare called for increased vigilance in complying with the Convention. Nevertheless, as a general rule, a measure that is a therapeutic necessity cannot be regarded as inhuman or degrading. That is, the treatment must be in accordance with a responsible body of professional opinion and be in the patient's best interests.*

In *R (on the application of PS) v RMO (DR G) and SOAD (DR W)* [2003], the court held that it was not a breach of article 8 of the Convention to require a patient detained for treatment to take medication for his mental disorder as it could be justified as necessary for the patient's health and for the protection of others from harm.

Treatment under the provisions of the Mental Health Act 1983 is defined as *nursing, psychological intervention and specialist mental health habilitation, rehabilitation and care,* the purpose of which is to *alleviate or prevent a worsening of the disorder or its symptoms* (Mental Health Act 1983, sections 145(1) and (4)). This recognises a treatment as a whole approach to mental disorder and allows for the treatment of a wide range of symptoms, including the force-feeding of a patient refusing to eat and the taking of blood samples to monitor therapeutic levels of medication.

Compulsory treatment for a patient's mental disorder is allowed where it is given by, or under the direction of, the approved clinician.

Case study 6.9: Force-feeding as treatment for mental disorder

In B v Croydon HA *[1995], B, who suffered from a psychopathic disorder, was compulsorily detained in hospital under section 3 of the 1983 Act. One of her symptoms was a compulsion to harm herself. She stopped eating, with the result that her weight fell to a dangerous level, and it was decided to feed her by nasogastric tube. B went to court arguing that the health authority should not tube-feed her without her consent.*

The court found that the word 'treatment' in section 63 of the 1983 Act referred to actions calculated to alleviate or prevent a deterioration of the mental disorder from which the patient was suffering. This included acts that prevented the patient from harming herself and so tube-feeding constituted treatment and could be carried out lawfully without B's consent.

Safeguards

Some treatment under the 1983 Act may only be given where provisions safeguarding patients have been met. There are three categories of safeguard.

- Treatments that require consent and a second opinion, including psychosurgery: these require both the consent of the patient and an agreeable second opinion from a doctor appointed by the Mental Health Act Commission (Mental Health Act 1983, section 57).
- Treatments that require consent or a second opinion, including the giving of medication for mental disorder beyond three months from when it was first administered: these require either the consent of the patient or an agreeable second opinion from an appointed doctor (Mental Health Act 1983, section 58).

In the case of electroconvulsive therapy (ECT):

- treatment cannot be given without the consent of a capable patient;
- treatment cannot be given without agreement from an appointed doctor where the person is incapable.

The second-opinion appointed doctor will not be entitled to authorise ECT for an incapable patient where:

- there is a valid and applicable advance decision refusing ECT;
- an attorney with authority under an LPA refuses consent;
- a deputy with authority Refuses consent.

(Mental Health Act 1983, section 58A)

The nurse as consultee

When asked to sanction treatment for a patient, second-opinion appointed doctors must consult with two people, one a nurse and one who cannot be a doctor or a nurse, about the patient's condition.

Activity 6.2 *Reflection*

The nurse's role as consultee

Imagine that you are to act as consultee for a patient whose treatment is being considered by a second-opinion appointed doctor. Note down the topics you are likely to discuss with the doctor before they decide on the suitability of treatment for the patient.

Now read below for further information.

The nurse will have had direct knowledge of the person's history and condition, and be in a position to comment on the issues affecting the patient including:

- the proposed treatment and the patient's ability to consent to it;
- other treatment options;
- the way in which the decision to treat was arrived at;
- the facts of the case, progress, etc.;
- the view of the patient's relatives on the proposed treatment;
- the implications of imposing treatment upon a non-consenting patient;
- the reasons for the patient's refusal of treatment;
- any other matter relating to the patient's care on which the consultee wishes to comment.

Patients who initially consent to treatment may withdraw that consent. Treatment would have to cease unless it could be justified as urgent as set out in section 62.

Independent Mental Health Advocacy service

An Independent Mental Health Advocacy service was established under the 1983 Act by an amendment introduced by the Mental Health Act 2007.

There is a duty to instruct an independent mental health advocate (IMHA) where a patient is a qualifying patient. A patient is a qualifying patient if they are:

- detained under the Mental Health Act (other than sections 4, 5(2), 5(4), 135 or 136);
- subject to guardianship; or
- a community patient; or
- discussing with a registered medical practitioner or approved clinician the possibility of being given treatment under section 57; or
- under 18 and not detained and discussing with a doctor or approved clinician the possibility of being given ECT.

The role of the IMHA is to help obtain information about and improve the patient's understanding of:

- the provisions of this Act;
- any conditions or restrictions to which he or she is subject;
- what (if any) medical treatment is given, proposed or discussed;
- why it is given, proposed or discussed;
- the authority under which it is, or would be, given; and
- the requirements of this Act which apply to giving the treatment to him or her.

To fulfil their role the IMHA may:

- visit and interview the patient in private;
- visit and interview the person professionally concerned with his or her medical treatment;
- require the production of and inspect any records relating to his or her detention or treatment or aftercare service and records held by a local social services authority which relate to him or her.

Qualifying patients in Wales

The Welsh government has extended the range of patients entitled to the assistance of an independent mental health advocate under the provisions of the Mental Health (Wales) Measure 2010 and the Mental Health (Independent Mental Health Advocates) (Wales) Regulations 2011. They expand the Independent Mental Health Advocacy scheme to include all patients subject to compulsion under the Mental Health Act 1983, and those in hospital informally.

All individuals subject to the 1983 Act are able to receive independent help and support from an advocate if they wish to. There is a statutory duty to ensure advocacy help and support is available for all inpatients. The aim is to assist inpatients to make informed decisions about their care and treatment, and support them in getting their voices heard.

Rehabilitation and aftercare

Leave of absence

Testing a patient's response to treatment by allowing controlled periods away from hospital is an important element of the rehabilitation process. An approved clinician may grant a detained patient a leave of absence from hospital. The leave may be subject to any conditions the approved clinician considers necessary (Mental Health Act 1983, section 17). The period of leave is at the responsible clinician's discretion and can range from hours to seven days, or longer if the use of a community treatment order is deemed unsuitable. A patient may be recalled to hospital if they do not fulfil the conditions set out when the leave was granted, without the need to undergo a new detention application.

Community treatment orders

Where long-term leave of over seven days is contemplated, the responsible clinician must first consider the use of a community treatment order. This order allows an approved clinician to test the rehabilitation of a patient detained for treatment by discharging the patient subject to their being recalled to hospital if they do not continue with treatment in the community.

A patient subject to a community treatment order is known and referred to in law as a *community patient*. A community patient cannot be made to take treatment by force in the community. Where compulsory treatment is deemed necessary, recall to hospital would be necessary.

The responsible clinician may make a community treatment order for a patient detained under the Mental Health Act 1983 for treatment under sections 3, 47 and 48 of the 1983 Act if they are satisfied that the following criteria are met and an AMHP agrees that a community treatment order is appropriate for that patient.

- The patient must need medical treatment for their mental disorder for their own health or safety, or for the protection of others.
- It must be possible for the patient to receive the treatment they need without having to be in hospital.
- The patient may be recalled to hospital for treatment should this become necessary.
- Appropriate medical treatment for the patient must be available while living in the community.
- The responsible clinician must state the conditions of the order that have been agreed with the AMHP.
- Where the patient does not comply with the conditions, this can be taken into account when considering a recall to hospital.
- The responsible clinician may also recall a community patient to hospital if:
  - they require medical treatment in hospital for mental disorder; and
  - there would be a risk of harm to the health or safety of the patient or to other persons if they were not recalled to hospital for that purpose.

Aftercare

Patients detained for treatment under the Mental Health Act 1983 have a right to aftercare under section 117 of the Act. It is the duty of the health and social services to provide any aftercare services they consider necessary for the patient. As aftercare is a right, the services provided cannot be charged for. The provision of aftercare must continue as long as the health and social services consider the patient requires it. The decision to end aftercare services must be a joint one.

Case study 6.10: Aftercare is an individual right owed to a patient discharged after a period of detention for treatment

In R v Ealing District HA Ex p. Fox *[1993], a man successfully argued that his health authority had breached its duty to provide aftercare when it accepted that its doctors did not wish to care for the patient.*

The court held that the health authority had not discharged its statutory obligations by merely accepting its own doctors' opinions. It had a duty to make arrangements itself with other health authorities or the private sector; if it failed, it should have referred the matter back to the Secretary of State for Health.

Guardianship

Under the Mental Health Act 1983, section 7, guardianship provides an alternative to detention for compulsory treatment by requiring a person with a mental disorder to:

- live at an address specified by the guardian;
- provide access to people named by the guardian, such as a doctor, nurse or social worker;
- attend any place the guardian may specify for medical treatment, occupation, education or training.

No treatment may be given to the patient without consent. Guardianship is administered by the local social services authority. They will name a social worker as guardian or accept a person known to the patient, such as a relative who is suitable and willing to act in the role.

The use of guardianship has been declining, despite the Mental Health Act Commission's attempt to encourage its use.

Implementation of the Mental Health Act 1983 in Wales

The Mental Health (Wales) measure sets out provisions for the implementation of the Mental Health Act 1983 in Wales in six key areas.

- Places a duty on health boards and local authorities to deliver local primary mental health support services across Wales to provide assessment of a person's mental health and, where appropriate, provide treatment for their mental ill health within primary care.
- Creates a duty requiring care and treatment planning and care coordination for all persons receiving care and treatment with secondary mental health services.

- The measure imposes duties on service providers, health boards and local authorities to act in a coordinated manner to improve the effectiveness of the mental health services they provide to an individual. This requires a care and treatment plan for all service users aged 18 and over who have been assessed as requiring care and treatment within secondary mental health services. Each care and treatment plan will:
  - be developed by a care coordinator in consultation with the service user, and the delivery of the care and treatment identified in the plan will be overseen by the care coordinator;
  - outline the expected outcomes of services, and how those outcomes are to be achieved;
  - be in writing;
  - be kept under review and may be updated to reflect any changes in the type of care and treatment which may be required by the service user over time.
- Care coordinators must work with the relevant patient and the patient's mental health service providers to agree the outcomes which the provision of mental health services for the patient are designed to achieve, including:
  - finance and money;
  - accommodation;
  - personal care and physical well-being;
  - education and training;
  - work and occupation;
  - parenting or caring relationships;
  - social, cultural or spiritual;
  - medical and other forms of treatment including psychological interventions.
- Requires secondary mental health services to have in place arrangements to ensure the provision of timely access to assessment for previous service users:
  - to enable individuals who have been discharged from secondary mental health services, but who now believe that their mental health is deteriorating to such a point as to require care and treatment again, to refer themselves back to secondary services directly, without needing to first go to their general practitioner or elsewhere for a referral.
- Extends the group of 'qualifying patients' under the Mental Health Act 1983 entitled to receive support from an independent mental health advocate, so that all patients subject to the formal powers of that Act are able to receive IMHA support if they request it. Requires all patients receiving care and treatment for mental health problems in hospital to have access to independent and specialist mental health advocacy.

Mental health law in Scotland

Mental health law in Scotland is set out under the provisions of the Mental Health (Care and Treatment) Scotland Act 2003 and applies to those who have a mental illness, learning disability or a related condition.

The 2003 Act is underpinned by ten guiding principles that must be taken into account by those who take action under its provisions (see Box 6.1).

Box 6.1: Mental Health Care and Treatment (Scotland) Act 2003 Guiding Principles

Non-discrimination People with mental disorder should, wherever possible, retain the same rights and entitlements as those with other health needs.

Equality All powers under the Act should be exercised without any direct or indirect discrimination on the grounds of physical disability, age, gender, sexual orientation, language, religion or national or ethnic or social origin.

Respect for diversity Service users should receive care, treatment and support in a manner that accords respect for their individual qualities, abilities and diverse backgrounds and properly takes into account their age, gender, sexual orientation, ethnic group and social, cultural and religious background.

Reciprocity Where society imposes an obligation on an individual to comply with a programme of treatment of care, it should impose a parallel obligation on the health and social care authorities to provide safe and appropriate services, including ongoing care following discharge from compulsion.

Informal care Wherever possible, care, treatment and support should be provided to people with mental disorder without the use of compulsory powers.

Participation Service users should be fully involved, so far as they are able to be, in all aspects of their assessment, care, treatment and support. Their past and present wishes should be taken into account and they should be provided with all the information and support necessary to enable them to participate fully. The information should be provided in a way that makes it most likely to be understood.

Respect for carers Those who provide care to service users on an informal basis should receive respect for their role and experience, receive appropriate information and advice, and have their views and needs taken into account.

Least restrictive alternative Service users should be provided with any necessary care, treatment and support both in the least invasive manner and in the least restrictive manner and environment compatible with the delivery of safe and effective care, taking account where appropriate the safety of others.

Benefit Any intervention under the Act should be likely to produce for the service user a benefit that cannot reasonably be achieved other than by the intervention.

Child welfare The welfare of a child with mental disorder should be paramount in any interventions imposed on the child under the Act.

As well as a requirement on health and social care professionals to take account of the principles when applying the 2003 Act, patients also benefit from the following.

- A named person, chosen by the patient to support them and to protect their interests in any proceedings under the Act. If no one is chosen by the service user the primary carer is the named person. If there is no primary carer, then the nearest relative will be the named person.
- Advocacy: Every person with a mental disorder has the right of access to independent advocacy. Health boards and local authorities must ensure that independent advocacy services are available. The right to access advocacy applies to all mental health service users, not just to people who are subject to powers under the new Act.
- Advance statements: People can make advance statements, setting out how they would wish to be treated, if they become unwell and unable to express their views clearly at some point in the future. The tribunal and any person responsible for giving treatment under the 2003 Act must take an advance statement into account when making decisions.
- Mental Health Tribunal, which has replaced the Sheriff Court as the forum for hearing cases considering care plans, deciding on compulsory treatment orders and carrying out reviews.
- The Mental Welfare Commission protects the rights of service users and promotes the effective operation of the 2003 Act by:
    - monitoring how the Act is working;
    - encouraging best practice;
    - publishing information and guidance;
    - carrying out visits to patients;
    - carrying out investigations, interviews and medical examinations, and inspection of patient records.

Main compulsory powers

Although the guiding principles call for informal care and treatment and the adoption of a least restrictive approach, three compulsory powers are available under the civil provisions of the 2003 Act.

Emergency detention (part 5 of the 2003 Act)

Allows a person who appears to be suffering from a mental disorder to be detained in hospital for up to 72 hours where hospital admission is required urgently to allow the person's condition to be assessed. It can only take place if recommended by a doctor and, when possible, the agreement of a mental health officer.

Short-term detention (part 6 of the 2003 Act)

Allows a person suffering from a mental disorder to be detained in hospital for up to 28 days. It requires a recommendation by an approved doctor and the agreement of a mental health officer. Short-term detention can be extended beyond 28 days where there is a pending application for a compulsory treatment order

Compulsory treatment order (CTO)

This order has to be approved by a tribunal. A mental health officer has to apply to the tribunal and the application must include two medical recommendations and a plan of care detailing the care and treatment proposed for the patient.

The patient, the patient's named person and the patient's primary carer would be entitled to have any objections that they have heard by the tribunal.

The order lasts for 6 months initially but can be extended for a further 6 months, and after that for 12 months at a time. It can be based in a hospital or community.

In community settings the order can include requirements setting out where the patient should live, attend for services at particular times or attend for treatment.

Compulsory treatment (part 16 of the 2003 Act)

A person subject to an emergency detention cannot be treated without consent unless it is urgently required or they lack decision-making capacity and can be treated under the Adults with Incapacity (Scotland) Act 2000 (see Chapter 5).

A person subject to short-term detention or compulsory treatment order can be given treatment without consent under part 16 of the Act.

Medical treatment is widely defined under the 2003 Act and includes:

- nursing;
- care;
- psychological intervention;
- habilitation (including education, and training in work, social and independent living skills);
- rehabilitation.

There are safeguards for neurosurgery for mental disorder (sections 234–6), electroconvulsive therapy (sections 237–9) and drug treatments given for more than two months (sections 240–2).

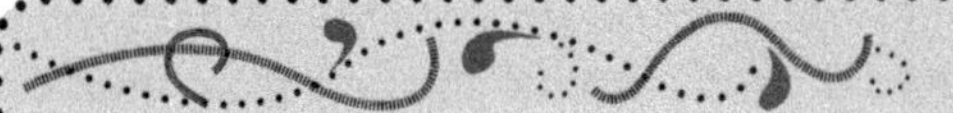

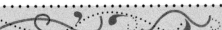

Chapter summary

- Mental healthcare is regulated through the provisions of the Mental Health Act 1983 as amended by the Mental Health Act 2007.
- The fundamental aim of the 1983 Act is to strengthen the rights of patients made subject to its compulsory powers through five key principles that all have a liberal thrust.
- The provisions of the Mental Health Act 1983 only apply to people who suffer from a mental disorder.
- Mental disorder is defined as any disorder or disability of the mind.
- Only people who are, or appear to be, suffering from a mental disorder and who actively resist admission to hospital are considered to be subject to compulsory powers under the 1983 Act.

continued . . .

- Approved mental health professionals (AMHPs) include nurses and social workers who have been approved by the local authority as having appropriate competence in dealing with people who have mental disorders.
- Detained patients must be informed of the conditions of detention and their right to appeal or complain once in hospital; managers usually delegate this duty to a registered nurse.
- A person can enter hospital for assessment and treatment of their mental disorder as an informal admission, without the need to be detained.
- Admission and treatment under the Mental Health Act 1983 are dealt with separately.
- Some treatment under the 1983 Act may only be given where provisions safeguarding patients have been met.
- An approved clinician may grant a detained patient a leave of absence from hospital.
- Where long-term leave, over seven days, is contemplated, the responsible clinician must first consider the use of a community treatment order.
- Guardianship provides an alternative to detention for treatment.
- The Code of Practice to the Mental Health Act 1983 provides clear guidance about your role and duties under the Act.
- The requirements of the Act and its Code of Practice must be followed to ensure that patients are cared for with respect and with due regard for their fundamental rights and freedoms.

Activities: Brief outline answers

Activity 6.1: Evidence-based practice and research (page 136)

You will see that the detention conditions for compulsory admission do reflect the requirements of *Winterwerp v The Netherlands* [1979]. For example, section 2 of the Mental Health Act 1983, Ordinary Admission for Assessment, requires that:

- the person is suffering from a mental disorder;
- the illness is of a nature or degree that warrants detention in hospital for assessment;
- it is in the interests of his own health or safety or protection of others;
- the application must be founded upon the recommendation of two doctors, one of whom must be recognised as having experience in the diagnosis and treatment of mental disorder under section 12 of the Mental Health Act 1983.

Further reading

The acknowledged authoritative guide to mental health law is the *Mental Health Act Manual* listed below. It should be available on every mental health unit. It is, however, as complex as it is comprehensive.

Jones, R (2007) *Mental Health Act Manual.* London: Sweet and Maxwell.

A far more readable book on mental health law is this book:

Brown, R, Barber, P and Martin, D (2008) *Mental Health Law in England and Wales: A guide for approved mental health professionals.* Exeter: Learning Matters.

To understand mental health law in the context of health policy generally, we recommend you read:

Bartlett, P and Sandland, R (2007) *Mental Health Law: Policy and practice.* Oxford: Oxford University Press.

A good introduction to the subject can be found in:

Marphy, R and Wales, P (2014) *Mental Health Law in Nursing.* London: Sage (Learning Matters).

Useful websites

The implementation of the Mental Health Act 1983 in England differs from that in Wales and each has its own advice and code of practice.

The England code can be obtained at:

www.gov.uk/government/publications/mental-health-implementation-framework

For Wales, go to:

www.wales.nhs.uk and search on Mental Health Act

Scotland has its own mental health law and details can be found at:

www.scotland.gov.uk/Publications/2004/01/18753/31686

For information and guidance on the implementation of the Mental Health (Care and treatment) (Scotland) Act 2003:

www.mwcscot.org.uk/the-law/mental-health-act

Welsh Government Mental Health (Wales) Measure 2010 website for information and guidance on mental health law in Wales:

http://wales.gov.uk/topics/health/nhswales/healthservice/mental-health-services/measure/?lang=en

Appendix 6.1 Civil detention provisions under Mental Health Act 1983, part 2, as amended

Section no. and purpose	Method	Conditions for detention	Duration	Can the patient apply to MHRT?	Can nearest relative apply to MHRT?	Automatic MHRT referral?	Do consent to treatment rules apply?
Section 4: Emergency admission for assessment	Application by AMHP or nearest relative founded on one medical recommendation	As for section 2, but AMHP or nearest relative must certify that it is of urgent necessity for the patient to be admitted and complying with section 2 would involve undesirable delay	72 hours; can be converted to ordinary admission for assessment if a second medical recommendation is received during this time	No, but an appeal under section 2 can begin	No	No	No
Section 2: Ordinary admission for assessment	Application by AMHP founded on two medical recommendations, one of which is from an approved clinician	Person is suffering from mental disorder of a nature or degree that warrants the detention of the patient in a hospital for assessment followed by medical treatment for at least a limited period; and person ought to be so detained in the interests of his or her own health or safety or with a view to the protection of other persons	28 days, not renewable; will be extended to the date of the hearing where a nearest relative is being displaced by the county court	Yes, within first 14 days	Yes	No	Yes

(Continued)

Appendix 6.1 (Continued)

Section no. and purpose	Method	Conditions for detention	Duration	Can the patient apply to MHRT?	Can nearest relative apply to MHRT?	Automatic MHRT referral?	Do consent to treatment rules apply?
Section 3: Admission for treatment	Application by AMHP founded on two medical recommendations, one of which is from an approved clinician	Person is suffering from mental disorder of a nature or degree that makes it appropriate for them to receive medical treatment in a hospital; and it is necessary for the health or safety of the patient or for the protection of other persons that they should receive such treatment; and it cannot be provided unless they are detained under this section; and appropriate medical treatment is available	6 months; can be renewed under section 20 for a further 6 months, then yearly	Yes, within first 6 months, then once in each period of detention	Yes	Yes, if a completed appeal has not occurred in first 6 months	Yes
Section 5(2)	Report from a doctor or approved clinician in charge of the patient's treatment	In-patient in a hospital who appears to a registered medical practitioner or approved clinician in charge of their treatment to need detention under this part of this Act	72 hours, not renewable	No	No	No	No

Section no. and purpose	Method	Conditions for detention	Duration	Can the patient apply to MHRT?	Can nearest relative apply to MHRT?	Automatic MHRT referral?	Do consent to treatment rules apply?
Section 5(4)	Report from a nurse of the prescribed class	Appears to a nurse of the prescribed class that (a) a patient who is receiving treatment for mental disorder as an in-patient in a hospital is suffering from mental disorder to such a degree that it is necessary for his or her health or safety or for the protection of others for him or her to be immediately restrained from leaving the hospital; and (b) it is not practicable to secure the immediate attendance of a practitioner or clinician to furnish a report under section 5(2)	6 hours, not renewable	No	No	No	No

Appendix 6.2 Detention provisions for people with mental disorder who commit offences

Section no. and purpose	Duration	Application to MHRT?	Nearest relative application to MHRT?	Automatic referral to MHRT?	Do consent to treatment provisions apply?
Section 35: Remand to hospital for psychiatric report	28 days; may be renewed by the court for further periods of 28 days to a maximum of 12 weeks	No	No	No	No
Section 36: Remand to hospital for treatment	28 days; may be renewed by the court for further periods of 28 days to a maximum of 12 weeks	No	No	No	Yes
Section 37: Hospital order by the court	6 months, renewable for further 6 months, then yearly	In second 6 months, then in each period of detention	In second 6 months and then each period of detention	After 3 years if the patient remains in hospital and has not made an appeal of their own	Yes
Section 37: Guardianship order by the court	6 months, renewable for further 6 months then yearly	Within first 6 months, then in each period of detention	Within first year then yearly	No	No

Section no. and purpose	Duration	Application to MHRT?	Nearest relative application to MHRT?	Automatic referral to MHRT?	Do consent to treatment provisions apply?
Sections 37/41: Hospital order with restriction	Without limit of time; discharge and leave of absence restricted by the Home Office	In second 6 months, then in each period of detention	No nearest relative	If one has not been held, Home Secretary will refer the case to the MHRT every 3 years	Yes
Section 38: Interim hospital order	12 weeks; may be renewed in 28-day periods to a maximum of 1 year	No	No	No	Yes
Section 45A: Hospital and limitation direction	Without limit of time	In first 6 months, second 6 months, then yearly	No	Home Secretary will refer case every 3 years if one has not been held	Yes
Section 46: Transfer to hospital of patient in custody during Her Majesty's pleasure	Without limit of time	Within first 6 months, then once in each period of detention	No	Home Secretary will refer case every 3 years if one has not been held	Yes
Section 47: Transfer to hospital of a person serving a prison sentence	6 months, a further 6 months, then a year at a time	Within first 6 months, then once in each period of detention	No	Hospital managers will refer case every 3 years if one has not been held	Yes

(Continued)

Appendix 6.2 (Continued)

Section no. and purpose	Duration	Application to MHRT?	Nearest relative application to MHRT?	Automatic referral to MHRT?	Do consent to treatment provisions apply?
Sections 47/49: Transfer with restrictions	Restriction lapses on earliest release date from prison	In second 6 months after transfer, then yearly	No nearest relative	Home Secretary will refer case every 3 years if one has not been held	Yes
Section 48: Transfer of other prisoners for urgent treatment	According to treatment needs of the patient	Within first 6 months, then once in each period of detention	No	Home Secretary will refer case every 3 years if one has not been held	Yes
Sections 48/49: Transfer with restriction	Restriction will lapse on earliest release date	In second 6 months, then each period of detention	No nearest relative	Home Secretary will refer case every 3 years if one has not been held	Yes
Section 136: Police power in places to which the public have access	72 hours, not renewable	No	No	No	No
Section 135: Warrant to enter and search for a person with mental disorder	72 hours, not renewable	No	No	No	No

Chapter 7
Protecting the vulnerable adult

NMC Standards for Pre-registration Nursing Education

This chapter will address the following competencies:

Domain 1: Professional values

2. All nurses must practise in a holistic, non-judgemental, caring and sensitive manner that avoids assumptions, supports social inclusion; recognises and respects individual choice; and acknowledges diversity. Where necessary, they must challenge inequality, discrimination or exclusion from access to healthcare.
3. All nurses must support and promote the health, well-being, rights and dignity of people, groups, communities and populations. These include people whose lives are affected by ill health, disability, ageing, death and dying. Nurses must understand how these activities influence public health.
4. All nurses must work in partnership with service users, carers, families, groups, communities and organisations. They must manage risk, and promote health and well being while aiming to empower choices that promote self-care and safety.
6. All nurses must understand the roles and responsibilities of other health and social care professionals and seek to work with them collaboratively for the benefit of all who need care.

Domain 2: Communication and interpersonal skills

7. All nurses must respect individual rights to confidentiality and keep information secure and confidential in accordance with the law and relevant ethical and regulatory frameworks, taking account of local protocols. They must also actively share personal information with others when the interests of safety and protection override the need for confidentiality.

Domain 3: Nursing practice and decision-making

8. All nurses must be able to recognise and interpret signs of normal and deteriorating mental and physical health and respond promptly to maintain or improve the health and comfort of the service user, acting to keep them and others safe.
9. All nurses must be able to recognise when a person is at risk and in need of extra support and protection and take reasonable steps to protect them from abuse.

Chapter aims

By the end of this chapter you will be able to:

- define a vulnerable adult;
- outline the types of abuse suffered by a vulnerable adult;
- discuss the legal provisions in place to protect vulnerable adults from abuse;
- examine how the provisions of the Safeguarding Vulnerable Groups Act 2006 offer protection to vulnerable adults.

Introduction

This chapter considers how the law can be employed by health and social care professionals to protect vulnerable adults from abuse. It is essential that we begin with an agreed definition of a vulnerable adult and then consider what is meant by abuse and the forms it may take. The chapter then summarises the powers available to health and social care authorities to protect vulnerable adults from harm. The chapter ends by looking at the vetting and barring scheme introduced by the Safeguarding Vulnerable Groups Act 2006 that seeks to ensure that unsuitable people are prevented from working with adults who are vulnerable.

We saw in Chapter 4 that a key principle of human rights law is the duty on state governments to have laws and policies in place that prevent one person violating the human rights of another. Since 2000 the government departments responsible for health and social care in England, Scotland and Wales have issued policy documents requiring multi-agency working led by local social services departments to prevent, identify, investigate, respond to and ameliorate the abuse of vulnerable adults in all settings and to take appropriate action against perpetrators of abuse.

The extent of the problem is significant and the figures are generally under-reported. A study of abuse and neglect of older people in 2006 reported that about 227,000 people aged 66 years and over in the UK had experienced mistreatment involving a care worker, a family member or a close friend (O'Keeffe et al., 2007). A third of those who reported mistreatment had sought help from either a health professional or a social worker. There has also been an increase in the number of cases of physical and financial abuse referred to social services (Association of Directors of Adult Social Services, 2009). Undoubtedly you will come across vulnerable adults who could be subject to abuse and it is important that you are aware of how the law protects those who are at risk. Nurses are well placed to recognise those people who have non-accidental injuries and to raise concerns about the welfare of vulnerable people (NMC, 2015a). Standard 17 of *The Code* requires that you:

- raise concerns immediately if you believe a person is vulnerable or at risk and needs extra support and protection.

To achieve this *The Code* (2015a) requires you to:

- take all reasonable steps to protect people who are vulnerable or at risk from harm, neglect or abuse;
- share information if you believe someone may be at risk of harm, in line with the laws relating to the disclosure of information; and
- have knowledge of and keep to the relevant laws and policies about protecting and caring for vulnerable people.

Activity 7.1 ***Reflection***

What is a vulnerable adult?

Before reading on, jot down what you consider to be the factors that would make an adult vulnerable to abuse.

Read on for answers to this activity.

Vulnerable adults

A vulnerable adult is defined under the Protection of Freedoms Act 2012 as

> *any adult to whom an activity which is a regulated activity relating to vulnerable adults is provided. Therefore any adult receiving a regulated activity such as nursing or personal care is considered vulnerable because of that activity. It is not based on a person's age, condition or behaviour.*

The Police Act 1997 (Enhanced Criminal Record Certificates) (Protection of Vulnerable Adults) Regulations (2002) contains a slightly broader definition of a vulnerable person as

> *someone aged 18 years or over who has either a dependency upon others in the performance of, or a requirement for assistance in the performance of basic functions. It also includes someone with a severe impairment in the ability to communicate with others; or has a reduced ability to protect themselves from assault, abuse or neglect due to a learning or physical disability, a physical or mental illness, which may be chronic or otherwise and including an addiction to alcohol or drugs, or a reduction in physical or mental capabilities.*

Both of these definitions would include adults who are at risk of abuse from other people but also includes those who need to be protected from themselves by being removed from a dangerous situation. The inclusion of a risk of exploitation encompasses those who may be vulnerable to financial or sexual abuse.

Abuse

Abuse is the violation of an individual's human or civil rights by any other person or persons (DH, 2000). There are different types of abuse, which may consist of single or repeated acts and which can take place in different settings. Abuse may be planned or unplanned; it may be intentional or the result of negligence or ignorance.

Activity 7.2 — *Team working*

In a group, discuss what acts can constitute abuse, taking into account the Department of Health (2000) definition in relation to a breach of a person's human and civil rights.

Read on for answers to this activity.

Types of abuse

Physical abuse

Physical abuse includes hitting or slapping a person, misusing medication, and subjecting the person to undue restraint or inappropriate sanctions.

Case study 7.1: Physical abuse

Simon Hack was a care worker who was said to have a pathological hatred of women. He had committed over 100 assaults on women in his care before he was arrested and then convicted of actual bodily harm. He received a sentence of four years in prison.

Financial abuse

A vulnerable person can also be abused financially through theft, fraud, pressure around wills, property or inheritance, and misuse or misappropriation of benefits.

Case study 7.2: Financial abuse by a carer

In R v Hinks *[2001] a man of limited intelligence was persuaded by his carer to make a series of transfers from his bank account to her own. The carer maintained that the transfers had constituted a gift. The jury held that accepting such a large sum from a vulnerable adult was dishonest and convicted the carer of theft.*

Sexual abuse

Sexual abuse includes rape and sexual assault or sexual acts to which the vulnerable adult has not or could not consent or was pressured into consenting.

Case study 7.3: Sexual abuse by a member of staff

In Re SKR *[1994], a 27-year-old woman was indecently assaulted at a day centre by a member of staff. He inserted his finger into her vagina and asked her to touch his genitals. The woman had learning difficulties and a schizoaffective disorder which got worse after the incident. She developed severe depression, became more aggressive and regressed to child-like activities at times.*

Psychological abuse

Psychological abuse can include threats of harm or abandonment, blackmail, humiliation, verbal or racial abuse, isolation or withdrawal of services or supportive networks.

Case study 7.4: Blackmail as a form of psychological abuse

In R v Collard *[2002], Collard had made a number of demands for money from a 65-year-old man, threatening to tell of an allegation of indecent assault if he failed to pay. The victim paid a total of £74,000, the bulk of his life savings. He then committed suicide. Collard was sentenced to four years' imprisonment for blackmail.*

Institutional abuse

Institutional abuse may take the form of poor or unsatisfactory professional practice or ill-treatment or gross misconduct.

Case study 7.5: Abuse within an institution

In 2007, the Healthcare Commission highlighted several sex attacks and other assaults by staff members on people in the care of a primary care trust. It described widespread institutional abuse, such as impoverished and unsatisfactory living conditions with some people in cramped rooms with only three or four hours of activity a week. There were failures in management and leadership in the service.

The abuse was found to be prevalent in most parts of the service. It was mainly due to lack of awareness, lack of specialist knowledge, lack of training and lack of insight. It was exacerbated by

continued . . .

low morale among staff, shortages of staff, inadequate supervision and lack of leadership. The Commission's investigators said that in most cases the way people were cared for encouraged dependency rather than independence and that the views of people with learning disabilities or their relatives were seldom taken into account.

(Fleming, 2007)

Abuse through neglect

Abuse through neglect can take the form of neglect and failure to act in the best interest of the vulnerable person. For example, this may include ignoring healthcare needs or withholding the necessities of life, such as medication or adequate nutrition.

Case study 7.6: Neglect of a vulnerable adult

A husband left his wife with three pork pies and some water when she got wedged down the side of the bed. The man admitted neglect and ill-treatment and said he could not free his wife because of his bad back. The pork pies were still sitting on the mattress in their packet when police arrived at the couple's flat. The court heard how he failed to look after his wife properly when he should have been caring for her because she lacked capacity. For a period of four months he had failed to obtain his wife's medication for her epilepsy. The court said that the fact she was uncooperative and unable to do things at her husband's request was a marker that she needed care from him and from outside agencies. The man was given a 36-week prison sentence suspended for two years and will be supervised by a probation officer.

(Western Mail, 2008)

Self-neglect covers a wide range of behaviour such as neglecting to care for one's personal hygiene, health or surroundings and includes behaviour such as hoarding.

Case study 7.7: Man was left to live in squalor after errors assessing his mental capacity

A man was left in squalor after his care team failed to adequately assess his mental capacity to look after himself at home.

Health and social care professionals were so fixated on the man's wishes to live independently that they failed to carry out a capacity assessment of his ability to look after himself which would have revealed that he was unable to cope with everyday tasks like feeding himself and cleaning. As a

continued . . .

result, he was two-and-a-half stone underweight, his teeth were rotten and his bedclothes had not been washed in months. At one point his family were so concerned for him that they brought him to live with them.

(McNicoll, 2014)

Discriminatory abuse

Discriminatory abuse includes forms of harassment, slurs or similar treatment because of race, gender and gender identity, age, disability, sexual orientation or religion.

Case study 7.8: Discriminatory abuse

In R v Bell *[2001] a man was given an eighteen month sentence for a racially aggravated assault. Bell subjected an elderly neighbour to a physical attack and racial abuse.*

Organisational abuse

This includes neglect and poor care practice within an institution or specific care setting such as a care home, or in relation to care provided in one's own home. This may range from one-off incidents to on-going ill-treatment. It can be through neglect or poor professional practice as a result of the structure, policies, processes and practices within an organisation.

Case study 7.9: Organisational abuse

The Winterbourne View hospital inquiry was commissioned following a BBC Panorama broadcast in 2011 that exposed organisational physical and psychological abuse of people with learning disabilities and challenging behaviour at the hospital. The undercover footage showed staff repeatedly assaulting and harshly restraining patients under chairs. Staff gave patients cold punishment showers, left one outside in near zero temperatures and poured mouthwash into another's eyes. They pulled patients' hair and forced medication into patients' mouths. Victims were shown screaming and shaking, and one patient was seen trying to jump out of a second floor window to escape the torment, and was then mocked by staff members. The publicly funded hospital was shut down as a result of the abuse that took place.

(DH, 2012b)

Domestic violence

The Home Office has changed the definition of domestic abuse to an incident or pattern of incidents of controlling, coercive or threatening behaviour, violence or abuse by someone who is or has been an intimate partner or family member regardless of gender or sexuality. It therefore includes: psychological, physical, sexual, financial, emotional abuse and so called 'honour' based violence (Home Office, 2012a, b).

It is clear that the Home Office does not limit the definition of domestic abuse to intimate partners but extends the definition to encompass other family members as well.

Modern slavery encompasses slavery, human trafficking, forced labour and domestic servitude.

Where does abuse take place?

Abuse of vulnerable adults can take place in many different settings, such as the person's own home, a care home, a hospital, a day centre or even a public place. Of the estimated half a million elderly people regularly suffering abuse, the majority, 67 per cent, are abused in their own home with 22 per cent of incidents occurring in care homes and a further 5 per cent in hospital (House of Commons Health Committee, 2004).

All local adult protection policies have a reporting requirement. You may become concerned that a vulnerable adult is being abused, or is at risk of abuse, as a result of one or more of the following:

- direct disclosure by the vulnerable adult;
- a complaint or expression of concern by another person; or
- observing the behaviour of the vulnerable adult.

It is important at this stage that you do not discuss concerns about abuse with the alleged perpetrator. You must also take care not to disturb or destroy articles that may be used in evidence during a criminal investigation or ultimate prosecution.

If abuse is suspected or reported, you will be expected to act in accordance with your local adult protection policies and procedures.

- Take reasonable steps to ensure the adult is in no immediate danger.
- Seek treatment for the abused adult if required.
- Obtain permission from the vulnerable adult before disclosing confidential information about them (see Chapters 5 and 12).
- Where appropriate, discuss your concerns with your manager or person responsible for overseeing the care of the vulnerable adult.
- Consider the need to inform the vulnerable adult's GP or doctor.
- If, after discussion, abuse or neglect is still considered to be a possibility, a referral should be made to social services.
- Following discussion with your mentor or manager, contact the police if it is believed that a crime may have been committed.

- Where a child is also at risk, local child protection procedures should be followed.
- Records must be kept of all concerns and discussions about the adult, the decisions made and reasons for these decisions.
- Abuse can often be a culmination of events. It is important to maintain appropriate records of concerns, whether or not further action is taken at the time.

Vulnerable adults have the right to decide how and with whom they live. A person who is able to make decisions is entitled to refuse protection. However, if the person lacks mental capacity to make this decision or there is an overriding public interest, such as where other vulnerable adults are at risk, the need for referral should be considered. Wherever possible, the vulnerable adult should be informed that a referral will be made and the reasons for it.

Local agencies involved in the care and protection of vulnerable adults, such as commissioners, providers and regulators of health and social care services, the police, local housing and education departments, and voluntary and private sector organisations are required to work in partnership to ensure that robust procedures are in place to protect those at risk of abuse. As the lead agency, social service authorities (and where a criminal offence may have been committed, the police) have a responsibility to make enquiries into concerns about the welfare of a vulnerable adult. Their primary aim is to prevent abuse where possible, but if preventative measures fail, a robust set of legal powers can be used to deal with incidents of abuse effectively.

We have already seen in Chapters 5 and 6 that a range of provisions is available to protect people with mental health problems or people who lack decision-making capacity from abuse.

A dilemma arises, however, when vulnerable persons place themselves at risk of harm but are capable of making their own decisions and do not suffer from a mental disorder.

Scenario: Should autonomy have limits?

Mrs Smith, 75, lives alone in a very large house with over 100 cats. She spends her money on cat food that she has taken to eating herself. She has lost considerable weight, and has a severe outbreak of ringworm caught from the cats, treatment for which she refuses. Cat excrement and empty food tins are everywhere. Neighbours have complained of the smell to the local council. Mrs Smith refuses to give up the cats. She refuses to leave her house. She refuses any medical treatment. She has decision-making capacity and there is no indication of a mental disorder.

In a group, consider what action, if any, could be taken against Mrs Smith.

It is probable that your discussions have focused on the right of individuals to live their lives as they please, free from interference from the state. You may argue that Mrs Smith is entitled to express her autonomy as she sees fit and that she should be left alone. Where you have concerns they may initially focus on the welfare of the cats and perhaps the involvement of the RSPCA or the SSPCA. Another argument for action may focus on the environmental health issue complained of by neighbours and enforcement action by the local council. Some of you may argue that in an extreme case such as this the only realistic way to rehouse the cats and clear the mess is to temporarily remove Mrs Smith to a more suitable place.

Should there be provision to allow a person to be removed from their home and taken to a hospital or appropriate place?

Safeguarding vulnerable adults

The Care Act 2014 created a statutory duty to protect vulnerable adults and the Act's statutory guidance at 14.2 sets out when the duty applies. The Care Act 2014 now defines a vulnerable adult as one who

> *has needs for care and support whether or not a local authority is meeting any of those needs and; is experiencing, or at risk of, abuse or neglect; and as a result of those care and support needs is unable to protect themselves from either the risk of, or the experience of abuse or neglect.*

Local authorities have statutory adult safeguarding duties under the Care Act 2014. When a nurse has concerns about the abuse or neglect of a vulnerable adult they must report the matter to their local authority adult safeguarding team.

The statutory adult safeguarding duty of local authorities is widely defined under the Care Act 2014 and it applies equally to those adults with care and support needs regardless of whether those needs are being met, regardless of whether the adult lacks mental capacity or not and regardless of the setting (DH, 2014).

Duty to safeguard vulnerable adults

Safeguarding is defined as protecting an adult's right to live in safety, free from abuse and neglect (DH, 2014). It requires people and organisations working together to prevent and stop the risks and experience of abuse or neglect.

To achieve this, local authorities must work with their relevant partners to protect adults. Local authorities must also co-operate with such other agencies or bodies as it considers appropriate in the exercise of its adult safeguarding functions, including nursing services.

In common with all local authority partners, nurses are required to apply the six principles that underpin all adult safeguarding work as set out in Box 7.1.

Box 7.1: Key principles of adult safeguarding

1. **Empowerment**: People are supported and encouraged to make their own decisions and informed consent.
2. **Prevention**: It is better to take action before harm occurs.

3. **Proportionality**: The least intrusive response appropriate to the risk presented.
4. **Protection**: Support and representation for those in greatest need.
5. **Partnership**: Local solutions through services working with their communities. Communities have a part to play in preventing, detecting and reporting neglect and abuse.
6. **Accountability**: Accountability and transparency in delivering safeguarding.

(DH, 2014)

The requirement to work with local authorities to prevent and take action against adult abuse underpins the nurse's professional duty to raise concerns if a patient is at risk (NMC, 2015a).

As well as an individual professional duty on nurses to promote the safeguarding of adults there is also an organisational duty to prevent and ameliorate adult abuse that might occur within the nursing service. This duty is imposed by the Care Quality Commission (CQC), the statutory regulator for healthcare in England.

The CQC introduced revised fundamental standards that came fully into force on 1 April 2015. The standards are underpinned by the Health and Social Care Act 2008 (Regulated Activities) Regulations 2014 giving them legal force.

Regulation 13 of the Health and Social Care Act 2008 (Regulated Activities) Regulations 2014 requires nursing services to safeguard the users of their services from abuse and improper treatment.

Abuse for the purpose of the 2014 regulations means:

- any behaviour towards a service user that is an offence under the Sexual Offences Act 2003;
- ill-treatment whether of a physical or psychological nature of a service user;
- theft, misuse or misappropriation of money or property belonging to a service user; or
- neglect of a service user.

To meet the requirements of regulation 13 nursing services must ensure they take appropriate steps to impose a zero tolerance approach to abuse, including neglect and subjecting service users to degrading treatment, and to prevent service users from being abused by staff or others with whom they come into contact when using the services, and that includes visitors to the practice.

In addition, the nursing service must take appropriate steps to ensure a zero tolerance approach to unlawful discrimination or restraint and to unnecessary or disproportionate restraint or deprivation of liberty.

Where any form of abuse is suspected or reported even by a third party from outside the service then the NHS trust is required to take timely and appropriate action to investigate and refer on to an appropriate body such as the police, CQC or local authority under their adult safeguarding procedures (CQC, 2014).

In situations where service users do suffer abuse or are placed at risk of any form of abuse then it is open to the CQC to move directly to prosecution without having to first serve a warning notice on the nursing service.

If the CQC consider breaches of other regulations have led to abuse, or be a major contributory factor in not preventing abuse, they can again move directly to prosecution without serving a warning notice as well as taking action for breaches of the other regulations (CQC, 2014).

Safeguarding a vulnerable adult's liberty

The deprivation of liberty safeguards were introduced in the spring of 2009 in response to a European Court of Human Rights ruling that a man who lacked decision-making capacity had been detained in hospital on the arbitrary decision of his doctor (*HL v United Kingdom (45508/99)* [2005]). To meet the requirements of the European Convention on Human Rights (1950), article 5, a deprivation of liberty can only be lawful if it is authorised by a procedure set out in law. The Mental Capacity Act 2005 was amended to allow for a person to be lawfully deprived of their liberty where this is authorised by the Court of Protection under section 16 of the 2005 Act or authorised by the deprivation of liberty safeguard procedures under schedule A1 of the Act in hospitals or care homes.

Activity 7.3 *Critical thinking*

In groups write down what care, treatment or intervention might amount to a deprivation of liberty.

Once you have done that read on.

When the safeguards were first introduced the threshold for a deprivation of liberty was set at a relatively high level and was limited to situations where a high degree or intensity of restraint or restriction was used in the care of the person. This included situations where:

- Restraint, including sedation, was used to admit a person or care for a person who was resisting.
- Professionals exercised complete and effective control over the person's care and movement for a significant period.
- Professionals exercised control over assessments, treatment, contacts and residence.
- The person was prevented from leaving if they made a meaningful attempt to do so.
- Refusing a request by carers for the person to be discharged to their care.

(Ministry of Justice, 2008b)

A more inclusive test for determining a deprivation of liberty

In *Cheshire West and Chester Council v P* [2014] the Supreme Court considered the current authorisation process for the deprivation of liberty safeguards and the test for determining whether care and treatment amounted to a deprivation of liberty.

The Supreme Court held that the right to liberty is a human right guaranteed to all. Chapter 4 explained that human rights are universal and are guaranteed to everyone, including those who lack the capacity to make decisions about care and treatment. The right to liberty guaranteed by article 5 of the European Convention on Human Rights (1950) must therefore apply equally to everyone whether or not they have a physical or mental disability. The Supreme Court held that to protect vulnerable adults who lack capacity it was necessary to have a test for determining a deprivation of liberty that was more inclusive and that focused on the confinement of that person in a care setting.

Acid test for identifying a deprivation of liberty

The Mental Capacity Act 2005 section 64 states that a deprivation of liberty has the same meaning as in article 5(1) of the European Convention on Human Rights. The European Court of Human Rights requires three elements be considered when identifying a deprivation of liberty:

1. Objective element:
   - The person is confined in a particular restricted space for a not negligible length of time.
2. Subjective element:
   - The person has not consented to the restrictions or lacks capacity to consent to the restrictions.
3. Deprivation of liberty is one for which the state is responsible.
   (*HL v United Kingdom (45508/99)* [2005])

When considering the objective element, the Supreme Court in *Cheshire West* held that the key acid test was that the patient was under continuous supervision and control and was not free to leave. All three parts of the test must be present for the objective element to be satisfied.

The Supreme Court's approach returns to the original ruling by the European Court of Human Rights in *HL v United Kingdom (45508/99)* [2005] that led to the introduction of the deprivation of liberty safeguards. The Supreme Court held that an assessment of the objective element of a deprivation of liberty must be based on the acid test of whether the person is under continuous supervision and control and not free to leave.

Continuous supervision and control

The threshold for what amounts to continuous supervision and control has been set relatively low by the Supreme Court.

Case study 7.10: Continuous supervision and control

In Cheshire West and Chester Council v P *[2014] seven Supreme Court Justices agreed that a 38-year-old man with learning disabilities, placed in local authority care to meet his need for 24-hour care, was deprived of his liberty because although the care home tried to ensure his life was as normal as possible he was in reality under continuous supervision and control and not free to leave. This included a range of measures required to control his occasional aggressive outbursts and manage his habit of eating his incontinence pad. He could not go anywhere or do anything without their permission or assistance and support.*

Activity 7.4 — *Decision-making*

Two girls, aged 17 and 18 and suffering from moderate learning disabilities, were looked after by the local authority, one in foster care, the other in a small residential unit for adolescents with complex needs. Each had occasional outbursts of challenging behaviour, but attended a further education college during the day and led a reasonably full social life. The sisters did not express any wish to leave their accommodation but when they did go out they were accompanied by staff. They had never tried to leave without permission, but their carers said that should they ever do so they would be stopped to protect them from harm.

Does the situation amount to continuous supervision and control and not free to leave?

Once you have come to a decision then read on.

It is arguable that the restrictions imposed on the sisters were no more severe than a parent might impose in the same circumstances and their life was as near normal as their disabilities allowed.

The Supreme Court, however, held, by a majority, that it was not the sisters' parents but the state that was imposing the restrictions. As each was subject to continuous supervision and control and was not free to leave the place where they lived then they were being deprived of their liberty. That the restrictions were imposed to ensure their care needs were met and that the sisters did not object to them was irrelevant in the view of the Supreme Court. They were entitled to the same degree of liberty as everyone else (*P&Q [by their litigation friend, the Official Solicitor] v Surrey County Council* [2014]). The deputy president of the Supreme Court held that:

> *If it would be a deprivation of my liberty to be obliged to live in a particular place, subject to constant monitoring, only allowed out with close supervision, and unable to move away without permission even if such an opportunity became available, then it must also be a deprivation of liberty of a disabled person. The fact that my living arrangements are comfortable, and indeed make my life as enjoyable as it could possibly be, should make no difference. A gilded cage is still a cage.*
> (*Cheshire West and Chester Council v P* [2014] at paragraph 46)

It is clear that the Supreme Court has set a low threshold for finding that a person is subject to continuous supervision and control and not free to leave.

Nurses must promote the human rights of all patients

As a result of the Supreme Court judgment in *Cheshire West and Chester Council v P* [2014] nurses must now view the deprivation of liberty safeguards as a positive tool to promote the human rights of those whose care and treatment amounts to a deprivation of liberty.

As patients who lack decision-making capacity are properly considered vulnerable the Supreme Court requires that nurses err on the side of caution in deciding if a patient is being deprived of their liberty. That is, to presume that care and treatment amounts to a deprivation of liberty where the acid test is met.

The safeguards must be applied to adults in hospital under continuous supervision and control and not free to leave. This is likely to include patients who lack capacity because of dementia, learning disabilities and other forms of mental disorder even where they do not object to being in hospital. Nurses must now ensure that such patients are able to benefit from the protection given to them by the safeguards, particularly the periodic independent check on whether the arrangements for their care and treatment continues to be in their best interests.

The need for such checks should be viewed positively as a means of promoting human rights.

Authorising a deprivation of liberty

The deprivation of liberty safeguards protect patients in hospitals and people in care homes registered under the Care Standards Act 2000.

They apply to people aged 18 and over who:

- suffer from a mental disorder; and
- lack the capacity to give consent to the arrangements made for their care; and
- for who such care is considered by independent assessments to be necessary in their best interests to protect them from harm.

Such people will include, for example, those with profound learning disabilities, older people suffering from dementia and some people who have suffered trauma such as a head injury.

- Whenever a hospital or care home identifies a person who lacks capacity that is or appears to be deprived of their liberty they are be required to apply to the supervisory body to authorise the deprivation of liberty.
- Where a person is in a care home the supervisory body will be the local authority for the area where the person resides.
- Where the person is in a hospital the supervisory body will be the local authority in England and in Wales, the relevant local health board.

It is unlawful to deprive someone of liberty under the Mental Capacity Act 2005 without such an authorisation. The only exceptions would be in an emergency or where the Court of Protection orders a deprivation of liberty (Mental Capacity Act 2005, sections 4A and 4B).

To assist with the proper and timely implementation of the deprivation of liberty safeguards nurses have a duty under the Mental Capacity Act 2005, section 42 to have regard to the Deprivation of Liberty Safeguards Code of Practice.

Activity 7.5 *Research*

Download a copy of the Deprivation of Liberty Safeguards Code of Practice from **http://goo.gl/9SCEaW**

Keep it with you and refer to it as you work through the following section.

Deprivation of liberty safeguards

The deprivation of liberty safeguards prevent arbitrary decisions that deprive vulnerable people of their liberty and so comply with the European Convention on Human Rights. The safeguards provide:

- a representative who will look after the interests of the person and who can ask for a review of the authorisation;
- monitoring of the person's care and treatment by the supervisory body;
- a review of authorisation by the supervisory body; and
- a right of appeal to the Court of Protection.

The safeguards are not intended as an alternative to compulsion under the Mental Health Act 1983.

Applying the safeguards

To apply the safeguards a managing authority seeks authorisation from a supervisory body to deprive the relevant person of their liberty (see Box 7.2 for a definition of the terms used by the deprivation of liberty safeguards).

A person will only be deprived of their liberty if assessments show that:

- they are 18 or older;
- they have a mental disorder;
- they lack capacity to decide on their residence;
- there are no refusals to a deprivation of liberty;
- there are no conflicts with the person's status under the Mental Health Act 1983; and
- it is in their best interests to protect them from harm to be deprived of their liberty; and
- there is no less restrictive alternative.

Box 7.2: Definition of terms used by the deprivation of liberty safeguards

Relevant Person: The person being deprived of their liberty.

Managing Authority: The hospital or care home responsible for the care of the relevant person who request an assessment of deprivation of liberty.

Supervisory Body: The primary care trust, local authority or Welsh minister responsible for assessing the need for and authorisation of a deprivation of liberty.

Assessors: Persons instructed to carry out the deprivation of liberty safeguard assessments on behalf of the supervisory body.

Relevant Person's Representative: Maintains contact with relevant person and represents and supports them in relation to the safeguards.

Family and Carers: Have a right to be consulted, involved in the assessments and provided with information about the safeguards.

Independent Mental Capacity Advocate: Instructed to act as consultee where the relevant person has no one else who can be consulted. Will provide help to the relevant person and their representative about the continued use of the safeguards.

Court of Protection: Provides an appeals process that enables a review of lawfulness of deprivation of liberty.

Types of authorisation

A standard authorisation is requested by a managing authority when it appears likely that a person will be accommodated in circumstances amounting to a deprivation of liberty. If the person meets the criteria the authorisation is issued by the supervisory body and can be for up to twelve months duration.

An urgent authorisation is possible where a standard authorisation cannot be made in advance, and it is necessary in the best interests of the person to deprive them of liberty. A managing authority can issue an urgent authorisation for a maximum of 7 days.

Deprivation of liberty safeguard assessments

Mental health assessment

The purpose of the mental health assessment is to establish that the relevant person is suffering from a mental disorder within the meaning of the Mental Health Act 1983. This is necessary to meet the requirements of the European Convention on Human Rights, article 5(1), that states the limited circumstances under which a person can be deprived of their liberty in accordance with the law. One such derogation is where the person is of unsound mind. To be of unsound mind the person must be shown by objective medical evidence to be suffering from a mental disorder (*Winterwerp v The Netherlands* [1979]).

To ensure these requirements are met the mental health assessor must be a doctor who is approved under section 12 of the Mental Health Act 1983 or a registered medical practitioner who has at least three years' post qualifying experience in the diagnosis and treatment of mental disorder.

As doctors must be instructed to carry out the mental health assessment they cannot be best interests assessors.

Best interests assessor

The best interests assessor cannot be the same person as carries out the mental health assessment.

The purpose of the assessment is to establish whether a relevant person is being deprived of their liberty and if so whether it is in the person's best interests, necessary to prevent harm and proportionate to the likelihood and seriousness of the harm.

As with any assessment under the Mental Capacity Act 2005, the best interests assessor should seek the views of those interested in the care and welfare of the person such as family carers, other close relatives or an advocate already working with the person and any donee or deputy representing the person.

If there is none available to consult then the assessor has a duty to instruct an independent mental capacity advocate to act for the relevant person.

If the best interests assessment supports deprivation of liberty the assessor must state the maximum authorisation period in each case to a maximum of 12 months.

Professionals eligible to carry out a best interests assessment will be drawn from:

- approved mental health professionals;
- registered social workers;
- registered nurses;
- occupational therapists; and
- psychologists.

Mental capacity assessment

The purpose of the mental capacity assessment is to establish whether the relevant person lacks capacity to consent to the arrangements proposed for their care or treatment. The assessment is carried out in accordance with the requirements of the Mental Capacity Act 2005 and its Code of Practice (Department for Constitutional Affairs, 2007).

In England the assessment must be undertaken by an assessor who is eligible to carry out either a mental health or best interests assessment (The Mental Capacity (Deprivation of Liberty: Standard Authorisations, Assessments and Ordinary Residence) Regulations 2008). This requirement does not apply to Wales.

Age assessment

The age assessment establishes if the relevant person is 18 or over. In most cases, this is likely to be straightforward but if there is any doubt then age should be established by a birth certificate or other evidence that the assessor considers reliable. If it is not possible to verify if the person is aged 18 or over the assessor can base their assessment on the best of their knowledge and belief.

The age assessment is undertaken by the best interests assessor.

Eligibility assessment

The eligibility assessment considers the person's status with regard to the Mental Health Act 1983.

A person is not eligible for a deprivation of liberty authorisation if they are detained as a hospital in-patient under the Mental Health Act 1983, or the authorisation would be inconsistent with an obligation placed on them under the Mental Health Act 1983, such as a requirement to live somewhere else. This provision only affects people who are on leave of absence from detention under the Mental Health Act 1983 or who are subject to guardianship, supervised community treatment or conditional discharge.

Similarly if the relevant person is objecting to admission to hospital for the treatment of a mental disorder then they can only be admitted under the provisions of the Mental Health Act 1983.

The regulations for England require that this assessment is undertaken by:

- a mental health assessor who is also a section 12 doctor; or
- a best interests assessor who is also an approved mental health professional.

This is not the case in Wales (The Mental Capacity (Deprivation of Liberty: Standard Authorisations, Assessments and Ordinary Residence) Regulations 2008).

No refusals assessment

The purpose of the no refusals assessment is to establish whether an authorisation for deprivation of liberty would conflict with another existing authority for decision-making for that person.

A standard authorisation cannot be given where, for example, the relevant person has made an advance decision to refuse treatment that remains valid and is applicable to some or all of the treatment that is the purpose for which the authorisation is requested. Similarly if any part of the proposal to deprive the person of their liberty conflicts with a valid decision of an attorney under a personal welfare lasting power of attorney or court appointed deputy under the Mental Capacity Act 2005 then a standard authorisation cannot be given.

The no refusals assessment can be undertaken by a professional who the supervisory body is satisfied is eligible to be a best interests assessor.

Timeframe for assessments

All assessments for standard authorisation must be completed within 21 days from when the assessors are instructed unless there has been a prior urgent authorisation, when they must then be completed within 5 days of receipt of instructions.

Authorising detention

Where any of the assessments conclude that the person does not meet the criteria for an authorisation to be issued, the supervisory body must refuse the request for authorisation and inform all the people concerned that the person may not lawfully be deprived of their liberty.

Where the assessment concludes that the person meets the criteria for detention then they must authorise a deprivation of liberty. The authorisation must be in writing and include the purpose of the deprivation of liberty, the time period, any conditions recommended by the best interests assessor and the reasons that each of the assessment criteria are met.

A copy of the authorisation must be given to the hospital or care home managers, the person concerned and all interested persons consulted by the best interests assessor (The Mental Capacity (Deprivation of Liberty: Standard Authorisations, Assessments and Ordinary Residence) Regulations 2008).

Duration of the authorisation to deprive liberty

The duration of any authorisation will be assessed on a case-by-case basis, taking account of the individual's circumstances. Where the best interests assessor concludes that deprivation of liberty is necessary to protect the person from harm they will be required to recommend the time period of the authorisation. The maximum period for an authorisation would be 12 months but shorter periods may be recommended and on expiry of the time period the assessment process will begin anew.

Duty of care home and hospital managers

Care home and hospital managers will have a duty to ensure that the person concerned and their representative understand what the authorisation means and how they may appeal or request a review. They must also ensure that any conditions attached to the authorisation are met. For example, steps to be taken to keep contact with family or to ensure the cultural or faith-based needs of the person are met.

Managers also have a duty to monitor the individual's circumstances for any change that may require them to request that the authorisation is reviewed, such as the person regaining capacity.

Relevant person's representative

A relevant person's representative is provided for all persons subject to standard authorisation under the safeguards. They are appointed by the supervisory body when standard authorisation is given. Their role is to maintain contact with the relevant person and represent and support the relevant person in all matters relating to the operation of the deprivation of liberty safeguards.

It is part of the role of the best interests assessor to recommend a suitable person to act as the person's representative subject to the requirements of the safeguards. If the relevant person has capacity to choose his own representative then this must be who the best interests assessor recommends.

If the best interests assessor is unable to identify a suitable person then the supervisory body must appoint a professional representative in accordance with the requirements of the safeguards (The Mental Capacity (Deprivation of Liberty: Standard Authorisations, Assessments and Ordinary Residence) Regulations 2008). Until this can be arranged an independent mental capacity advocate is appointed to act for the person. An independent mental capacity advocate can also be asked to assist a relevant person and their representative when a review of deprivation of liberty or application to the Court of Protection is being undertaken. A paid or professional representative is not entitled to an independent mental capacity advocate.

Reviews

A review of the authorisation of a person's deprivation of liberty may be requested at any time by the relevant person, their representative or the managing authority.

A review must be requested by the managing authority if it appears:

- The person no longer meets all of the qualifying requirements.
- The person is ineligible because he is now objecting to receiving mental health treatment in hospital.
- The reason why the person meets a qualifying requirement is not the reason stated in the authorisation.
- There is a change in the person's situation, and as a result it is appropriate to vary the conditions of the authorisation.

Court of Protection

In accordance with the European Convention on Human Rights, article 5(4), anyone deprived of their liberty is entitled to speedy access to a court for a review of its lawfulness. The Court of Protection provides this review under the safeguards.

If standard authorisation is in place the Court of Protection can decide:

- whether the relevant person meets the qualifying requirements;
- the duration of the authorisation;
- the purpose of authorisation;
- the lawfulness of any conditions attached to the authorisation;
- vary or terminate authorisation; or
- direct the managing authority or supervisory body to vary or terminate the authorisation.

Impact of the *Cheshire West* case on the use of the deprivation of liberty safeguards

The introduction of a more inclusive test for determining when a person is being deprived of their liberty has seen a tenfold increase in applications for deprivation of liberty safeguards authorisations with some 137,540 applications made to the year ending March 2015 compared to some 13,700 in the year ending March 2014 (Health and Social Care Information Centre, 2015).

Protecting vulnerable adults from unsuitable staff and carers

A new employment vetting and a reformed criminal record regime, under the Protection of Freedoms Act 2012, has been introduced by the government to ensure respect for the civil liberties of individuals while at the same time providing adequate protection for vulnerable groups from harm from those who care for them.

Regulated activity

The Protection of Freedoms Act 2012 redefines regulated activity that will require people to be vetted.

The six categories are those who provide:

- healthcare;
- relevant personal care;
- social work;
- assistance with cash, bills or shopping;
- assistance in the conduct of a person's own affairs;
- conveyance (transportation).

Anyone working in a regulated activity, including nurses, must have an enhanced criminal record check together with a barred list check.

Family, personal and non-commercial arrangements will be outside the scope of regulated activity.

Regulated activity: vulnerable adults

Regulated activity includes healthcare and relevant personal care. That is, the provision of healthcare in any setting by a healthcare professional or by a person acting under the direction or supervision of a healthcare professional. Healthcare includes all forms of healthcare provided for individuals, whether relating to physical or mental health. It also includes palliative care and procedures that are similar to forms of medical or surgical care but are not provided in connection with a medical condition (Protection of Freedoms Act 2012, section 66).

A healthcare professional is a person who is a member of a profession regulated by a body under the National Health Service Reform and Health Care Professions Act 2002. An example would be a district nurse. Those acting under the supervision or direction of a healthcare professional will include healthcare support workers in a hospital or care home.

Relevant personal care concerns the provision of:

- physical assistance to or prompting and subsequently supervising a person who is in need of it by reason of age, illness or disability;
- help with eating or drinking (including parenteral nutrition);
- toileting (including care relating to intimate hygiene);
- washing or bathing;
- dressing;
- oral care;
- care of skin, hair or nails;
- instruction, advice or guidance;
- assistance in relation to general household matters to a person who is in need of it by reason of age, illness or disability; and
- assistance in the conduct of an adult's own affairs such as anything done on behalf of the person by virtue of a lasting power of attorney under the Mental Capacity Act 2005.

Disclosure and Barring Service (DBS)

The Disclosure and Barring Service (DBS) provides both a vetting and barring service (DfE et al., 2011). The vetting and barring scheme is limited to applications to fill vacancies in an area that includes regulated activity, such as a person applying to a university to be a student nurse and a student nurse applying for work as a registered nurse once qualified (Home Office, 2011).

A person will be automatically barred from working with vulnerable groups for serious offences such as rape, wilful neglect and ill-treatment. Employers will continue to face criminal sanction if they knowingly employ someone who is barred from working with vulnerable groups in regulated activity.

A person who is barred under the scheme will commit a criminal offence if they engage in regulated activity.

Employers and regulatory bodies, such as the NMC, will continue to have a duty to report individuals who could pose a risk of harm to children or vulnerable adults to the new barring body (Griffith and Tengnah, 2009).

Chapter summary

- Abuse is defined as the violation of an individual's human or civil rights by any other person or persons.
- Abuse can take many forms and can take place in a variety of settings including health settings.
- You are required to report suspected incidents of abuse according to the local adult protection policy for your area.
- The Safeguarding Vulnerable Groups Act 2006 strengthens arrangements for safeguarding vulnerable adults.
- An Independent Safeguarding Authority now assesses the suitability of people engaged in regulated or controlled activity with vulnerable adults through a vetting and barring scheme.
- Regulated activity covers a wide range of activities that provide the opportunity for close contact with vulnerable adults and includes nursing.
- The numbers of prosecutions for ill-treatment and wilful neglect by nurses and other care workers has risen considerably since the Francis report into the Mid Staffordshire hospital scandal.
- The Criminal Justice and Courts Act 2015, section 20 now makes it an offence for a nurse to ill-treat or wilfully neglect any person in their care.
- The Criminal Justice and Courts Act 2015, section 21 creates an offence that applies to care providers where the ill-treatment or wilful neglect is due to a gross breach of their duty to the patient.
- The offences are not meant to penalise errors, hinder clinical judgement or hinder decisions about particular treatments.
- Nurses have a duty to report abuse against vulnerable adults.
- Nurses must be familiar with the multi-agency adult protection policy for their area.
- Nurses must apply the six principles underpinning adult safeguarding.
- Abuse may be physical, psychological, financial, sexual or neglect.
- Nursing services have a duty to safeguard patients from abuse and improper treatment that might arise when the person is receiving care and treatment.

continued . . .

- Deprivation of liberty safeguards came into force in April 2009.
- The Supreme Court ruling in *Cheshire West and Chester Council v P* [2014] will see many more patients benefit from the protection of the deprivation of liberty safeguards.
- The acid test for determining the objective element of a deprivation of liberty is whether the person is subject to continuous supervision and control and is not free to leave.
- A nurse is required to err on the side of caution and finds that a person is being deprived of their liberty where the acid test is met even though the patient does not object to the benevolent care and treatment being provided in their best interests.
- Following assessment a standard authorisation will allow a supervising body to authorise deprivation of liberty in a hospital or care home for up to 12 months.
- There will be a system of review and appeal available to the person or their representatives against the authorisation.

Further reading

To fully understand the approach to protecting vulnerable adults in your region it is essential that you read the policy document that applies to that region.

For England, read **Department of Health and Home Office** (2002) *No Secrets: Guidance on developing and implementing multi-agency policies and procedures to protect vulnerable adults from abuse.* London: The Stationery Office.

For Wales, read **Welsh Assembly Government** (2000) *In Safe Hands: Implementing adult protection procedures in Wales.* Cardiff: WAG.

For Scotland, read *Adult Support and Protection (Scotland) Act* (2007).

Useful websites

Action on elder abuse has extensive information and case studies at: **www.elderabuse.org.uk**

Further information on the vetting and barring schemes in England and Wales may be found at: **www.gov.uk/government/organisations/disclosure-and-barring-service/about**

That for Scotland can be found at: **www.disclosurescotland.co.uk**

Chapter 8
Consent and children

NMC Standards for Pre-registration Nursing Education

This chapter will address the following competencies:

Domain 1: Professional values

1. All nurses must practise with confidence according to *The Code: Professional standards of practice and behaviour for nurses and midwives* (NMC, 2015a), and within other recognised ethical and legal frameworks. They must be able to recognise and address ethical challenges relating to people's choices and decision-making about their care, and act within the law to help them and their families and carers find acceptable solutions.
2. All nurses must ... be aware of their own values and beliefs and the impact this may have on their communication with others. They must take account of the many different ways in which people communicate and how these may be influenced by ill health, disability and other factors, and be able to recognise and respond effectively when a person finds it hard to communicate.

Domain 2: Communication and interpersonal skills

2. All nurses must use a range of communication skills and technologies to support person-centred care and enhance quality and safety. They must ensure people receive all the information they need in a language and manner that allows them to make informed choices and share decision-making.
3. All nurses must ... be aware of their own values and beliefs and the impact this may have on their communication with others. They must take account of the many different ways in which people communicate and how these may be influenced by ill health, disability and other factors, and be able to recognise and respond effectively when a person finds it hard to communicate.
8. All nurses must respect individual rights to confidentiality and keep information secure and confidential in accordance with the law and relevant ethical and regulatory frameworks, taking account of local protocols. They must also actively share personal information with others when the interests of safety and protection override the need for confidentiality.

continued . . .

Domain 3: Nursing practice and decision-making

4. All nurses must ascertain and respond to the physical, social and psychological needs of people, groups and communities. They must then plan, deliver and evaluate safe, competent, person-centred care in partnership with them, paying special attention to changing health needs during different life stages, including progressive illness and death, loss and bereavement.

Chapter aims

By the end of this chapter you will be able to:

- state the three developmental stages a child passes through to become an autonomous adult;
- outline how the law bestows parental responsibility for a child;
- describe the extent of a person with parental responsibility's right to consent to treatment for a child;
- analyse the test for Gillick competence;
- examine the requirements for a valid consent from a child who is 16 or 17 years old;
- judge when it is lawful to restrict a child's liberty in order to provide care and treatment.

Introduction

This chapter considers how the law of consent applies to children and young persons under 18 years old. It points out that in terms of the law children progress through three developmental stages on the path to becoming autonomous adults. Very young children rely on a person with parental responsibility to consent for them and the chapter outlines who has parental responsibility and the extent and limits of their decision-making authority. The chapter goes on to consider how a nurse would assess a child for Gillick competence, which gives sufficiently mature children the right to make their own consent decisions. Leading on from this, the rights of young people aged 16 or 17 to consent is highlighted. The chapter concludes with some of the dilemmas faced by nurses and other health professionals such as when a parent disagrees with the treatment their child should receive or where a child refuses to stay in hospital to have treatment.

Nurses have patients of all ages and it is essential that any care or treatment delivered to them is done within the law. Consent is an essential element of the lawfulness of treatment. It provides a defence to criminal assault and the tort or civil wrong of trespass to the person (*F v West*

Berkshire HA [1990]). Consent in a health context also has a more fundamental objective. Lord Mustill, in *Airedale NHS Trust v Bland* [1993], wondered why it was that doctors and nurses could with impunity perform acts on people that would be crimes if done by ordinary citizens. He held that

> *[t]he reason why the consent of the patient is so important is not that it furnishes a defence in itself, but because it is usually essential to the propriety of medical treatment.*
> (*Airedale NHS Trust v Bland* [1993], Lord Mustill at 889)

Unless a valid consent is present or consent is dispensed with by operation of law, such as in an emergency, the acts of nurses would lose their immunity.

The nature of consent

Consent is a state of mind in which a person agrees to the touching of their body as part of an examination or treatment (*Sidaway v Bethlem Royal Hospital* [1985]). It has a clinical and legal purpose. The clinical purpose recognises that the success of treatment depends very often on the cooperation of the patient. The legal purpose is to underpin the propriety of the treatment and furnish a defence to the crime and tort of trespass. For capable adults, the law recognises the right to self-determination, which includes the right to consent to or refuse medical treatment even if this would lead to their death.

Children reach the age of majority or adulthood at 18. However, while the courts acknowledge that no minor or child under 18 is a wholly autonomous being, they do recognise the right of the minor to consent to medical treatment as they develop and mature with age.

Consent and children

Kennedy and Grubb (1998) argue that children pass through three developmental stages on the journey to becoming fully autonomous adults:

- the child of tender years;
- the Gillick-competent child;
- children 16 and 17 years old.

The child of tender years

Early Roman law allowed a father to literally have the power of life or death over his child. The overwhelming power a father had was gradually removed during the nineteenth century by Talfourd's Act, the Custody of Infants Act 1839 and the Matrimonial Causes Act 1857. Yet children were still seen to be in the custody of their parents, who retained considerable power over them. For example, parents could demand that a child in care be handed back when they were old enough to earn a wage (*Barnado v McHugh* [1891]).

The relationship between a child and a parent was formalised in the Children Act 1989. This Act allows parents to have parental responsibility for their children, which includes a right to consent to treatment.

Parental responsibility

The concept of parental responsibility replaced the notion of parental rights.

Parental responsibility is defined as all the rights, duties, powers, responsibility and authority that, by law, a parent of a child has in relation to the child and its property (Children Act 1989, section 2). These are not defined or specified in the Act. In essence, the Act empowers a person to make most decisions in a child's life, including consenting to medical treatment on the child's behalf.

Parental responsibility may be shared and generally decisions about a child can be made independently. In most cases, only the consent of one person with parental responsibility is needed to proceed with treatment.

Activity 8.1 *Reflection*

Parental responsibility

- List all the people you think might have parental responsibility for a child.
- From that list select the person who you think would have automatic parental responsibility by law.

An outline answer is given at the end of the chapter.

Automatic parental responsibility

Parental responsibility is conferred automatically on the mother of the child and the father if he was married to the mother at the time of the birth (Children Act 1989, section 2). If unmarried parents subsequently marry, the child's father gains parental responsibility for his children (Family Law Reform Act 1987, section 1).

In recognition of the changing demographic of the family and to encourage both parents to play a full part in the upbringing of their child, the Children Act 1989 was amended in December 2003 to allow unmarried natural fathers to have automatic parental responsibility if they become registered as the child's father under any of the birth registration statutes from that date.

Acquired parental responsibility

If a father is not married to his child's mother and was not registered as the child's father from December 2003, he may still acquire parental responsibility under an agreement with the mother or by order of the court (Children Act 1989, section 3). Parental responsibility may also be acquired by others, such as those in possession of an emergency protection order or a care order, but only for the duration of the order.

Step-parents

Since December 2005, a step-parent who is married to a child's natural parent can acquire parental responsibility either by agreement with the natural parents or by order of the court (Children Act 1989, section 4A).

Delegation of parental responsibility

The Children Act 1989, section 2(9), allows a person with parental responsibility to arrange for someone else to exercise it on their behalf. This delegation need not be in writing and allows carers such as schools, nannies and childminders to make delegated decisions on behalf of a person with parental responsibility for the child. For example, a nurse may visit a young child to find him or her in the care of a grandmother. As long as the nurse is satisfied that the grandmother is acting with the authority of a person with parental responsibility, such as the child's mother, she may accept the grandmother's consent as permission to treat the child.

Carers

The Children Act 1989 allows those who have care for a child, but not parental responsibility, to do what is reasonable in all the circumstances to promote or safeguard the child's welfare (Children Act 1989, section 3(5)). In terms of medical treatment, what is reasonable would generally require the consent of a person with parental responsibility unless it was an emergency or the treatment was trivial.

The extent of parental responsibility

Although a person with parental responsibility can generally make decisions independently, the freedom of each to act alone is not unfettered.

The court held in *Re J* [2000] that there is a small group of important decisions made on behalf of a child that should not be carried out or arranged by one parent alone, even though they have parental responsibility under the Children Act 1989.

Activity 8.2 — *Critical thinking*

Limits to parental responsibility

In relation to a child, what kind of decisions do you think should not be made by one parent alone? Please do not read the next part unless you want to know the answer.

Now read below for further information.

Where the agreement of each person with parental responsibility is not forthcoming, the decision must not be made without the specific approval of the court. As held in *Re B (A Child)* [2003], the important decisions include:

- sterilisation of a child;
- changing a child's surname;
- circumcision of a child;
- a hotly disputed immunisation.

Authority to intervene

In *KD (A Minor) (Ward: Termination of Access)* [1988], the House of Lords held that the best persons to bring up a child are the natural parents. Their view is that public authorities cannot improve on nature and parents are given the exclusive privilege of bringing up a child with the decisions of devoted and responsible parents being treated with respect.

However, a parent's right to consent is not absolute. Parents' rights exist only for the benefit of the child and must be exercised in the child's best interests. The courts, through their inherent jurisdiction, exercise a supervisory role over parental decision-making and can overrule a parental decision that is not in the best interests of the welfare of the child.

Under the private law provisions of the Children Act 1989, section 8, the court also has the power to settle a dispute between two or more people with parental responsibility.

Private law is not a question of child protection and so the threshold criterion of significant harm does not have to be engaged for the court to have jurisdiction.

As long as there is a dispute between people regarding an issue of parental responsibility for a child, the court can intervene to settle the issue.

Private law orders

The Children Act 1989, section 8, gives the court powers to resolve disputes regarding an issue of parental responsibility for a child. The orders available are:

- **residence order**, which settles with whom a child should live and bestows parental responsibility on that person where necessary;
- **contact order**, which settles contact arrangements with a child; contact can be as widely interpreted as the court sees fit and ranges from telephone and email contact to visits and holidays;
- **prohibited steps order**, which prohibits an action without the permission of the court;
- **specific issues order**, which allows the court to settle a specific issue in relation to the parental responsibility of a child.

Where the health and welfare of a child are at issue, the courts have been prepared to use these orders in a creative way.

Case study 8.1: Using a residence order to bestow parental responsibility

In B v B (A Minor) (Residence Order) *[1992], a child lived with her grandmother at the request of her mother but found that the child's school and GP would not accept the grandmother's consent for such things as school outings and routine treatments such as immunisations. The court granted the grandmother a residence order, because the welfare of the child required her to have parental responsibility, even though where the child lived was not an issue.*

Prohibited steps and specific issues orders are also used by the courts to settle issues concerning a child's healthcare. In *J (A Minor) (Prohibited Steps Order: Circumcision)* [2000], the English mother of J, aged five, was granted a prohibited steps order preventing his Muslim father from making arrangements to have him circumcised without a court order, because ritual circumcision was an irreversible operation that was not medically necessary and had physical and psychological risks, and in such cases the consent of both parents was essential.

Case study 8.2: Authorising medical treatment through a specific issues order

In Camden LBC v R (A Minor) (Blood Transfusion) *[1993], a child's parents refused to allow him to have a blood transfusion for the treatment of B-cell lymphoblastic leukaemia because of their religious beliefs. The court found that, where the life of a child was at risk, it was essential to act urgently. The private law requirements of the Children Act 1989, section 8, could be used to seek a specific issues order. This procedure allows the matter to be brought before a High Court judge, who could order the treatment without delay and without transferring parental responsibility.*

Authorising treatment against the wishes of a child's parents is reserved for the most serious cases. In *A&D v B&E* [2003], the High Court accepted that, in general, there is wide scope for parental objection to medical intervention. The court considers medical interventions as existing on a scale. At one end are obvious cases where parental objection would have no value in child welfare terms, for example urgent life-saving treatment such as a blood transfusion.

At the other end are cases where there is genuine scope for debate and the views of the parents are important. These would not raise questions of neglect or abuse that would trigger child protection proceedings. Although an NHS trust can obtain leave to apply for a specific issues order (Children Act 1989, section 8) it is unlikely that leave would be granted in the face of unified parental opposition to this type of treatment.

Case study 8.3: Urgent and non-urgent treatment

In Re P (A Minor) *[1981], the court directed that a termination could proceed on a 15-year-old child despite the genuinely held objections of her parents on religious and other grounds.*

In Re B (A Child) *[2003], the Court of Appeal held that, while it was prepared to settle a dispute between two parents on the issue of childhood immunisations, it would not do so where the dispute was between a parent and the health authorities.*

The best interests test

The right of a parent to exercise their right to consent to treatment for a child is subject to them acting in the child's best interests. Chapter 2 stressed that the courts are also required to act in the best interests of the welfare of a child whenever a case is brought before them.

Consent to treatment for a child of tender years is provided by a person with parental responsibility for the child, usually a parent. However, the decision of the parent must be in the best interests of the welfare of the child and can be overridden by a court exercising its inherent jurisdiction to act in the child's best interests.

The Gillick-competent child

The matter of whether a child under 16 has the necessary capacity to consent to medical examination and treatment was decided by the House of Lords in *Gillick v West Norfolk and Wisbech AHA* [1986]. In this case, a mother objected to Department of Health advice that doctors could give contraceptive advice and treatment to children under 16 without parental consent. The court held that a child under 16 had the legal capacity to consent to medical examination and treatment, including contraceptive treatment, if they had sufficient maturity and intelligence to understand the nature and implications of that treatment.

A child who a nurse considers has the maturity and intelligence to consent to treatment is known as Gillick competent. Wheeler (2006) argues that an urban myth has emerged over the use of the term Gillick competence. It suggests that Mrs Gillick wishes to disassociate her name from the assessment of a child's maturity and intelligence, so carrying the implication that the text should be renamed Fraser competence (see overleaf).

Changing an established legal test would be unusual and cause confusion. Wheeler is clear that Mrs Gillick *has never suggested to anyone that she disliked being associated with the term Gillick competence* (Wheeler, 2006, p808). Gillick competence is the correct term and is still used by judges deciding cases concerning children.

The test for Gillick competence

Activity 8.3 *Reflection*

Before reading the next part for further information, make a list of the factors you think should be taken into account when deciding whether a child has sufficient maturity and intelligence to make a healthcare decision.

In determining whether a child has sufficient maturity and intelligence to make a decision, nurses need to take account of the child, their chronological, emotional and mental age, and their intellectual development, as well as their ability to reach a decision. The aim of the Gillick principle is to reflect the transition of a child to adulthood. The legal capacity to make decisions is conditional on the child gradually acquiring maturity and the ability to make decisions. The degree of maturity and capacity therefore depends on the gravity of the decision. A relatively young child would have sufficient maturity and intelligence to be capable of consenting to a plaster on a small cut. Equally, a child who had the capacity to consent to dental treatment or the repair of broken bones may lack capacity to consent to more serious treatment (*Re R (A Minor) (Wardship Consent to Treatment)* [1992]).

Case study 8.4: Gillick competence for life-saving treatment

In Re L (Medical Treatment: Gillick Competence) *[1998], a critically injured 14-year-old Jehovah's Witness had refused to consent to life-saving medical treatment because it would involve blood transfusions. The hospital authority wanted to carry out the treatment without her consent. The question for the court was whether L was competent to withhold consent within the rule in Gillick.*

The court found that, despite her maturity, L was still a child and her beliefs had been developed through her sheltered upbringing within the Jehovah's Witness community. She knew she would die without treatment but had not been informed of the likely nature of her death. She was not Gillick-competent and it was in her best interests for the treatment to be carried out.

With regard to contraceptive advice and treatment, there is much to be understood by the child if they are to have capacity to consent. The practitioner giving the advice or treatment would need to be satisfied that not only was the advice understood, but that the child had sufficient maturity to understand what was involved. This would include moral and family questions, such as the future relationship with parents, longer-term problems associated with the emotion of pregnancy or its termination, and the health risks associated with sexual intercourse at a young age.

Where the practitioner giving the advice or treatment is satisfied that the child is Gillick-competent, the consent of the child is as effective as that of an adult. This consent cannot be overruled by a parent.

Fraser guidelines

Giving contraceptive advice and treatment to a child under 16 years of age gives rise to a concern that a practitioner may be accused of procuring sexual intercourse with a child under 16 years, which is a criminal offence (Sexual Offences Act 2003). To protect nurses from such accusations, Lord Fraser in *Gillick* issued guidance to ensure that contraceptive advice and treatment were only given on clinical grounds. There might be exceptional cases when, in the interests of the child's welfare, a nurse might give contraceptive advice and treatment without the permission or even knowledge of the parents. You must be satisfied:

- that the girl understood the advice;
- that you could not persuade her to tell or allow you to tell her parents;
- that she was likely to have sexual intercourse with or without contraceptive treatment;
- that, unless she received such advice or treatment, her physical or mental health was likely to suffer;
- her best interests required such advice or treatment without the knowledge or consent of her parents.

It is essential that this guidance is followed in practice to avoid any possibility of criminal conduct.

The defence offered by Lord Fraser's guidance has been extended by the Sexual Offences Act 2003, section 13. This provides a defence against aiding, abetting or counselling a sexual offence if the purpose is to:

- protect the child from sexually transmitted infection;
- protect the physical safety of the child;
- protect the child from becoming pregnant;
- promote the child's emotional well-being by the giving of advice, unless the purpose is to obtain sexual gratification or to cause or encourage the relevant sexual act.

Case study 8.5: Giving sex and contraceptive advice without the knowledge of parents

In R (Axon) v Secretary of State for Health *[2006], the court held that there was no reason why the rule in Gillick should not apply to other proposed treatment and advice.*

The approach of a health professional to a young person seeking advice and treatment on sexual issues without notifying his or her parents should be in accordance with Lord Fraser's guidelines. There was no infringement of the rights of a young person's parents if a health professional was permitted to withhold information relating to the advice or treatment of the young person on sexual matters.

Children aged 16 and 17 years old

Children who have attained the age of 16 years have a right to consent to medical examination and treatment by statute. The Family Law Reform Act 1969, section 8, provides that:

- the consent of a minor who has attained the age of 16 years to any surgical, medical or dental treatment, which, in the absence of consent, would constitute a trespass to his person, shall be as effective as it would be if he were of full age; and where a minor has by virtue of this section given an effective consent to any treatment it shall not be necessary to obtain any consent for it from his parent or guardian;
- in this section 'surgical, medical or dental treatment' includes any procedure undertaken for the purposes of diagnosis, and this section applies to any procedure (including, in particular, the administration of an anaesthetic), which is ancillary to any treatment as it applies to that treatment.

The provisions allow a child of 16 or 17 years to give consent as if they were of full age, that is, an adult. Where such consent is given, it is as effective as that of an adult. It cannot be overruled by the child's parent or guardian.

The courts have adopted a very narrow construction of the provisions of section 8 of the 1969 Act. A child to whom the provisions apply can only consent to treatment or examinations that are therapeutic or diagnostic (*Re W (A Minor) (Medical Treatment Court's Jurisdiction)* [1992]). It does not allow consent for the donation of organs or blood. Even the giving of blood samples is excluded (separate provision is made for these under section 21(2) of the Family Law Reform Act 1969).

Contraceptive advice and treatment is considered a legitimate and beneficial treatment under section 5 of the National Health Service Act 1977 and section 41 of the National Health Service (Scotland) Act 1978. Children who have attained 16 years can consent to contraceptive advice and treatment, including termination of pregnancy.

The assessment of the capacity of a 16- or 17-year-old child to consent to treatment would be in accordance with the provisions of the Mental Capacity Act 2005 and its Code of Practice.

Activity 8.4 *Team working*

What happens if a child refuses consent to treatment?

You will have gathered so far that a competent child under 18 years can make treatment decisions and consent to treatment even though the person with parental responsibility objects. Imagine that the same competent child decides to refuse to consent to treatment. Discuss in a group the rights of the competent child to refuse treatment and what action can be taken when such a refusal happens. During the discussion, please make some notes of the issues raised.

An outline answer is given at the end of the chapter.

Parents and consent

Although both the courts and Parliament allow children to make treatment decisions for themselves as they mature, no minor, that is a child under 18 years, is a wholly autonomous being (*Re M (A Child) (Refusal of Medical Treatment)* [1999]). If a child under 18 refuses medical examination or treatment, the law does allow others to consent even if the child has capacity. Lord Donaldson summed up the position thus:

> *I now prefer the analogy of the legal 'flak jacket' which protects you from claims by the litigious whether you acquire it from your patient, who may be a minor over the age of 16 or a 'Gillick competent' child under that age, or from another person having parental responsibilities which include a right to consent to treatment of the minor.*
>
> *Anyone who gives you a flak jacket (i.e. consent) may take it back, but then you only need one and so long as you continue to have one you have the legal right to proceed.*
> (*Re W (A minor) (Medical Treatment Court's Jurisdiction)* [1992],
> Lord Donaldson MR at 641)

Where a child with capacity consents to medical examination or treatment, it cannot be overruled by a parent. However, where the same child refuses to consent, you may obtain it from another person with parental responsibility who has the right to consent to treatment on the child's behalf. (Note the exception to this rule under Mental Health Act 1983, section 131.)

Activity 8.5 *Team working*

Restricting a child's liberty

You may come across a situation where a competent child under 18 years refuses to remain in hospital. Discuss in a group what actions can be taken in such a situation. Make a note of the key points arising from your discussion.

Now read below for further information.

There may be occasions where a child refuses to remain in hospital for treatment. The Children Act 1989, section 25, allows the use of secure accommodation to restrict the liberty of a child.

Secure accommodation is not defined by the Children Act 1989. It depends on what use is made of the environment to restrict the liberty of a child, rather than having a pre-designated secure area. For example, locking the entrance to a ward, standing in a doorway or preventing a child leaving a room would be using accommodation in a secure way (*Re B (A Minor) (Treatment and Secure Accommodation)* [1997]).

The provisions of the Children Act 1989, section 25, apply to local authority homes, residential and nursing homes, and health and educational premises. The Act allows restriction without a court order for 72 hours in any 28-day period. A record must be kept of the nature and duration of the restriction. Where the period of restriction is going to be longer, a court order is required.

Conditions

Before restricting the liberty of a child you must be satisfied that he or she is 13 years or older and has:

- a history of absconding and is likely to abscond from any other description of accommodation; and
- if they abscond they are likely to suffer significant harm; or
- if they are kept in any other description of accommodation they are likely to injure themselves or other persons.

Case study 8.6: Restricting the liberty of a child

In Re B (A Minor) (Treatment and Secure Accommodation) *[1997], a 17-year-old child suffered from a cocaine/crack addiction and was pregnant. Complications developed in the pregnancy that were potentially fatal to the patient and to the foetus.*

However, B had a phobia about needles, doctors and any medical treatment, and wished to discharge herself from hospital. The hospital applied to the court for an order restricting her liberty by locking the door to the ward.

The court allowed the restriction of liberty and held that, while B had a right to refuse to give consent to medical treatment as she was over 16 years, that right could be overridden by the court or a person with parental responsibility for her. B's refusal carried little weight as it had been demonstrated that she could neither comprehend and retain information about her treatment, nor believe such information, and was unable to make a reasoned choice about her treatment.

The local authority and her mother having parental responsibility could take steps to protect her best interests, which could permit the use of reasonable force in order to administer the correct treatment.

The restriction of liberty was the essential factor in determining whether accommodation could be secure accommodation within the meaning of section 25 of the Children Act 1989, so that secure accommodation did not need to be previously designated but that each case would depend on its facts.

Therapeutic holding

In the course of your practice, you may come across children who need some form of immobilisation in order for a procedure to be undertaken. The aim is to undertake a painful or uncomfortable but necessary procedure effectively. In such a situation, the need for therapeutic holding should be carefully assessed and alternatives methods explored. Where a clinical procedure requires therapeutic holding, consent or assent should be sought if practicable. Those with parental responsibility should be informed of the possible use of therapeutic holding and their agreement sought if possible.

Activity 8.6 *Group work*

You may have come across a situation where a child actively resisted a clinical procedure. In a group discuss what actions can be taken and make some notes of the key points you have discussed.

Go to **www.rcn.org.uk** and download a copy of the RCN document entitled *Restrictive Physical Intervention and Therapeutic Holding for Children and Young People: Guidance for nursing staff* (2010).

Compare what you have discussed with the guidance from the RCN.

As this activity will be based on your own thoughts and reflections, no outline answer is given.

Children and research

The provision for children to consent for research, apart from clinical trials for new medicines, is based on common law (as discussed earlier in this chapter). Therefore, where children have sufficient understanding and intelligence to understand what is proposed, their consent alone to participate in research is sufficient. Where a child is deemed incompetent to consent to participate in research, the person with parental responsibility can consent on their behalf. As a sign of good practice, research is normally undertaken with the consent of the person with parental responsibility and/or the child depending on the competence of the child.

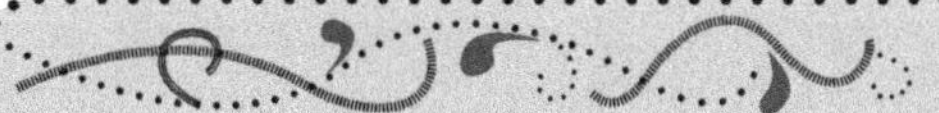

Chapter summary

- Consent is a state of mind in which a person agrees to the touching of their body as part of an examination or treatment.
- The courts acknowledge that no child under 18 is a wholly autonomous being.
- But the law recognises the right of a child to consent to medical treatment as they develop and mature with age.
- Children pass through three developmental stages to becoming a fully autonomous adult: the child of tender years, the Gillick-competent child and the 16- and 17-year-old child.
- A person with parental responsibility is generally entitled to consent to treatment on behalf of a child.
- There is a small group of important decisions made on behalf of a child that should not be carried out or arranged by one parent alone.
- Parents' rights exist only for the benefit of the child and must be exercised in the child's best interests.
- Where those with parental responsibility strongly oppose the giving or withholding of treatment by a health professional to a child, the matter will need to be referred to the court for a decision.

continued . . .

- The court may use a permissive declaration to authorise the withholding of certain treatment at the discretion of the team caring for the child.
- A child under 16 has the legal capacity to consent to medical examination and treatment if they have sufficient maturity and intelligence to understand the nature and implications of that treatment.
- Children who have attained the age of 16 have a right to consent to medical examination and treatment under the Family Law Reform Act 1969, section 8.
- If a child under 18 refuses medical examination or treatment, the law does allow others to consent even if the child has capacity.
- Where a child with capacity consents to medical examination or treatment, it cannot be overruled by a parent.
- There may be occasions when a child refuses to remain in hospital for treatment and the Children Act 1989, section 25, can be used to restrict the liberty of a child.

Activities: Brief outline answers

Activity 8.1: Reflection (page 187)

Parental responsibility is defined as the rights duties, powers duties and responsibilities which by law a parent has in relation to a child (Children Act 1989, section 3):

- mother has automatic parental responsibility on the birth of the child (Children Act 1989, sections 2(1) and (2));
- father has parental responsibility if he was married to the child's mother at the time of the birth (Children Act 1989, section 2(1)); *or*
- if he subsequently married the mother of his child (Children Act 1989, section 2(3) and Family Law Reform Act 1987, section 1); *or*
- if he became registered as the father of the child after 30 December 2003 (Children Act 1989, section 4(1)(a)); *or*
- he and the child's mother make a parental responsibility agreement that is made and recorded in the form prescribed by the Lord Chancellor (Children Act 1989, section 4(1)(b)).
- the court on his application orders that he shall have parental responsibility (Children Act 1989, section 4(1)(c)); *or*
- he obtains a residence order (Children Act 1989, section 12 read with section 4); *or*
- he is appointed as the child's guardian and the appointment takes effect (Children Act 1989, section 5).

Others who can acquire parental responsibility

- Step-parent if they are married to a parent with parental responsibility by agreement of the parents or order of the court.
- A person in possession of a residence order which could include the father of the child (Children Act 1989, section 12).
- A person appointed as the child's guardian once the appointment takes effect; this could include the father of the child (Children Act 1989, section 5).

- A person, other than a police officer, who is in possession of an emergency protection order (Children Act 1989, section 44(4)(c)).
- A person who has adopted a child (Adoption Act 1976, section 12 or Adoption & Children Act 2002, section 46).

A local authority may additionally acquire parental responsibility

- By obtaining a care order (Children Act 1989, section 31).
- By obtaining a freeing for adoption order (Adoption Act 1976, section 18) or a placement order (Adoption & Children Act 2002, section 21).

Activity 8.4: Team working (page 194)

- No child under 18 years is wholly autonomous.
- If a child under 18 years refuses medical examination or treatment, the law does allow others to consent even if the child has capacity.
- Where a child with capacity consents to medical examination or treatment, it cannot be overruled by a parent.
- However, where the same child refuses to consent, you may obtain it from another person with parental responsibility who has the right to consent to treatment on the child's behalf.

Further reading

A very useful booklet on a wide range of consent issues with children is provided by the General Medical Council:

General Medical Council (2007) *0–18 Years: Guidance for all doctors.* London: GMC (can be downloaded from www.gmc-uk.org/guidance/ethical_guidance/children_guidance_index.asp).

To help children and parents understand the rights they have to make decisions about treatment, the Department of Health has two useful explanatory booklets:

Department of Health (2001) *Consent: A guide for children and young people.* London: DH.

Department of Health (2001) *Consent – What You Have a Right to Expect: A guide for parents.* London: DH.

To help you meet the legal requirements for consent and children we recommend this booklet from the Department of Health:

Department of Health (2001) *Seeking Consent: Working with children.* London: DH.

Useful websites

The Medical Protection Society is an organisation that supports health professionals when they face litigation. They have a range of advice sheets on the topic of children and consent:

www.medicalprotection.org/uk/factsheets/consent-children

The Scottish Law website has a very useful explanation of the provisions for consent and children in Scotland:

www.scottishlaw.org.uk/journal/mar2001/sclubgilmar01.pdf

Chapter 9
Safeguarding children

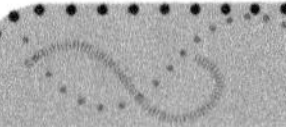

NMC Standards for Pre-registration Nursing Education

This chapter will address the following competencies:

Domain 1: Professional values

2. All nurses must practise in a holistic, non-judgemental, caring and sensitive manner that avoids assumptions, supports social inclusion; recognises and respects individual choice; and acknowledges diversity. Where necessary, they must challenge inequality, discrimination or exclusion from access to healthcare.
6. All nurses must understand the roles and responsibilities of other health and social care professionals, and seek to work with them collaboratively for the benefit of all who need care.

Domain 2: Communication and interpersonal skills

1. All nurses must build partnerships and therapeutic relationships through safe, effective and non-discriminatory communication. They must take account of individual differences, capabilities and needs.
4. All nurses must recognise when people are anxious or in distress and respond effectively, using therapeutic principles, to promote their well-being, manage personal safety and resolve conflict ... They must know when to consult a third party and how to make referrals for advocacy, mediation or arbitration.

Domain 3: Nursing practice and decision-making

9. All nurses must be able to recognise when a person is at risk and in need of extra support and protection and take reasonable steps to protect them from abuse.

Chapter aims

By the end of this chapter you will be able to:

- describe the five principles of the Children Act 1989;
- define significant harm;
- explain the role of the nurse in protecting children;
- describe the powers available to safeguard children from abuse.

Introduction

This chapter examines the law relating to the safeguarding of children at risk of significant harm. The chapter begins by considering the disturbing nature of child abuse and its many forms. It then goes on to consider the key principles set out in the Children Act 1989 that aim to promote the welfare and safety of children. The chapter then considers the legal arrangements in place when things go wrong and children need protection from significant harm.

The United Nations Convention on the Rights of the Child (1989) requires the government to have regard to the full spectrum of human rights for all children and to consider children in legislative and policy decisions. The Convention defines a child as a person under the age of 18 years. In the UK the age of majority, at which a person reaches adulthood, was reduced from 21 to 18 years by the Family Law Reform Act 1969. People under 18 are often referred to in law as minors.

Article 19 of the United Nations Convention says that children have the right to be protected from abuse and the UK provides this protection through the Children Act 1989.

Nurses have a key role in the identification of children who may have been abused or who are at risk of abuse. They are also well placed to recognise when parents or other adults have problems that might affect their capacity to fulfil their roles with children safely.

Nurses must know when to refer a child for help as a 'child in need' (Children Act 1989, section 17) and how to act on concerns that a child is at risk of significant harm through abuse or neglect (Children Act 1989, section 31(10)).

Child abuse

Activity 9.1 *Research*

The extent of child abuse

Before you continue to read the rest of this chapter, look at the annual summary of the most up-to-date child protection register statistics for England, Northern Ireland, Wales and Scotland (**www.nspcc.org.uk**). You do not need to read the whole document, just look at some of the key statistics to give you an idea of the extent of child abuse in the UK and the nature of the abuse.

Now read below for further information.

An estimated 300 million children worldwide are subjected to violence, exploitation and abuse. In Europe in 2003, the United Nations Children's Fund (2003) reported that two children die from abuse and neglect every week in Germany and the UK, and three a week in France. In the UK available figures show that there are 32,100 children on child protection registers as being at risk of abuse (Creighton, 2006).

A child protection register is a list of children who are at risk of abuse. The register acts as an alert that these children need special consideration.

Activity 9.2 *Reflection*

Forms of abuse

Note down what you consider abuse to mean. Make a list of the types of activity with children that you would consider to be abusive.

Now read below for further information.

The following are the categories of abuse listed on the registers.

- **Neglect** – the persistent failure to meet a child's basic physical and/or psychological needs, which is likely to result in the serious impairment of the child's health or development.

Case study 9.1: Neglect of a child

In R v Banu *[1995], the parents of a child were jailed for three years after they admitted neglect as they had starved the child of adequate nourishment over a period of four months.*

- **Physical abuse** – involves hitting, shaking, throwing, poisoning, burning, scalding, drowning, suffocating or causing other physical harm to a child.

Case study 9.2: Physical abuse

In R v Barraclough *[1992], a mother was sentenced to two years' detention for repeated attacks on her young child that resulted in a fractured skull.*

- **Sexual abuse** – involves forcing or enticing a child or young person to take part in sexual activities. The activities may involve physical contact or non-contact activities such as those in Case study 9.3.

Case study 9.3: Sexual abuse

In R v G *[1999], a brother received a jail sentence of seven years for the persistent sexual abuse of his sisters in the form of indecent assaults and rape.*

And in R v B *[2001], a man was sentenced to nine months' imprisonment for taking indecent photographs of a child.*

- **Emotional abuse** – persistent emotional ill-treatment of a child such as to cause severe and persistent adverse effects on the child's emotional development.

Case study 9.4: Emotional abuse

In Re B (Children) (Emotional Welfare: Interim Care Order) *[2002], the Court of Appeal upheld an interim care order on two children on the grounds of emotional abuse when their father had made persistent threats to their lives during an acrimonious period of separation from their mother.*

The category of concern is important as it requires nurses to identify evidence of a risk of significant harm before a child's name is placed on the register. In *R v Hampshire County Council* [1999], the Court of Appeal held that, before a child was placed on the child protection register there had to be evidence of significant harm, or a risk of such harm, in relation to the category of abuse under which the child was to be registered. For emotional abuse, nurses would have to be satisfied on the evidence before them that a child is at risk of suffering persistent or severe emotional ill-treatment or rejection. It is not enough to identify a stressful family situation – there must be evidence of a risk of significant harm to the child.

The Children Act 1989

The aim of the Children Act 1989 was to provide an effective legal framework for the safety and protection of children. It enshrines five main principles.

1. The welfare principle.
2. Keeping the family together.
3. The non-intervention principle.
4. Avoidance of delay.
5. Unified laws and procedures.

The welfare principle

The welfare principle states that, when a court determines any question with respect to the upbringing of a child or the child's property, the child's welfare shall be the court's paramount consideration (Children Act 1989, section 1).

Activity 9.3 — *Critical thinking*

Defining key terms

'Welfare' and 'paramount' are two terms that stand out in the courts' duty to children under the Children Act 1989. Note down what you consider the terms 'paramount' and 'welfare' to mean.

Now read below for further information.

'Paramount' means more than the child being the first of a list of considerations by the court. In *J v C* [1970], the court held that 'paramount' means

> *[m]ore than placing the child's welfare first. It connotes a process where the course to be followed will be that which is most in the interests of the child's welfare.*

It is the only consideration of the court, and the duty to consider the welfare of the child will be reflected in the court's decision.

'Welfare' is not statutorily defined by the Children Act 1989 and the court is able to exercise its discretion in each case. It is not uncommon for the court to speak of acting in the best interests of the child. The Court of Appeal will only overrule a decision on the welfare principle where it considers it to be plainly wrong (*G v G (Minors: Custody Appeal)* [1985]).

Case study 9.5: The welfare principle

In Re W (A Minor) (Residence Order) *[1992], a couple agreed before their child was born that she would live with her father. Two days after the birth a parental responsibility agreement gave the father parental rights, but the mother then changed her mind and applied for the return of the child. When the judge declined to move the baby pending a welfare officer's report and final determination of the case, the mother appealed. The Court of Appeal held that, although there was no presumption that any child of any age was better off with one parent than the other, it was a rebuttable fact that a tiny baby's interests were best served by being with its mother. The judge was plainly wrong to leave the question of the child's placement until the final hearing, as the child was less than a month old and her welfare required that she should be with her mother.*

In child protection proceedings, the court must consider a checklist of factors to help it determine what would be in the best interests of the child's welfare (Children Act 1989, section 1(4)). The checklist encourages the court to consider all factors in a holistic way and can help people with a child protection role, such as nurses, to focus on the relevant issues.

Activity 9.4 — *Team working*

Coming to a decision on welfare

You have already written what the term 'welfare' means. Imagine that you have been asked to decide on the best interests of a child's welfare. In a group discuss what factors you would take into account in making such a decision. For example, will you allow the child to express his or her wishes?

Now read on for further information.

The welfare checklist requires the court to have regard to the following.

- **The ascertainable wishes and feelings of the child.**

These will be considered in the light of the child's age and understanding (*Gillick v West Norfolk and Wisbech AHA* [1986]). Unless the child can show sufficient maturity and understanding to exercise a wise choice on the issues, the court will appoint a children's guardian, an independent officer of the Children and Family Court Advisory and Support Service experienced in working with children and families, to represent the interests of the child (*Re S (A Minor) (Representation)* [1993]).

- **The child's physical, emotional and educational needs.**

The court is required to take a wide-ranging view of the needs of the child that goes beyond material and monetary needs. As Lord Justice Griffiths (at 637) stated in *Re P (Adoption: Parental Agreement)* [1985], *Anyone with experience of life knows that affluence and happiness are not necessarily synonymous.*

- **The likely effect of any change in circumstances.**

The court must consider the impact of change on the child and is encouraged to avoid unnecessary disruption to the life of the child. In *Re B (Minors) (Residence Order)* [1992], the mother of four children left the family home leaving them with their father. She later returned and removed one of the children. The Court of Appeal held that an order for the return of the child to his father and siblings could be made in order to minimise the effect of a change of circumstances on the child.

- **The age, sex, background and any characteristics of the child that the court considers relevant.**

The age and sex of the child will not conclusively determine the welfare of the child but can be influential. In *Re S (A Minor) (Custody)* [1991], a mother was granted custody of a child, even though she had previously assaulted the child, then disappeared for several weeks leaving the very young child with its father. The Court of Appeal held that there was no presumption that one parent was to be preferred over the other for the purposes of looking after a child. Although it might be expected that young children, especially girls, would remain with their mothers, where there was a dispute over custody this was merely a consideration rather than a presumption.

- **The harm suffered or that a child is at risk of suffering.**

In *Re G (Children) (Same Sex Partner)* [2006], the court refused to allow a woman and her two children to relocate from the Midlands to Cornwall when her relationship with her same sex partner broke down. The court held that, in the case of a same sex relationship where the care of the children was shared, the children would not distinguish between one woman and another on the grounds of a biological relationship. Therefore, it was necessary for the court in making its determination on the welfare of the children to balance the harm to the children of not allowing the move against the future harm to the children if they were not able to have the relationship with the estranged partner that they needed for their welfare.

- **How capable each parent, and any other person is of meeting the child's needs.**

In *Humberside County Council v B* [1993], the Court of Appeal held that a court had been wrong to issue an interim care order against the parents who both suffered from schizophrenia. The court concluded that the magistrates had failed to consider the capability of the parents when determining the welfare of the child.

- **The range of powers available to the court under this Act.**

This provision requires the court to consider how best to provide for the child's welfare. It is not confined to considering the order requested by the local authority and can instead substitute a different order or no order at all. In *Re O (A Child) (Supervision Order: Future Harm)* [2001], the court substituted a supervision order in place of the care order sought by the local authority as, on the evidence, what was required to protect the child was support and a watching brief on the family, where the mother suffered from recurring episodes of mental health problems that might result in future risk of harm to the child.

Courts must clearly demonstrate that they have considered each element of the welfare checklist when making a decision about the welfare of the child.

Keeping the family together

The Children Act 1989 has a presumption that a child is best looked after within a family where both parents play an equal part. Where difficulties occur, families should be supported to carry out that role unless it is clearly against the best interests of the welfare of the child. Before the introduction of the Children Act 1989, social services departments were seen as needlessly adversarial and the removal of children from the family was the main solution to problems within the family.

Now a range of family support mechanisms and the involvement of other family members are used to provide a nurturing and protective environment for children. In the first five years of the Children Act 1989 there were some 20,000 fewer children in the care system.

Children in need

To encourage work with families, local authorities have a duty to promote the welfare of a child in need by providing appropriate services (Children Act 1989, section 17). The aim is to promote the upbringing of such children by their families.

Activity 9.5 *Team working*

A child in need

In a group, discuss what you consider the meaning of a child in need to be. Write down key points that will indicate that a child is in need. Please do not read the text below until you have completed this exercise.

Now read on for further information.

A child in need is one that

> *[i]s unlikely to achieve or maintain a reasonable standard of health or development without the provision of services by a local authority or their health or development is likely to be significantly impaired or further impaired without the provision of services by a local authority or they are disabled.*
> (Children Act 1989, section 17(10))

The definition includes children at risk of abuse but can also include other children. For example, a child who is disabled may meet the definition of a child in need but is not necessarily at risk of abuse. The duty to children in need is key to preventative work with particularly vulnerable children, and nurses are ideally placed to help identify children who would benefit from intervention by the local authority. Good practice requires the local authority to assess need in an open way that involves the child and their carers, and families have a right to receive sympathetic support and sensitive intervention in their lives (DH, 1997).

The non-intervention principle

The Children Act 1989, section 1(5), provides that a court shall not make an order unless it considers that doing so would be better for the child than making no order at all. The non-intervention or no order principle is one of the most innovative principles of the Act (Bainham, 1990). It requires the court to be satisfied that any order it issues will make a positive contribution to the welfare of the child. This helps avoid unnecessary state intervention and preserves the integrity and independence of the family. As Justice Wall stated in *Re DH (A Minor) (Child Abuse)* [1994]:

> *Parents should be free wherever possible to bring up their children without interference from courts or other statutory body.*
> (at 707)

Where nurses are involved in child protection proceedings, they must take note of the no order principle and the initial presumption of the court that no order will be issued. It will be for the agencies involved to rebut this presumption by demonstrating that the grounds for an order are met and that such an order is necessary to promote the welfare of the child.

Avoidance of delay

Delays in child care cases are considered detrimental to the child concerned. Children require stability and prolonged litigation is damaging. Under the Act, courts may be accessed according to the degree of complexity of the case. In applications for care and supervision orders, courts are required to draw up a timetable for disposal of the case. There is a presumption that a full hearing will take place in 12 weeks. The Court of Appeal held in *B v B (Minors) (Residence and Care Disputes)* [1994] that practitioners had a duty to avoid delay in child cases. Where nurses are asked to provide reports or statements as proof of evidence they must do so without unnecessary delay.

Unified laws and procedures

The Children Act 1989 unifies the laws and procedures relating to the welfare of children. Previously there existed distinct private and public law systems. Now there exists one set of laws that includes provision for both private law matters, where there are disputes within families that cannot be resolved without recourse to the law, and public law matters, which allow for the protection of children suffering significant harm.

The Act introduced a three-tier court system in which cases could be moved according to complexity in order to avoid delay.

Magistrates' courts

Children Act cases are heard by the Family Proceedings Court. The bench is drawn from magistrates on the criminal bench and from the youth court. All applications for care or supervision orders under the Children Act 1989 start in the Family Proceedings Court.

County courts

County courts deal with a wide variety of civil cases, including family proceedings. Cases are normally heard by a judge, and some 50 county courts are designated care centres where specially nominated care judges hear care order applications transferred from the magistrates' courts. A number of county courts are family hearing centres, which deal with contested private law hearings, such as with whom a child should live, and adoption applications, while divorce county courts are able to hear applications relating to children arising out of divorce proceedings.

Any county court may make orders under the Children Act 1989 in the course of other family proceedings, such as when orders need to be made regarding children following an application by a parent for a non-molestation order under the Family Law Act 1996.

The High Court's civil jurisdiction

The family division of the High Court hears family proceedings, including Children Act and adoption cases, and appeals from the Family Proceedings Court. Where urgent cases need to be considered, the court operates a service out of court hours and there is always a High Court judge on call.

Case study 9.6: Need for an urgent judgment

In Re M (A Minor) (Medical Treatment) *[1997], Justice Johnson was on call on a Friday evening when the duty clerk informed him of an application for leave to give a 15-year-old girl a heart transplant against her wishes. With the assistance of the official solicitor, his Lordship was able to gather the necessary evidence and make a ruling in the early hours of Saturday morning. Where there is great urgency, decisions can be made quickly outside normal court hours.*

The aim of the five principles of the Children Act 1989 is to ensure that matters of concern regarding children are managed sensitively and with appropriate speed for the benefit of the welfare of the child. This, suggests Dame Butler-Sloss (2003), ensures that the child is viewed by the law and practitioners as a person, not an object of concern.

Significant harm

Prior to the Children Act 1989, there were some 17 routes into care. The welfare principle alone is not robust enough to act as the threshold for state intervention in family life. The minimum requirement that has to be fulfilled before state intervention in a family's life is the risk of significant harm to the child.

Activity 9.6 — *Critical thinking*

Significant harm

In a group, discuss what factors you would take into account when determining if a child is suffering or is likely to suffer significant harm. Remember to look at factors that may cause significant harm now and factors that could cause significant harm in the future. Separate your list into present harm and future harm. Some factors may be present in both lists.

Now read below for further information.

Significant harm is the threshold criterion below which state intervention with families cannot be justified. That is, the child is suffering or likely to suffer significant harm (Children Act 1989, section 31(2)).

The phrase is expressed in the present and the future tense. The present tense refers to harm suffered at the time immediately preceding intervention by the child protection authorities.

Case study 9.7: Applying the threshold criterion

In Re M (A Minor) (Care Order: Threshold Conditions) *[1994], a court held that the significant harm criterion no longer applied after a father killed the mother of the child who was now being looked after by an aunt. The father was serving life in prison and was therefore no longer a risk to the child.*

continued . . .

In Northamptonshire County Council v S *[1993], the court held that the significant harm criterion still applied even though the children had been removed from their abusive parents and put in the care of their grandparents, as the grandparents had no legal authority over the children and so their parents could remove them at any time. Only where there have been significant changes in circumstances can the court ignore the original circumstances in which action was taken by the child protection authorities.*

The future tense element of the threshold criterion relies on speculation about the likelihood of harm. That is, there must be a real possibility of harm to the child.

It need not be proved that the child is more likely to be harmed than not. The standard of proof is the normal civil standard based on the balance of probabilities, not the criminal standard requiring evidence beyond reasonable doubt (*Re H (Minors) (Sexual Abuse: Standard of Proof)* [1996]). However, the House of Lords states that the more serious the allegation the less likely it is to have happened and the more sceptical the courts should be of evidence to prove it. More evidence is required by the courts to prove more serious allegations.

It is not necessary to establish who caused harm to the child. If the harm is attributable to a third party it will only be actionable in care or supervision proceedings if it could reasonably have been prevented by the parent.

Case study 9.8: Preventable harm

In Lancashire County Council v W (A Child) (Care Orders: Significant Harm) *[2000], it could not be established whether the parents or a childminder caused injuries to the child. The court held that it did not matter whether it was the parents or the childminder as the childminder was under the supervision and control of the parents.*

To satisfy the threshold criterion for state intervention the harm must be significant. This definition incorporates physical and emotional harm and neglect. For example, in *Re O (A Minor) (Care Order: Education Procedure)* [1992], the court held that truanting amounted to harm that could be significant. Minor shortcomings in healthcare or minor deficits in physical, psychological or social development should not require compulsory intervention unless cumulatively they are having, or are likely to have, serious and lasting effects upon the child (DH, 1997). Where the harm relates to health or development, the child is compared with a similar child (Children Act 1989, section 31(10)). The need to use a standard appropriate to the child in question arises because some children have characteristics or developmental difficulties that mean they cannot be expected to be as healthy or well developed as others.

To meet the threshold criterion, the Children Act 1989 requires that the significant harm is attributable either to unreasonable care or to the child being beyond parental control.

Care refers to the physical and emotional support that a reasonable parent would give to the particular child having regard to their needs (*Re B (A Minor) (Care Order: Criteria)* [1993]). Where the child is beyond parental control the fault or innocence of the parents is irrelevant (*Re O (A Minor) (Care Order: Education Procedure)* [1992]).

Powers to safeguard children

Urgent intervention

The need for timely intervention is crucial to the proper protection of children at risk of significant harm.

Case study 9.9: Failure to act

In Z v United Kingdom *[2001], Z and his three siblings had been subjected to severe long-term neglect and abuse contrary to the European Convention on Human Rights 1950 (article 3), which granted freedom from torture or inhuman or degrading treatment. The behaviour of the family had been reported to the social services on several occasions, yet they had only acted five years after the first complaint, when the children were placed in emergency care at the insistence of their mother. The court held that the system had failed to protect Z and his siblings, as the state had clearly failed in its obligation to protect the children from ill-treatment of which it had, or ought to have had, knowledge.*

Activity 9.7 — *Team working*

Protecting children

Before you move on to the next part of this chapter, discuss in a group what actions can be taken and by whom in the following situations:

- a child is being abused and is in need of urgent intervention;
- a mother has walked on to a ward and taken her sick child away despite being told that the child was severely ill.

Now read below for further information.

Emergency protection orders

Protection for children in urgent need of intervention is provided by an emergency protection order under the Children Act 1989, section 44. The order is intended for use in an emergency rather than as a routine response to concerns about a child or a measure to coerce parents to cooperate with the local authority.

A court may make the order to any person where it is satisfied that there is reasonable cause to believe that the child is likely to suffer significant harm if they are not removed to accommodation provided by the applicant or if they remain where they are being accommodated. The applicant must convince the court of the urgency of the situation. Proof that a child has suffered significant harm in the past will not satisfy the grounds for the order. Emergency protection must be needed in the current circumstances the child faces, not past dangers.

A court may also grant an emergency protection order in cases where enquiries by the local authority or an authorised person (an officer of the National Society for the Prevention of Cruelty to Children (NSPCC)) are being unreasonably frustrated and they are unable to establish if the child is at risk of significant harm and need access to the child as a matter of urgency.

Effect of an emergency protection order

An emergency protection order operates as a direction to comply with a request to produce the child and can include a provision requiring a person to disclose information about the whereabouts of the child (Children Act 1989, section 48). It may authorise the applicant to enter and search for the child named in the order. Should another child be found on the premises, the order will apply to them as well. It is an offence to obstruct the execution of an order.

The emergency protection order authorises the removal of the child or prevents the child's removal from any hospital or other place. It allows the applicant to see the child and if necessary remove them from the home. The court may order that a doctor or a registered nurse accompany the applicant. If the child is produced unharmed, with no likelihood of significant harm, they should not be removed.

If the child is removed, parental responsibility is conferred on the applicant for the duration of the order. The order can last for up to eight days and can be renewed for up to a further seven days. Contact by those with parental responsibility cannot be prevented unless specifically directed in the order. There is no right of appeal against the order but the parents can apply to have it discharged after the initial 72-hour period has elapsed.

As an alternative to removing the child, a court may include an exclusion requirement in an emergency protection order. This allows a perpetrator to be removed from the home instead of the child. To grant the order the court must be satisfied that there is reasonable cause to believe that, if the person is excluded, the child will cease to suffer significant harm or enquiries will cease to be frustrated. There must be another person living in the home who is both able and willing to give the child the care he or she requires.

Police protection

In *X v Liverpool City Council & the Chief Constable of Merseyside Police* [2005], the court held that the removal of children from their family in an emergency should usually be carried out by means of an emergency protection order, as it requires a magistrate to scrutinise the evidence for action before granting an order.

Where such an order is not practical, a police officer may use their powers under the Children Act 1989, section 46. Where a constable has reasonable cause to believe that a child would be likely to suffer significant harm, they may remove the child to suitable accommodation or prevent the child's removal from any hospital, or other place, in which they are being accommodated. The power allows police officers to take immediate action without the need for a court order. A child made subject to the power cannot be kept in police protection for more than 72 hours and no parental responsibility is conferred on the police. A constable using the power must inform the local authority of the steps that have been taken and the reasons for them. If the child is capable of understanding, he or she must also be informed and the officer must take steps to discover the wishes and feelings of the child. As soon as is practicable, the constable will contact the child's parents and inform them of the use of the order and what further steps may be taken with respect to the child. Every police force has an officer designated to enquire further into cases where the police power has been used. Once that officer has completed their enquiries, the child should be released from police protection unless there is evidence to suggest a continued risk of significant harm. The 72-hour period is considered sufficient time to decide what further action needs to be taken to protect the child from significant harm. The designated officer may allow parents contact with a child in police protection if they consider it to be in the child's best interests to do so.

Duty to investigate

The use of an emergency protection order or police power begins a process of continued investigation and assessment of the child's welfare. A local authority has a duty to make such enquiries as they consider necessary to enable them to decide whether to take further action to protect a child from harm or promote the welfare of a child (Children Act 1989, section 47). This duty arises when they are informed that a child in their area is the subject of an emergency protection order or police protection.

The local authority must also investigate when they have reasonable cause to suspect that a child is at risk of significant harm. A local authority must treat as serious any allegations of abuse raised with them by nurses or teachers. In *Re E (Children) (Care Proceedings: Social Work Practice)* [2000], a local authority applied for care orders in respect of three children who had been physically ill-treated and showed signs of emotional disturbance. Social services had originally supported the children, but despite warnings from teachers and without proper consideration of the file, had decided to take no further action because of the parents' failure to cooperate. The case had been reopened after another referral from a concerned school and an emergency protection order was made in respect of two of the children and care proceedings were commenced in respect of all the children. It was clear to the court that the children had been left to suffer in totally inadequate conditions for many years. They recommended that every case file should have, at the top or on the front, a chronology recording every significant event. Lack of parental cooperation should never be a reason to close a case, but should inspire closer investigation of the case. The court also stressed that nurses, health visitors and teachers were important sources of information and any referrals by them must be treated with utmost seriousness.

The need to ensure effective interagency working to protect children has now been placed on a statutory footing with the introduction of the Children Act 2004.

Children Act 2004

The aim of the government's strategy for reforming children's services (DH, 2003d) is to ensure that children have the support they need to:

- be safe;
- stay safe;
- enjoy and achieve through learning;
- make a positive contribution to society;
- achieve economic well-being.

The Children Act 2004 provides the legal framework for this reform and it acknowledges that children can only be properly safeguarded if key agencies work together effectively.

Local Safeguarding Children Boards (LSCBs) now oversee the way agencies work together to safeguard and promote the welfare of children (Children Act 2004, section 31).

The investigation of allegations of abuse and subsequent intervention with the child and their family are now conducted in accordance with the policies and procedures established by the LSCBs (HM Government, 2006).

The Children Act 1989 places a duty on health, education and other services to help the local authority to carry out its enquiries under the Children Act 1989, section 47. Professionals, including nurses, who participate in these enquiries are assisted in fulfilling their roles by guidance set out in *Working Together to Safeguard Children* (HM Government, 2006).

Enquiries should always be carried out in such a way as to minimise distress to the child, and to ensure that families are treated sensitively and with respect. This includes the need to explain the purpose and outcome of the enquiries to the parents and child, and being prepared to answer questions openly where this would not affect the safety and welfare of the child (HM Government, 2006).

In the great majority of cases, children remain with their families following an inquiry into an allegation of abuse even though concerns about abuse or neglect have been substantiated. By encouraging cooperation and respect between agencies and families under investigation, it is hoped that constructive working relationships with families will be developed.

Where families refuse to cooperate with the assessment of a child, a child assessment order under the provisions of the Children Act 1989, section 43, may be sought.

Child assessment orders

A child assessment order may be sought where a child's health, development or treatment is a cause for real concern, but where the child is not regarded by the local authority to be in need of urgent intervention. The order is used where repeated attempts to examine and assess the child have failed. Before granting the order the court must be satisfied that there is reasonable cause to suspect that the child is at risk of significant harm, and that an assessment to determine this is unlikely to be made without the order (Children Act 1989, section 43(1)). When granting the order the court will state the date on which the assessment will commence and the order will expire seven days from that date. The effect of the order is to require the child to be produced for assessment. Where a child is of sufficient understanding to make an informed decision, they may refuse to submit to a medical or psychiatric examination or other assessment. Where a nurse is involved in an assessment under this order it will be essential for them to record the consent or refusal of the child to submit to the assessment process.

A child subject to an assessment order may only be kept away from home if it is necessary for the purposes of the assessment and only for the period specified in the order. The child cannot be kept away from home for the convenience of those operating the assessment.

Once the assessment is completed the local authority will decide how to proceed following discussions with those who have been significantly involved in the enquiries, and this includes the child and the parents.

Where it is judged that a child may continue to be at risk of suffering significant harm, a child protection conference will be convened (HM Government, 2006).

The aim of this conference is to enable those professionals most involved with the child and family, and the family themselves, to assess all relevant information and plan how best to safeguard and promote the welfare of the child.

The initial child protection conference is responsible for agreeing an outline child protection plan (HM Government, 2006) aimed at:

- ensuring the child is safe and preventing them from suffering further harm;
- promoting the child's health and development;
- supporting the family and wider family members to safeguard and promote the welfare of the child.

Where there is concern that a child continues to suffer or is at risk of suffering significant harm, the local authority (or NSPCC) may apply to the court for a care or supervision order (Children Act 1989, section 31).

Care or supervision orders

Care or supervision orders are the only route into care and there is no way to avoid these proceedings. The courts cannot use their wardship jurisdiction to compel local authorities to look after children (Children Act 1989, section 100). Similarly, a residence order that settles where a child should live cannot be granted in favour of a local authority (Children Act 1989, section 9(2)).

A court cannot make a care order on its own motion. It has no power to force a local authority to take a child into care.

A court may make a care or supervision order if:

- the child is, or is likely to, suffer significant harm; and
- the harm is attributable either to unreasonable care (present or potential) or to the child being beyond parental control.

Once the court has established that the threshold criterion has been satisfied, it is able to make a care or supervision order under the Children Act 1989, section 31, if it is in the best interests of the child's welfare to do so.

To reach a decision about the welfare of the child, the court will scrutinise any plan that the local authority has for the care of the child should the order be granted. This must include plans for continued contact with the child's parents, unless the application for the order specifically requests that all contact should be curtailed (*Re T* [1994]).

Once the order is made, the court hands over the care of the child to the local authority and it no longer has supervision over the local authority's exercise of the care order (*S (Children) (Care Order: Implementation of Care Plan)* [2002]).

In care and supervision proceedings, the court is being asked to make a long-term order for the protection of the child. The effects of the two orders are different, even though the grounds for granting them are the same. The choice of order depends on the amount of intervention needed to ensure the safety of the child.

A supervision order

Under this order a child would be placed under the supervision of the local authority or a probation officer. That person's duty would be to befriend, advise, assist and supervise the child.

Parental responsibility is not granted to the local authority and the child cannot be removed from the family home. The court can impose a wide range of health-related requirements in a supervision order that authorise medical examination and assessment and, in some cases, treatment for the child. A supervision order initially runs for a year and may be extended up to a maximum of three years (Children Act 1989, section 35(1) and part 1 of schedule 3).

A care order

Under a care order a local authority receives a child into its care and takes control of their life. The authority gains parental responsibility for the child and, although parents do not lose their parental responsibility, the local authority can control how they exercise it in relation to their child (Children Act 1989, section 33(2)).

Once the order is made, the local authority controls the care of the child absolutely, free from court scrutiny. The care order will be carried out in accordance with the care plan agreed by the court and, where necessary, this can include removing the child from the family home immediately or at a later date, where a lack of cooperation or continued risk of significant harm makes this necessary. A care order, which generally cannot be made in respect of a child over 17, or 16 if married, is usually in force until the child is 18 or a court grants an application to have it removed.

Care orders provide for longer term intervention in a child's life, in order to promote the child's welfare and protect the child from significant harm.

Chapter summary

- The United Nations Convention on the Rights of the Child requires the government to have regard to the full spectrum of human rights for all children and to consider children in legislative and policy decisions.
- The Convention says that children have the right to be protected from abuse and the UK provides this protection through the Children Act 1989.
- Nurses have a key role in the identification of children who may have been abused or who are at risk of abuse.
- In the UK, available figures show that there are 32,100 children on child protection registers as being at risk of abuse.
- The Children Act 1989 enshrines the five key principles of holding the child's welfare as paramount: the welfare principle; keeping the family together; only intervening where it would make a significant contribution to the welfare of the child; avoiding delay; and unifying laws and procedures.
- The minimum requirement that has to be fulfilled before state intervention in a family's life is the risk of significant harm to the child.
- Protection for children in urgent need of intervention is provided by an emergency protection order under the Children Act 1989.
- A constable who believes a child is suffering significant harm may remove them to suitable accommodation or prevent their removal from hospital, or another place.
- A local authority has a duty to make enquiries to enable them to decide whether to take further action to protect a child from harm or promote the welfare of a child.
- In reforming children's services, the government aims to ensure that children are able to be safe, stay safe, enjoy and achieve through learning, make a positive contribution to society and achieve economic well-being.
- A child assessment order may be sought where a child's health, development or treatment is a cause for real concern, but where the child is not regarded by the local authority to be in need of urgent intervention.
- Care or supervision orders are the only route into care and there is no way for a local authority to avoid these proceedings.
- A supervision order places a child or family member under the supervision of the local authority or a probation officer.
- With a care order a local authority receives a child into its care and takes control of their life by gaining parental responsibility for the child and by controlling how parents exercise their own parental responsibility in relation to the child.

Further reading

A good introduction to the topic of safeguarding can be found in:

Watson, G and Rodwell, S (2014) *Safeguarding and Protecting Children, Young People and Families: A guide for nurses and midwives.* London: Sage (Learning Matters).

For a fuller understanding of the powers available under the Children Act 1989 and the support for children in need we recommend the Department of Health guidance below:

Department of Health (1997) *Children Act 1989: Guidance and regulations.* London: HMSO.

The emphasis on multi-agency working and safeguarding children boards is explained by:

Department of Health (2003) *Every Child Matters (Cm 5860).* London: The Stationery Office.

For Wales, advice is given in:

Welsh Assembly Government (2004) *Safeguarding Children: Working together under the Children Act 2004.* Cardiff: WAG.

Useful websites

The Scottish government provides a wide range of advice, information and downloadable publications on its website at: **www.scotland.gov.uk/Topics/People/Young-People**

The procedures and policy aims for England and a wide range of further information may be found at: **www.everychildmatters.co.uk**

The NSPCC website provides statistics on the extent of their work with children at: **www.nspcc.org.uk**

Chapter 10
Negligence

NMC Standards for Pre-registration Nursing Education

This chapter will address the following competencies:

Domain 1: Professional values

1. All nurses must practise with confidence according to *The Code: Professional standards of practice and behaviour for nurses and midwives* (NMC, 2015a), and within other recognised ethical and legal frameworks. They must be able to recognise and address ethical challenges relating to people's choices and decision-making about their care, and act within the law to help them and their families and carers find acceptable solutions.
5. All nurses must fully understand the nurse's various roles, responsibilities and functions, and adapt their practice proactively to meet changing needs of people, groups, communities and populations.
8. All nurses must practise independently, recognising the limits of their competence and knowledge. They must reflect on these limits and seek advice from, or refer to, other professionals where necessary.

Domain 3: Nursing practice and decision-making

6. All nurses must practise safely by being aware of the correct use, limitations and hazards of common interventions, including nursing activities, treatments, and the use of medical devices and equipment. The nurse must be able to evaluate their use, report any concerns promptly through appropriate channels and modify care where necessary to maintain safety. They must contribute to the collection of local and national data and formulation of policy on risks, hazards and adverse outcomes.
10. All nurses must evaluate their care to improve clinical decision-making, quality and outcomes, using a range of methods, amending the plan of care, where necessary, and communicating changes to others.

Chapter aims

By the end of this chapter you will be able to:

- explain the tort of negligence;
- describe the elements of a negligence action;
- outline the extent of a nurse's duty of care;
- identify situations where carelessness becomes a crime.

Introduction

This chapter considers how the law imposes a minimum standard on the care you provide to your patients through the negligence law. It begins by highlighting the harm that can be caused to patients by the carelessness of nurses and goes on to outline the legal obligation to take care when providing care and treatment to patients. Leading on from this, the chapter considers the extent of your duty of care and the role of the courts in determining the standard of care required of you. The chapter ends by considering negligence as a criminal rather than civil action, when you may face jail if your carelessness results in a patient's death.

Nurses in the course of their duties can make careless mistakes that result in harm to patients in their care. Such mistakes might not be intentional, but the resulting harm can have a profound effect on the life of the patient. To discourage such carelessness and to provide a remedy for those harmed by the mistakes of others, the law imposes a standard of care on nurses that requires them to be careful when caring for patients.

Failing to meet that standard and harming a patient means that the nurse will be accountable for carelessness through the law of negligence.

Claims for compensation as a result of negligence in the NHS increased by 10.8 per cent in 2012/13. In 2012/13 the National Health Service Litigation Authority (NHS LA) received 10,129 claims for clinical negligence and 4,632 claims for non-clinical negligence against NHS bodies in England. About £1.309 billion was paid out in connection with clinical negligence claims in 2012/13, up from £863 million in 2011/12. The NHS LA estimates that it has further potential liabilities of over £22 billion (NHS LA, 2013).

For the nurse concerned it is undoubtedly a frightening prospect to face a negligence claim. As well as any damages that may be awarded, the nurse faces having their professional integrity and good name challenged in court and the prospect of further action being taken against them by their employer and regulatory body.

Negligence

Where a nurse acts in a careless way and causes an injury to another person, such as a patient, that careless nurse will be liable in negligence for any resulting harm.

Negligence may be defined as an omission to do something a reasonable man *[sic]* would do or to do something a prudent and reasonable man would not do (*Blyth v Birmingham Waterworks* [1856]).

Case study 10.1: Nurse's carelessness causes harm

A 13-year-old girl with Crohn's disease underwent a colectomy as her symptoms were not being controlled. After surgery she returned to the ward lying on her left side and was not turned nor had her position changed by the nurses caring for her until the following morning. She had remained in the same position for some 16 hours and when she tried to stand up found her left leg felt numb and weak and she had difficulty walking.

A lesion of the sciatic nerve had occurred with total interruption of the nerve supply to the skin and muscle of the leg. This serious and permanent injury causes pain and discomfort in the whole of the left leg and altered sensation in the foot and outer side of the leg. She can walk for only 5 minutes before needing a rest and cannot participate in any of the physical activities most young people take for granted. She has missed over two years of schooling and college because of the injury.

She argued that her injury was due to pressure palsy of the sciatic nerve resulting directly from the negligent failure of nursing staff to change her position over a 16-hour period.

The hospital trust settled the case for £400,000.

A person can claim for damages as a result of loss or harm they have suffered following a nurse's carelessness. Negligence is therefore best defined as actionable harm. If your act or omission causes harm, you could be liable for the civil wrong – known in law as a tort – of negligence. If no harm occurs as a result of the negligent act, a patient cannot bring an action against the nurse.

Activity 10.1 — *Reflection*

The scope of accountability in nursing

Imagine you have administered the wrong drug to a patient in your care. Fortunately, no harm was done.

- Can you still be held accountable for your actions?
- Who can hold you to account and why?
- What sanctions can be imposed on you?

When answering this question, consider the four spheres of accountability discussed in Chapter 3 (see page 47).

An outline answer is given at the end of the chapter.

Negligence as a tort has been developed in English law under the common law provisions. These are a series of judicial decisions and precedents that have the authority of tests that need to be satisfied if a case is to be successful. A tort is derived from the Norman French word meaning 'wrong' and is now legally defined as a civil wrong. If a member of the public, such as a patient, feels that a tort has been committed against them, they might seek redress from the court. In order to establish negligence in law, three conditions must be met:

- the person who is considered at fault for the negligence, such as the nurse, must owe the patient a duty of care;
- that duty of care must have been breached; this means that the nurse responsible fell below the standard of care expected of them;
- as a result of that breach in the standard of care, harm was caused to the patient.

All three conditions must be satisfied in order to establish liability in the law of negligence.

Duty of care

The first condition to be satisfied in a case of negligence is whether there is a duty of care owed to the individual patient. The tort of negligence does not impose a general duty to act carefully towards everyone. Instead, it lays down standards for particular circumstances and, if someone fails to reach those standards and damage is caused, that is negligence.

These situations are called 'duty situations' and the nature of the relationship gives rise to a duty of care. The courts have also described this duty as a duty to take care or a duty to be careful (*Bolitho v City and Hackney HA* [1998]). That is, there is a legal obligation to ensure that your acts or omissions do not cause harm to the person to whom you owe the duty.

The courts usually rely on previous cases – precedents – to guide them as to when a duty of care arises, and it is well established that the relationship between a health professional and a patient is one that gives rise to a duty of care (*Kent v Griffiths and Others* [2000]).

Your duty of care to the patient arises once you undertake the care and treatment of the patient and therefore assume responsibility for the acts and omissions that make up the nursing interventions you provide (Nathan, 1957).

In novel situations where there is no previous case to follow and it is less clear about whether a duty of care is owed, the court has established a three-stage test.

In *Caparo Industries Plc v Dickman* [1992], the House of Lords provided guidance for establishing a duty of care in novel circumstances. The court held that a duty of care will arise if the following criteria are satisfied.

- **It was reasonably foreseeable that someone would be harmed by a careless act or omission.**

The test is based on the reasonable foreseeability of harm. That is, would a reasonable person have foreseen that harm would have been caused by the act or omission in question? For example, in *Roe v Ministry of Health* [1954], a man was paralysed when a local anaesthetic was contaminated by a strong disinfectant due to microscopic cracks in the ampoule. The court held that the harm was not foreseeable as the situation was new and a reasonable person would not have foreseen it.

- **It is shown that there is a legal proximity between the parties.**

The need for a close or proximate relationship with the person harmed was established in *Donoghue v Stevenson* [1932], where a woman claimed damages after drinking ginger beer from a bottle that was contaminated by a decomposing snail. The manufacturer argued that, as there was no contract with Mrs Donoghue, who had not bought the drink, there was no duty of care. However, the court held that in law we owe a duty of care to our *neighbours*, whom the court described as

> *persons who are so closely and directly affected by my act or omission that I ought reasonably to have them in contemplation as being so affected when I am directing my mind to the acts or omissions in question.*

- That is, there is a relationship that gives rise to a duty of care – in this case between the manufacturer and consumer of a product. It also includes the nurse–patient relationship. Once you undertake the care and treatment of a patient, the relationship gives rise to a duty of care and continues until that relationship ends. For example, a capable adult patient can absolve you of your duty by refusing the treatment you offer to provide. **It is just and reasonable to impose a duty of care in these circumstances.**
- There are some circumstances where the courts believe that imposing a duty is not just and reasonable and so no duty of care arises. For example, in *JD v East Berkshire Community Health NHS Trust* [2003], parents who had unfounded allegations of child abuse made against them sued the trust for damages due to psychiatric harm. The court held that it was not just and reasonable to impose a duty in these circumstances as the nurse's paramount concern was the child, and if the nurse had suspicions they must be able to report it without having to worry about being sued by parents.

Activity 10.2 *Critical thinking*

Who in law is my neighbour?

While on duty on a ward, you accidentally spill some water in the main corridor. The wet floor is not clearly visible. To whom will you owe a duty of care in this situation? Answer this question by focusing on the neighbour principle.

An outline answer is given at the end of the chapter.

All three elements for establishing a duty of care will not always be separately identifiable. They may overlap or include other factors in some cases. They act as a guide to enable the court to decide whether a duty is owed. Similarly, you ought to take into account these factors when deciding whether you are in a duty situation.

Case study 10.2: A duty of care

In Kent v Griffiths and Others *[2000], a woman and her newborn baby suffered harm as a result of an ambulance taking some 30 minutes to arrive to take her to hospital instead of the promised 9 minutes. The ambulance service argued that they did not owe the patient a duty of care as they were an emergency service that provided a service to the public, not to individual patients.*

The court held that the ambulance service was part of the health service and owed a duty of care to the patient, as it was reasonably foreseeable that harm would be caused if they acted in a careless way. And, as they knew the name and address of the patient, they had a legal proximity in the same way as other health professionals had with their patients and it was, therefore, just and reasonable to impose a duty of care on the ambulance service towards their patients. By taking so long to arrive without reasonable excuse was careless and a breach of that duty of care.

The scope of the duty of care

The scope of the duty of care owed by a nurse to a patient is very wide and covers every facet of your involvement with the patient. Lord Diplock, in *Sidaway v Bethlem Royal Hospital* [1985], described it as a single comprehensive duty covering all the ways in which a nurse is called on to exercise their skill and judgement in the improvement of the physical and mental condition of the patient. The scope of your duty of care has already been found to include:

- the care given to your patients;
- giving advice to your patient or to another about the patient;
- explaining risks inherent in a procedure to patients;
- the standard of your handwriting when giving instructions regarding a patient;
- the standard of your record keeping in terms of legibility and content;
- the timing of a decision to act;
- seeking the assistance of others;
- failing to recognise the limits of your competence;
- failing to report substandard care.

Breach in the standard of care

Once it is established that the defendant owed a duty of care to the claimant, the second question is whether that duty was breached. That is, did the standard of care fall below that required by law?

Generally, the standard of care is based on the 'reasonable man' test. As cited earlier, in *Blyth v Birmingham Waterworks Co* [1856], it was held that negligence is the omission to do something a reasonable man would do or do something a prudent and reasonable man would not do. Both what you do and what you fail to do can be equally culpable when establishing negligence.

Case study 10.3: Negligence by omission

A man fell down the stairs leading to his flat upon returning home from a night out. He was found by a neighbour two hours later, slumped in vomit and unable to say anything intelligible. When he arrived at hospital he was resuscitated and a CT scan arranged but for various reasons, including a cancellation of the original booking, the scan was performed more than six hours later. The scan showed an acute subdural haematoma requiring urgent neurosurgery. A transfer to a different hospital was immediately arranged, but the ambulance did not arrive for another 4 hours. He was left with permanent cognitive and neuropsychological impairment, which prevented him from working.

The court found that both periods of delay had been negligent and awarded £454,858.65 in compensation.

John v Central Manchester and Manchester Children's University Hospitals NHS Foundation Trust *[2016] 4 W.L.R. 54*

In *Hall v Brooklands Auto Racing Club* [1933], the characteristics of a reasonable man were described by the court:

> *A reasonable man is sometimes described as the man in the street or the man on the Clapham omnibus or … the man who takes the magazines at home and in the evening pushes the lawn mower in his shirt sleeves.*
> (Lord Justice Greer at 244)

Activity 10.3 — *Critical thinking*

The reasonable man

What do you think the judge was trying to say about the standard of care generally required at law in his description of the reasonable man?

Now read the following paragraph for the answer.

By describing the reasonable man in this way Lord Justice Greer was emphasising that the standard of care generally expected in law is that of the ordinary or average person in that situation. That is, what would an ordinary person have done in the same circumstances?

For example, a reasonable person would know what adults learn from experience – that rivers are dangerous, that fires burn, etc. They would also take extra care if they knew that a person had a particular sensitivity, such as an allergy, or that a woman was pregnant. The reasonable person would also take greater precautions where the likelihood of harm was serious and would not ignore even a small risk if it could be avoided simply.

Case study 10.4: The reasonable man and the cricket ball

In Bolton v Stone *[1951], a woman was struck by a cricket ball when standing on a road some way from a cricket match. The court held that the cricketer had not been negligent, as a reasonable man would not have foreseen that such an exceptional cricket stroke would have not only travelled so far but then gone on to hit a pedestrian on a quiet country road.*

However, Lord Reid pointed out that he would have reached a different conclusion if he had thought that the risk had been other than extremely small, because a reasonable man considering the matter of safety would not disregard any risk unless it was extremely small.

Judging the skilled person

Where the person considered to be at fault for a negligent act or omission is a professional, skilled person, the law modifies the reasonable man test to take account of the skill involved. In *Bolam v Friern HMC* [1957], the court established that:

> *The test is that of the ordinary skilled person exercising and professing to have that special skill.*
>
> *A professional need not possess the highest expert skill as it is well established in law that it is sufficient if they exercise the ordinary skill of an ordinary competent professional exercising that particular skill or art.*

The test is well established in healthcare law and is known as the *Bolam* test. In *Bolitho v City & Hackney HA* [1998], the House of Lords described the *Bolam* test as the *locus classicus* (the traditional basis) of the test for the standard of care required of a doctor or any other person professing some skill or competence.

The test applies to any profession, including the nursing profession, and it was made clear in *Gold v Haringey HA* [1987] that

> *[n]o matter what profession it may be, the common law does not impose on those who practise it any liability for damage resulting from what in the result turned out to have been errors of judgment, unless the error was such as no reasonably well-informed and competent member of that profession could have made.*

The standard of care will, therefore, be determined by what a responsible body of professional opinion would have done in the same situation. In nursing practice the standard of care will be determined by what a responsible body of nursing opinion would have done in the same situation.

This approach allows for different schools of thought within a profession. As long as the practice conforms to a standard accepted by a responsible body of opinion, it meets the standard required in law.

Case study 10.5: Is there a best standard?

In Maynard v West Midlands RHA *[1984], two consultants treating a patient for a chest complaint thought she was suffering from tuberculosis, but also considered that she might be suffering from Hodgkin's disease. Before obtaining the result of a tuberculosis test, they performed an exploratory operation to see if she was suffering from Hodgkin's disease. It showed that she had tuberculosis, but the patient suffered damage to a nerve affecting her vocal cords, which caused a speech impairment – an inherent risk of the operation.*

The patient sued, claiming that the consultants had been negligent in deciding to carry out the operation before obtaining the result of the tuberculosis test, which would have taken seven weeks.

Expert medical evidence was called on both sides concerning whether the operation should have been carried out. The judge preferred the patient's expert evidence, which said the consultants should have waited, and awarded damages against the hospital.

On appeal, the House of Lords held that it was not sufficient to show that there was a body of competent opinion, which considered that a decision was wrong, if there also existed a body of professional opinion, equally competent, which supported the decision as being reasonable in the circumstances.

It had to be recognised that differences of opinion and practice existed in the health professions and therefore, although the court might prefer one body of opinion to the other, it was not a basis for a conclusion that there had been negligence.

The *Bolam* test imposes a higher standard of care on health professionals than is generally required when using the reasonable man test. The law requires a person professing to have a particular skill or art to exercise to the standard of the ordinary professional skilled to that level. Two important qualifications of the standard emerge from this principle.

First, the more a professional puts themselves forward as an expert, the higher is the standard expected of them. It is the post, not the person, that carries the duty. A ward sister is putting herself forward as a person with greater skill than a more junior grade member of the nursing staff. The law expects a higher standard of care from the ward sister than from her junior colleagues.

Case study 10.6: Higher standard when putting yourself forward as an expert

In Smith v Brighton and Lewes Hospital Management Committee *[1958], a woman lost her balance due to damage to a cranial nerve caused by receiving four injections of streptomycin above 30 prescribed by the doctor. Junior nurses had given the injections, but it was the ward sister who was held liable for negligence as it was found to be her role, as a person in a position of greater competence and expertise, to ensure that the stop date for the treatment was clearly marked on the medication administration chart.*

Second, the requirement to perform to the standard of the ordinary person exercising that skill means that there is a minimum level of competence below which no person can fall. Inexperience is, therefore, no defence to an allegation of negligence. If you profess to have a particular skill, you must perform to the standard of the ordinary nurse.

Case study 10.7: The standard of the average road user

In Nettleship v Weston *[1971], a learner driver was given lessons by an instructor who made sure the car was properly insured. Weston was a careful learner, but on the third lesson she failed to straighten out after turning left and struck a lamp standard, breaking Nettleship's kneecap.*

The court held that a learner driver owes a duty to their instructor to drive with proper skill and care, the test being that of the ordinary careful driver. It was no defence to say they were a learner doing their best. The duty of care owed by a learner driver was the same as that owed by every driver, and Weston was liable for damages.

An important way of ensuring that you do not carelessly harm a patient by practising beyond your competence is to acknowledge the limitations of your practice and seek more senior assistance. This will ensure that you benefit from the help and advice of that colleague. It will also demonstrate that you have discharged your duty of care towards your patient.

Should any harm now occur, it will be the senior professional who will be held liable for negligence, as they are putting themselves forward as an expert and a higher standard of care is expected of them. For example, in *Wilsher v Essex HA* [1988], a baby was born prematurely and was placed in a special baby care unit. The baby needed oxygen and the junior doctor inserting the catheter to measure blood gases was inexperienced and asked a senior colleague, a senior registrar, to check the catheter. The catheter was wrongly inserted into an umbilical vein instead of an artery and the baby was supersaturated with oxygen. He developed retrolental fibroplasia, which resulted in blindness. The court held that, as the junior doctor had asked a more senior doctor to check his work, he had discharged his duty of care to the senior doctor and could not be liable in negligence.

Activity 10.4 — *Critical thinking*

Unsure what to do?

What action would you take if you were unsure of how to carry out a nursing intervention on a patient in your care?

An outline answer is given at the end of the chapter.

Emergencies

One exception to the principle that a nurse will be judged according to the standard of reasonably experienced nurses in their field is provided by emergency treatment.

In relation to treatment decisions taken in an emergency, a nurse will not be found negligent simply because the reasonably competent nurse would have made a different decision, given more time and information.

In *Wilson v Swanson* [1956], the Supreme Court of Canada held that there was no negligence when a health professional had to make an immediate decision whether to treat, when the treatment was subsequently found to have been unnecessary.

Moreover, the standard of skill itself required in the execution of treatment may be somewhat lower. As Lord Justice Mustill commented in *Wilsher v Essex HA* [1988]:

> *An emergency may overburden the available resources, and, if an individual is forced by circumstances to do too many things at once, the fact that he does one of them incorrectly should not lightly be taken as negligence.*

The role of the courts in determining the standard of care

Generally, the courts are content to allow the profession to set the standard of care for a particular treatment or intervention. The essence of the *Bolam* test is that you act in accordance with a practice accepted by a responsible body of professional opinion. However, the court is the final arbiter of the professional standard of care and, although it must accept that there are different schools of thought about how to best provide treatment within a profession, it can reject a standard where it does not consider that the standard stands up to logical analysis (*Bolitho v City and Hackney HA* [1998]).

Activity 10.5 *Critical thinking*

Does the evidence stand up to logical analysis?

In *Hucks v Cole* [1968], Mrs Hucks was expecting her third child when she noticed a septic spot on her finger. She gave birth three days later in hospital and the following day a nurse noticed the spot and another one on her toe. The doctor prescribed a five-day course of tetracycline and sent a swab to pathology.

The pathologist's report stated that the bacteria was resistant to tetracycline but the doctor decided to stick to the five-day course he had prescribed.

Mrs Hucks was discharged at the end of the five days despite the septic spots not having healed and later developed fulminating septicaemia and was seriously ill.

At the trial, evidence was given by other doctors that they would not have changed the prescribed treatment.

Do you think that the doctor's actions stand up to logical analysis?

Now read below for the answer.

In the *Hucks v Cole* [1968] case, the judge held that, despite the evidence of the doctors, no reasonable doctor would have allowed a patient to continue with a course of treatment when they knew it to be ineffective. The standard of care suggested by the doctors did not stand up to logical analysis and would be rejected.

This was later approved by the House of Lords in *Bolitho v City and Hackney HA* [1998], when they held that

> *[where], in a rare case, it can be demonstrated that the professional opinion is not capable of withstanding logical analysis, the judge is entitled to hold that the body of opinion is not reasonable or responsible.*
> (Lord Browne-Wilkinson at 240)

It is essential, therefore, that you base your practice on sound evidence and research. You will not be exonerated because others too are negligent or common professional practice is slack (*Reynolds v North Tyneside HA* [2002]). You must keep your practice up to date and inform your practice by reference to improvements and amendments introduced through changes in the law.

Guidance on best practice and standard of care

To improve care standards, NHS trusts have policies and procedures to inform best practice. These are supplemented by guidance from bodies such as the National Institute for Health and Care Excellence (NICE), and professional organisations such as the Royal College of Nursing (RCN). Nurses are able to use these to inform their practice. For example, in *Sutton v Population Services Family Planning Programme* [1981], a nurse was found to be negligent when she failed to follow the correct procedure for referring a patient with a lump in her breast to a doctor.

However, the value of such guidance is only as good as the evidence upon which it is based. If it is not based on sound research, the court may reject it as not standing up to logical analysis.

Case study 10.8: Logical analysis

In Reynolds v North Tyneside HA *[2002], a woman who was admitted in labour was not given a vaginal examination for some six hours, at which point a prolapsed cord was discovered and an emergency caesarean was carried out. The child suffered cerebral palsy and sued. The hospital argued that its policy did not require the immediate vaginal examination of the woman; however, the pre-eminent textbook of the day suggested that such an examination was necessary where a woman was in labour.*

The court held that the hospital policy was not based on sound research evidence and did not stand up to logical analysis, and that there had been a breach in the standard of care causing harm to the child. The hospital was therefore negligent.

Causation: the breach in the standard of care caused harm

Once it is established that, due to the carelessness of the nurse, the standard of care required in law has been breached, it is necessary to consider what effect this had on the patient. This stage is known as 'causation' or the 'causal link'. It must be established that the breach in the standard of care caused the harm.

It is generally for the person who has suffered the wrong (the claimant) to prove causation. The claimant must prove on the balance of probabilities that care fell below the standard of a reasonably competent person and caused the harm. There is a distinction between causation in fact and causation in law.

Causation in fact is based on the 'but for test'. That is, but for your carelessness the patient would not have suffered harm.

Case study 10.9: A case of too much arsenic

In Barnett v Chelsea and Kensington Hospital Management Committee *[1969], a night watchman was taken to a cottage hospital complaining of stomach pain. The doctor had flu and told the nurse to ask the patient to go and see his GP. The patient subsequently died of arsenic poisoning before seeing his GP.*

The court decided that the doctor who had refused to see the man had acted irresponsibly, but was not negligent, as the doctor's actions did not contribute to the death of the night watchman. He had ingested so much arsenic that he would have died even if the doctor had seen him.

Causation in law requires the court to determine whether the defendant is liable as a matter of law. This is determined by the principle that the defendant will not be held liable in law if the damage is too remote from the original negligent act. For example, in *French v Chief Constable of Sussex* [2006], a police officer claimed damages for psychiatric harm caused when a fatal shooting occurred during an armed robbery. The officer argued that it was his employer's negligent handling of the robbery that had resulted in the fatal shooting and caused him psychiatric harm. The court rejected his claim, holding that, as he did not witness the shooting, the harm he suffered was too remote from the incident and was not reasonably foreseeable.

Res ipsa loquitur

While it is generally for the complainant to prove that a breach in the standard of care caused them harm, there is a principle that allows the burden of proof to shift in certain circumstances.

The principle of *res ipsa loquitur*, or 'the thing speaks for itself', applies when three key conditions are present. That is:

- there is no explanation for the accident;
- harm does not normally happen if care is taken; and
- the instrument causing the accident is in the defendant's control.

The principle, when it applies, requires the respondent to show that they did not act negligently by shifting the burden of proof from the complainant to the respondent.

Case study 10.10: *Res ipsa loquitur*

In Saunders v Leeds Western HA *[1993], an otherwise healthy four-year-old boy suffered a cardiac arrest and brain damage during a routine arthroplasty operation. The theatre team argued that his heart stopped abruptly without warning; however, expert evidence argued that an otherwise healthy child's heart does not simply stop. The judge held that the principle of* res ipsa loquitur *applied, as there was no reasonable explanation for the incident, expert evidence had shown that harm does not normally happen if care is taken and the instruments that caused the incident were under the control of the hospital. As the theatre could offer no other explanation for what had occurred, the judge found them negligent.*

Negligence as a crime

Negligence is generally associated with the civil law. It is the law's way of imposing a standard of care on professionals such as nurses, and it provides redress by way of compensation for those harmed by another's careless act or omission.

In extreme cases the negligent act of a nurse can cause the death of a patient. The nurse may then be liable to prosecution for manslaughter as a result of their gross negligence. In *R v Bateman* [1925], the court decided that gross negligence occurs when someone shows such disregard for the life and safety of other persons as to constitute a crime worthy of punishment. In healthcare the issue of gross negligence arose in *R v Misra & Srivastava* [2004], where two doctors were found guilty of gross negligence when they failed to heed the warnings of nurses that a patient was seriously ill. The patient subsequently died of toxic shock. The judge held that

> *[a] health professional would be told that grossly negligent treatment which exposed a patient to the risk of death, and caused it, would constitute manslaughter.*

This was the case in *R v Adomako* [1995], where the defendant, an anaesthetist, failed to notice for four minutes that an endotracheal tube had become disconnected during an operation. Although an alarm sounded, the tube was not checked until the patient suffered a cardiac arrest. An expert witness for the prosecution stated that a competent anaesthetist should have spotted the problem within 15 seconds. The House of Lords held that gross negligence would occur where a patient dies as the result of:

- a health professional displaying an indifference to an obvious risk of injury to the patient;
- a health professional being aware of the risk of injury to the patient but deciding to run the risk;
- a health professional's attempt to avoid a known risk was so grossly negligent that it deserves to be punished;
- a health professional displays inattention or a failure to avert a severe risk.

Based on these tests, a nurse could be convicted of manslaughter if the act or omission exposes the patient to the risk of death and subsequently causes the patient's death.

Where a nurse is found guilty of such an offence, they are likely to receive a custodial sentence.

Case study 10.11: Nurse's gross negligence

A nurse was found guilty of the gross negligence manslaughter of a six-year-old boy admitted to hospital with sickness and diarrhoea. The jury accepted that in failing to recognise his condition, she took no account of the important fact that he was struggling for oxygen; did not recognise that he was already in shock; failed to monitor his condition; and because of that delayed the start of effective treatment. Her care of the child was so exceptionally bad it amounted to a criminal offence. The child died 11 hours after he was admitted to hospital.

The nurse was sentenced to two years in prison suspended for two years.

(R v Amaro *[2015] (Nottingham Crown Court, 2 November))*

Accountability

As a registered nurse, you are not only accountable to the patient through the law of negligence. As shown in Chapter 3, you are also accountable to your employer through contract and to the NMC through the Nursing and Midwifery Order 2001. Even if you show that your carelessness did not cause harm, you are likely to face investigation by your employer and the NMC.

Under contract law, your employer will pay any damages for liability in negligence through the principle of vicarious liability. This requires that an employer is liable for the negligent acts or omissions of their employee in the course of their employment. The liability arises whether or not such an act or omission was specifically authorised by the employer.

In return for this protection, employers expect their employees to carry out their duties with due care and skill. They can hold you to account through reasonable disciplinary measures, which could include dismissal, if an investigation reveals misconduct.

Under the terms of your contract of employment, you owe your employer a duty of care and undertake to work with due skill and diligence. If you breach that duty by being negligent, it is open to the employer to sue you for the compensation they have had to pay to a patient (*Lister v Romford Ice and Cold Storage Co Ltd* [1957]).

It is essential, therefore, that you carry indemnity insurance to cover you for any damages for which you are personally liable. Currently, the easiest way of obtaining such insurance is to join a professional organisation such as the RCN or Unison.

The European directive on patient rights in cross-border healthcare (Council and Parliament Directive 2011/24/EU) sets out a set of shared operating principles for healthcare systems throughout the European Union (EU) to ensure patient trust in cross-border healthcare and so promote the free movement of people in the EU. These shared principles require the harmonisation of patients' rights throughout the European Union to guarantee a high degree of health protection.

The cross-border healthcare directive requires that member states:

- have national contact points that supply patients with standards and guidelines on quality and safety in healthcare, the regulation of registered health professionals and hospital accessibility for the disabled;
- have information on charges for health services;
- ensure access to health services is free from discrimination based on nationality;
- have in place a transparent complaints procedure;
- uphold the right to privacy with respect to personal data and health records;
- put in place a system of professional indemnity insurance or similar arrangement.

(Directive 2011/24/EU, article 4)

Health providers and individual health professionals, including nurses, are required to have in place professional indemnity insurance or a similar system of indemnity. The requirement will mean that a registered nurse will not be allowed to practise unless they have professional indemnity. The majority of nurses work for the NHS or private care providers and their employer is vicariously liable for any compensation awarded in a negligence action.

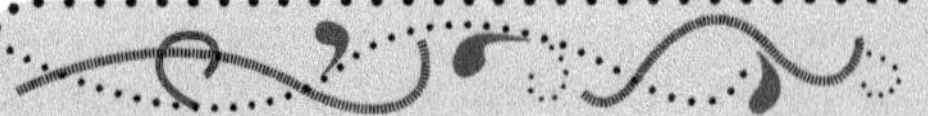

Chapter summary

- Although being sued for negligence is a rare event in nursing, increasing litigation is a real trend in healthcare with the current NHS liability bill exceeding £4 billion.
- Where a nurse acts in a careless way and causes an injury to another person, such as a patient, that careless nurse will be liable in negligence for any resulting harm.
- Negligence is best defined as actionable harm.
- In order to establish negligence in law, three conditions must be met: the nurse must owe the patient a duty of care; that duty of care must be breached; and, as a result, harm was caused to the patient.

continued . . .

- The relationship between a nurse and a patient is one that gives rise to a duty of care.
- This duty covers all the ways in which a nurse is called upon to exercise their skill and judgement in the improvement of the physical and mental condition of the patient.
- As a skilled professional you are expected to carry out your duties to the standard of the ordinary skilled person exercising and professing to have that special skill.
- The standard of care is determined by what a responsible body of professional opinion would have done in the same situation.
- The more a nurse puts themselves forward as an expert, the higher the standard expected of them.
- Inexperience is no defence to an allegation of negligence.
- The court can reject a professional standard where it does not consider that the standard stands up to logical analysis.
- The principle of *res ipsa loquitur* applies when there is no explanation for the accident, where harm does not normally happen if care is taken and where the instrument causing the accident is in the defendant's control.
- Grossly negligent treatment that exposes a patient to the risk of death, and causes it, constitutes manslaughter.
- For registered nurses, liability may extend to other spheres of accountability and may draw sanctions from the employer and the regulatory body.
- It is essential that you carry indemnity insurance to cover you for any damages for which you are personally liable.

Activities: Brief outline answers

Activity 10.1: Reflection (page 221)

You can still be held to account for your actions as there are four spheres of accountability generally attributed to a registered nurse.

Although the patient cannot sue for negligence as no harm occurred, you are still accountable to:

- society through the public law where you may face criminal prosecution;
- the employer through contract law for misconduct;
- the profession through the Nursing and Midwifery Order 2001 for professional misconduct.

Activity 10.2: Critical thinking (page 223)

The courts have held that in law you owe a duty of care to your neighbours who the court describe as:

- persons who are so closely and directly affected by your act or omission that you ought reasonably to have them in contemplation as being so affected when directing your mind to the acts or omissions in question.

In the case of an accidental spill, you would therefore owe a duty to those persons walking along that corridor because it is reasonably foreseeable that they could be harmed if they slipped on that water.

Activity 10.4: Critical thinking (page 228)

Given the decision in *Wilsher v Essex Health Authority* [1988] you would be well advised to seek the supervision of a more senior colleague. Should any harm now occur, it would be the senior professional who would be held liable for negligence as they have put themselves out as an expert and a higher standard of care would be expected of them.

Further reading

To appreciate the courts' approach to the standard imposed by a duty of care it is well worth reading the House of Lords' opinion in:

Bolitho v City and Hackney HA [1998] AC 232, which can be downloaded from **www.bailii. org/uk/cases/UKHL/1997/46.html**

A very interesting document by the Department of Health that strives to get health professionals to learn from the mistakes of others is well worth student nurses reading for its case studies and cautionary tales:

Department of Health (2003) *An Organisation with a Memory*. London: DH.

Useful websites

To keep up to date with negligence cases affecting health professionals, we recommend the following websites:

The British and Irish Legal Information Institute: **www.bailii.org**

The National Health Service Litigation Authority: **www.nhsla.com**

Chapter 11
Record keeping

NMC Standards for Pre-registration Nursing Education

This chapter will address the following competencies:

Domain 1: Professional values

1. All nurses must practise with confidence according to *The Code: Professional standards of practice and behaviour for nurses and midwives* (NMC, 2015a), and within other recognised ethical and legal frameworks. They must be able to recognise and address ethical challenges relating to people's choices and decision-making about their care, and act within the law to help them and their families and carers find acceptable solutions.

Domain 2: Communication and interpersonal skills

7. All nurses must maintain accurate, clear and complete records, including the use of electronic formats, using appropriate and plain language.
10. All nurses must keep information secure and confidential in accordance with the law and ethical and regulatory frameworks, taking account of local protocols.

Chapter aims

By the end of this chapter you will be able to:

- define a health record;
- outline the two purposes of a health record;
- describe what must be included in a record entry;
- discuss the elements of good record keeping;
- consider the role of audit in raising the standard of record keeping;
- compare and contrast the right of access to records of patients who are living with access to the records of patients who have died.

Introduction

In this chapter the importance of accurate record keeping to the safety of patients and protection of nurses is considered. The legal implications of records are explained and how you should write records to ensure that these legal requirements are met. By drawing on case law the chapter continues by highlighting the consequences for nurses of failing to meet those requirements.

Record keeping is a crucial aspect of a nurse's duty. It remains an instance where failing in this duty can lead to your name being removed from the professional register.

Case study 11.1: Struck off for failing to keep adequate records

A nurse manager was struck off by the NMC for poor record keeping when a conduct and competence committee found her fitness to practise impaired because she had:

- *Failed to ensure that the staff rota adequately met service users' needs.*
- *Failed to ensure that there was always a senior member of staff on duty.*
- *Failed to ensure adequate records were kept in staff files, in that some contained:*
    - *inadequate staff training records*
    - *inadequate Criminal Records Bureau checks*
    - *inadequate proofs of identification*
    - *incomplete and insufficient employment references.*
- *Failed to ensure adequate records were kept of service users, in that they contained insufficient information of:*
    - *dietary needs*
    - *historical backgrounds*
    - *risk assessments*
    - *weight charts*
    - *activity needs.*
- *Failed to ensure adequate records were kept of service users, in that the accident books were inadequately completed.*
  (NMC, 2011b)

What is a health record?

A health record is any electronic or paper information recorded about a person for the purpose of managing their healthcare (Data Protection Act 1998, section 68(1)(a)). Health records include a variety of patient records that are held or filed within a hospital practice, not just the main doctor's record. They include nursing records, health visiting records, X-rays, pathology reports, outpatients' reports, pharmacy records, etc. Together they form a record of the care and treatment a patient has received.

Activity 11.1 — *Reflection*

Purpose of record keeping

Why do you believe the NMC regards record keeping as such an important nursing duty? Write down what you consider to be the purpose of keeping nursing records.

Now read below for further information.

The purpose of record keeping

The primary purpose of keeping records is to have an account of the care and treatment given to a patient. This allows progress to be monitored and a clinical history to be developed. The clinical record allows for continuity of care by facilitating treatment and support. It is an integral part of care that is every bit as important as the direct care provided to patients.

As well as their clinical function, records have a very important legal purpose. Records provide evidence of your involvement with a patient. Therefore, they need to be sufficiently detailed to demonstrate this involvement.

Case study 11.2: The legal function of records

In Saunders v Leeds Western HA *[1993], a fit four-year-old child suffered cardiac arrest and brain damage during an arthroplasty operation. The theatre team argued that the patient's pulse had simply stopped abruptly. This was rejected by the court. As there was no evidence in the records of a sequence of events leading to the pulse stopping the court found the health authority liable in negligence.*

Remember that the standard of proof in civil cases is the balance of probability. That is, if the weight of evidence is 51 per cent in your favour the case is won. As a nurse's contact with patients is mainly on a one-to-one basis, records made at the time of, or soon after, seeing a patient often provides the necessary evidence to tip the evidence in your favour. For example, in *McLennan v Newcastle HA* [1992], a patient claimed she had not been told of the relatively high risk associated with her operation. The surgeon, however, had written in the notes at the time that the risks were explained and understood by the patient. This contemporaneous record persuaded the judge that the patient had probably been told about the risks and the case failed.

Legal implications of records

The Data Protection Act 1998 defines a health record very widely. In litigation that definition becomes wider still. The discovery process of a case allows any material document to be used as evidence. Any document that records any aspect of the care of a patient can be required as evidence before a court of law or before any of the regulatory bodies. There is no restriction on access to these documents. The rules of the court demand that all documents are produced (Rules of the Supreme Court Order 24). It is important, therefore, that nurses do not view record keeping as a mechanistic process. What you write does matter. In litigation the outcome is not based on truth but proof. If it is not in the notes it can be difficult to prove it happened. Cases are won and lost on the strength of records. The secret of success in court is preparation, so winning in court could be said to be:

- 96 per cent preparation;
- 2 per cent luck;
- 2 per cent law.

Next time you write in notes, remember that you may be relying on them as evidence in court. They are of little value to you if they do not contain the information necessary to demonstrate that you have discharged your duty of care to the patient with professional skill and diligence. Records are never neutral; they will either support or condemn you.

Activity 11.2 *Communication*

What should be recorded by nurses?

Write down the information you feel needs to be included in a patient's nursing record.

Now read below for further information.

What to include

Records need to be sufficiently detailed to show that you have discharged your duty of care. An evidence-based care plan and regular progress reports form the backbone of this detail. To be useful in evidence, however, the record needs to show much more. In *Marriott v West Midlands HA* [1999], a GP was found negligent when he failed to refer back to hospital a man who suffered a head injury in a fall and was still having headaches, lethargy and appetite loss a week later. As this was a home visit, the GP had not taken the man's records with him and was heavily hampered in court by not being able to recount the detail and results of the examination he carried out or why he decided not to refer the patient back to hospital.

It can be seen from *Marriott* that an incomplete or inaccurate record can be fatal to a case. In this instance, details of the examination were missing, but equally damning was the lack of evidence as to why the doctor decided to wait and see. Decisions about care must be included in the patient's record. If you decide that a particular form of treatment or care should be delayed, say so. If you decide to wait and see before you call for a doctor or other assistance, record why you decided to wait.

Decisions about care and treatment are often taken on a multidisciplinary basis. Your records must include the background to the discussion and its outcome. This will indicate the reason for the decision and corroborate the account of other team members. Records must also corroborate any other legal requirement or form completed by the patient in your presence. For example, if a patient signs a consent form, that should be recorded and details discussed should be included. Details of telephone calls made, even if unanswered, to the patient or to others about the patient, and discussions arising from them with date and time, should be included as should referrals to specialist practitioners. Where there are particular concerns, these telephone conversations should be confirmed in a letter.

Case study 11.3: Victoria Climbié Inquiry

Victoria Climbié died as the result of systematic abuse by her aunt (DH, 2003b). The Inquiry into her death focused on the transfer of the case from a neighbouring social services department. The social worker assigned to her case told the Inquiry that she had contacted the social services department, who told her the family had moved out of the borough, so the case was closed.

Social services denied the conversation took place and the department was still seeing Victoria and her aunt in December 1999 – fully four months after she was referred.

The social worker admitted that she could not remember exactly when the phone conversation had taken place, nor had she dated the entry about the phone call in Victoria's files.

She also had record entries with uneven spaces between them, leading the barrister to the Inquiry to suggest that the note about the phone call to social services was added after the girl's murder in an effort to explain away the fact that she had done nothing with this referral.

Team members occasionally have differences of opinion on patient care. Any expression of dissent you have with another nurse, doctor or pharmacist should be recorded, and included should be the facts leading to the disagreement, the reason why you object and, importantly, what follow-up action was taken.

Views of patients and relatives

A further essential entry must be the views of patients and their relatives. It is useful to differentiate the views of patients and relatives and your own entry by using quotation marks. For example, 'I'm in agony with the pain'. Relatives are an important source of progress or concern about patients. They know the patient well and notice changes in condition more quickly as a result. Their views must be recorded and responded to.

Case study 11.4: The concerns of relatives must be recorded

In a complaint against Hastings and Rother NHS Trust put by Mrs M and Mrs N (Health Service Commissioner, 1999), concerning a man who died from an intestinal obstruction, the Health Service Commissioner (the ombudsman) found that the concerns of a patient's relatives were not recorded in the nursing notes. This he found to be a significant oversight. In evidence, the nurses had stated that they would only record conversations with relatives where there was a real concern or anxiety raised.

The ombudsman, however, was clear that all concerns raised by relatives should be recorded. He held that relatives will often be the first to notice changes in a patient, because of their greater familiarity with the patient's normal state, and recording those concerns is necessary if they are to be properly taken into account. He found that the lack of information in the nursing records about the relatives' concerns must have increased the risk of a delay in acting in response to, or being alerted of, deterioration in the patient's condition.

Records must be written legibly

It is essential that all records, instructions, prescriptions or referrals for treatment be written legibly and indelibly. Records are the key communication tool between nurses. They allow for continuity of care. It is essential that record entries can be read and this begins with the clarity of the entry. Clarity requires ink that contrasts with the paper being used for entries. For white paper use black ink as this gives the greatest contrast and best clarity when copied. There is a growing trend to use different colour paper for medical, nursing and other entries in shared records. It is essential that the colour chosen facilitates copying. In litigation a record will be copied to each of the relevant parties. That means that, on average, some 20 copies will be made. Records are of little use as evidence if the writing cannot be read due to deterioration in clarity when photocopied.

The standard of your handwriting is also a requirement of your duty of care to a patient. If care is initiated by you through a care plan and harm results because others could not read your writing, liability in negligence is likely to arise.

Case study 11.5: A doctor with poor handwriting

A good analogy is the case of Prendergast v Sam and Dee *[1989], in which an illegible prescription resulted in the patient being given the wrong drug and this caused harm. The pharmacist was held to be 75 per cent liable for that harm. For his poor handwriting, the GP was found to be 25 per cent liable. The Court of Appeal held that there is a duty to write clearly so that busy or careless staff can read your instructions.*

Legibility extends to the signature of the person who made the entry. Identifying the people and therefore witnesses involved in an incident is crucial to building a successful case. As well as a signature, the name in print or block capitals and grade of the person writing should be noted at least once in the notes during the course of the record. As a useful back-up, the human resources department or GP practice will often hold a signature bank with forwarding addresses, especially if there is a frequent turnover of staff, so that staff who have left can be identified should they be required as a witness to an incident at a later date.

Writing with indelible ink or typeface is essential for two reasons. First, the record must stand the test of time. It may be many years before it is referred to again and a faded record is of little value as evidence. It is usual for several years to pass before an incident goes to court to be decided. Cases generally take three to six years to resolve and can often go on for much longer.

Case study 11.6: Twenty-one years before a case came to court

In Reynolds v North Tyneside HA *[2002], a woman argued that she had suffered cerebral palsy as a result of the negligent mismanagement of her mother's labour some 21 years earlier. The patient's records and hospital policy were central to the case. In this instance, the patient's records were in good condition and properly completed. They showed that staff attending the birth had acted according to hospital policy. It was the hospital policy that was found to be incorrect and the court found for the woman.*

Second, the credibility of your record as evidence is enhanced by its being made at the time of the incident. Credibility is essential to the reliability of the record as evidence of what occurred. Using indelible ink or typeface reassures the court that the entry has not been subsequently altered in any way. You must, therefore, avoid using pencil or a computer entry system that does not use a time stamp or some other method to ensure that the entry cannot be altered without a trace. Altering a record is seen as a serious matter and can result in prosecution, dismissal and removal from the nursing register.

Case study 11.7: Student who altered record is jailed

A student who faked her birth delivery figures at a Southampton hospital to boost her hopes of qualifying as a midwife was jailed for six months (Hampshire and Isle of Wight Counter Fraud Team, 2007). The student altered computer records at the hospital to show that she had gained sufficient experience to qualify in her profession. Using colleagues' passwords, she changed the details to convince her supervisor that she had overseen almost 30 births more than she actually had.

Records must be clear and unambiguous

Records are an essential tool in the continuity of care. Care to be implemented and progress made must be clearly stated. The record is also likely to be read by non-nursing and non-medical persons. Under the Data Protection Act 1998, patients have the right to access records and obtain an explanation of their contents. The Human Rights Act 1998 (schedule 1, part 1, article 8) gives a separate right of access both to patients and in some respects to relatives, where this affects their right to respect for a private and family life. In *Gaskin v UK* [1990], the European Court of Human Rights emphasised the need for specific justification for preventing individuals from having access to information that forms part of their private and family life.

Access to health records

A legal right of access to health records is given to living people, whether their records are computerised or manually created (handwritten), under the provisions of the Data Protection Act 1998 and its regulations. The right of access applies equally to all records regardless of when they were made. Limited statutory rights of access to the records of deceased patients still exist in the Access to Health Records Act 1990.

Access rights under the Data Protection Act 1998

Patients have a right to be informed as to whether personal data about them is being processed, including being obtained, recorded or held, and why (for more detail, see Chapter 12 on confidentiality). Patients have a right of access to health records that:

- are about them and from which they can be identified;
- consist of information relating to their physical or mental health or condition;
- have been made by or on behalf of a health professional in connection with their care.

Where access is agreed, the health record must be communicated to the patient in an intelligible form. That will often require the person responsible for the record meeting with the patient to explain the content and any technical or cryptic remarks or abbreviations that may be within it. Patients are entitled to a permanent copy of the information and this must also be accompanied by an explanation of any terms that are unintelligible to them. Where the person considers that the record or part of it is inaccurate, they can seek a correction.

You are not obliged to accept the patient's opinion or version of events, but you must ensure that the record indicates the patient's view and provide them with a copy of the correction or appended note. These arrangements must indicate why the alteration was made to avoid any allegation of tampering with the record.

If the person remains dissatisfied with their record, they may take the matter to court. The courts have the power to require that inaccurate data and any expression of opinion based on them are corrected or removed. The court may also require that the records be supplemented by a statement of the true facts, and that third parties be notified of any corrections.

Applications for access

Nothing in the Act prevents nurses from giving patients access to their records on an informal and voluntary basis, provided no other provisions of the Act preventing disclosure are breached.

Indeed, the Data Protection Act 1998 calls for you to work in partnership with patients in an open and informal way, so that, if access to a record is requested, there are no surprises for patients. Formal applications for access must be in writing and accompanied by the appropriate fee.

Any patient is entitled to seek access to their health records. Where the patient is a child, any person with parental responsibility may apply independently. Where the child's parents live apart and have parental responsibility, they may individually apply to see their child's record. Where this occurs the other parent does not need to be told.

In *Gillick v West Norfolk and Wisbech AHA* [1986], the House of Lords held that, where a child is competent to make their own decisions about treatment, they are entitled to the same degree of confidentiality as an adult patient. Where access to a competent child's record is requested, it can only be granted if the child consents.

Competent children and young people may, of course, seek access to their own health records, and any patient may authorise a third party, such as a relative or legal representative, to seek access on their behalf.

Requests for access are made to the person in charge of keeping the records, known under the Data Protection Act 1998 as the data controller. The decision about disclosure is made by the appropriate health professional. This person would be the health professional currently or most recently responsible for the nursing care of the patient. Access must be given promptly and, in any event, within 40 days of receipt of the fee and a clear request. Where access is given, there is no obligation to give access again until a reasonable time interval has elapsed. There is no legal guidance on how long this would be and it must be assessed on a case-by-case basis. For example, if the patient has received no further treatment in the intervening period, a grant of access would seem unreasonable.

Information that cannot be disclosed

The right of access does not include information that would identify some other person mentioned in the record. This information cannot be released unless:

- the third party is a health professional who has compiled or contributed to the health records or who has been involved in the care of the patient;
- the other individual gives consent to the disclosure of that information; or
- it is reasonable to dispense with that third party's consent.

Where the record includes information from other identifiable sources, it is advisable to distinguish this information in the records when the information is entered, in order to avoid inadvertent disclosure. It is still necessary to disclose as much of the information in the records as is possible, but you must ensure that you:

- omit names and identifying particulars from the records before disclosure; and
- ensure that the information is genuinely anonymous.

You are not required to approach a third party for consent to disclosure, although you may wish to in some circumstances.

Harm

Access must not be given to any information that, in the opinion of the appropriate health professional, would be likely to cause serious harm to the patient or another person. The decision about likely harm must be taken by the appropriate health professional. This exemption does not justify withholding comments in the records because patients may find them upsetting.

Case study 11.8: Refusal to grant access to a health record

In R (on the application of S) v Plymouth City Council *[2002], a mother whose son was the subject of guardianship under the Mental Health Act was refused access to his health and social services record. She argued that she needed access to decide if she should accept or object to his continued guardianship order. The court granted access and it then emerged that the record contained uncomplimentary remarks about the woman.*

Children

The Act does not allow disclosure of information prohibited in legislation concerning adoption records and reports, statements of a child's special educational needs and parental order records and reports. None of these exemptions apply where the disclosure is required by law, or where it is necessary for the purposes of establishing, exercising or defending legal rights.

Access to records of deceased patients

The Data Protection Act 1998 does not cover the records of deceased patients. Statutory rights of access are granted within the provisions of the Access to Health Records Act 1990.

Any person with a claim arising from the death of a patient has a right of access to information covered by the 1990 Act, where this information is directly relevant to that claim. The information that can be accessed is, however, restricted to that covered by the Access to Health Records Act 1990, that is, manually created (handwritten) health records made since 1 November 1991.

Use of jargon and abbreviations

The temptation to use jargon and abbreviations as a form of professional shorthand is compelling for busy overworked health staff. However, the risk of miscommunication increases dramatically by using this shorthand.

Activity 11.3 *Team working*

Abbreviations and jargon

In a group, write down individual lists of abbreviations and technical jargon you have used or read during your clinical placements. Now pass the lists among the other group members and ask them to explain what they understand by the terms and abbreviations. Did you all come to the same definitions and meaning of the terms?

An outline answer is given at the end of the chapter.

A combination of shorthand instructions and poor handwriting led to the death of a patient. The patient was taking 2 mg of warfarin daily. When reviewed, the GP wrote 'same' on the card. The receptionist mistook the 's' as a 5 and the rest of the word as mg, resulting in the patient being given 5 mg of warfarin daily. He died from a massive haemorrhage some three weeks later (Marsh and Narain, 2003).

Although under considerable work pressure, nurses must not use abbreviations or jargon. The risks are too great and misinterpretation by staff and patients is common.

Case study 11.9: Misinterpretation of abbreviations

Wright (2003) reported an incident where a member of nursing staff who, when he saw DOA on a patient's notes, told the enquiring relative that the patient was 'dead on arrival' at hospital. This was the meaning of the acronym in A&E, where he usually worked. On the ward, however, DOA meant 'date of admission' and the patient was very much alive.

Jargon is also used to convey offensive remarks unrelated to patient care. Brindley (2003) reported that a GP wrote 'She's mad', along with a cartoon drawing, on a set of notes. Other cryptic acronyms are more offensive. Examples include CLL or 'chronic low life', FLK for 'funny-looking kid', often explained by JLD or 'just like dad'. The temptation to use such acronyms is always there.

Remember, in litigation your records will be subject to rigorous scrutiny. There is no right to withhold any part of the record from the court. Having to explain under cross-examination that the entry GPO meant you thought the patient was 'good for parts only' will be at best embarrassing and at worst fatal to your case. Evidentially, the first impression the court has of you is from your notes. Cryptic comments have no place in records. If records are not professional, the assumption is that neither is your care and your credibility as a witness is greatly diminished.

Records must be accurate

To confirm the chronology of record entries, each entry must be identified with date (day, month and year) and time (using the 24-hour clock) and signed with the professional's name printed legibly underneath the signature together with their position. Initials for entries must not be used, as it is vital to be able to identify the member of staff if a complaint is made.

Case study 11.10: Ten minutes of unexplained delay

In Richards v Swansea NHS Trust *[2007], a child suffered from cerebral palsy and argued that it was as the result of delaying, at the time of his birth, the emergency caesarean that had occurred some 50 minutes after it was considered necessary. Professional guidance states that it must occur within 30 minutes and the judge was content to grant the trust a period of 40 minutes, but the trust and care team had to justify the extra 10-minute delay. As they were unable to demonstrate what call on their time there was during that 10-minute period, the judge said he had no alternative but to find for the patient.*

Errors

All alterations must be made by scoring out with a single line that does not completely obscure the error. Correcting fluid must not be used. This removes any suggestion of wrongdoing or attempting to cover up an incident. The struck-out error should be followed by the dated, timed and signed correct entry. No blank lines or spaces that could facilitate entries being added at a later date should be left between entries.

Pressure of work

It may be argued that pressure of work was such that it reduced the nurse's ability to maintain the usual standard of care. Such situations have been called 'battlefield situations', in which resources are so stretched that a court has to accept that the expected level of the standard of care has to be reduced (*Wilsher v Essex HA* [1988]). In these situations, the court can order the disclosure of other patients' records to see how busy the ward was at the time.

Case study 11.11: Pressure of work

In Deacon v McVicar *[1984], a woman argued that she had received negligent care causing her harm. The hospital argued that the evening of the incident was a singularly busy one, with several emergency cases draining available resources. The court ordered that the records of all other patients on the ward that evening be released to the court to see how busy the unit was. They showed that it was an exceptionally busy evening with many emergencies overstretching the staff and resources available.*

Contemporaneous record entries

Record entries need to be written at the time of, or as soon as possible after, the events to which they relate. Contemporaneous recording is vital as it adds to the reliability of the entry and means that, with the leave of the court, you can refer to the record when giving evidence. Contemporaneous altering of a record contributed to a finding of negligence in *Kent v Griffiths and Others* [2000]. Here, an emergency ambulance took some 30 minutes to arrive at an address, but the crew recorded the duration of the journey as 9 minutes. The judge held that the record had been contemporaneously falsified and found for the patient.

The record should demonstrate the chronology of events and of all significant consultations, assessments, observations, decisions, interventions and outcomes. Reports and results should be seen, evaluated and signed by the practitioner before being filed in the patient's records. This is the key to a good record. This is what a lawyer is going to try to pull apart in order to win a case. If the patient's condition remains the same, say so. In one case, a record entry stated *6.30 a.m. sleeping peacefully, 8.40 a.m. dead* (Wright, 2003). In the cold light of a courtroom, such an entry makes it look like the patient was not being properly monitored.

Records are never neutral

To be of use in evidence your records need to be thorough, otherwise they will act to your detriment. Records are never neutral; they will either support or condemn you.

Case study 11.12: The incomplete record

In S (A Child) v Newcastle and North Tyneside HA *[2001], the negligent management of the latter stages of labour resulted in severe cerebral palsy. The judge's annoyance at the standard of record keeping is clear from his comments:*

> It is important to emphasise at this early stage that unhappily the evidence was, in certain important respects, incomplete. The clinical records of this labour are not full and no records at all appear between 4 a.m. and 10.15 a.m. Each of these might be regarded as critical periods. Unhappily whoever did take over from [the midwife] singularly failed to complete the partogram, that is the record of the labour, which is effectively devoid of useful information.

The importance of personal details

The patient's personal details are every bit as important as the care plan and progress entries. The Audit Commission (2002) found that the average NHS trust wastes some £20,000 per year on redirected mail due to incorrectly addressed home or GP details that have been recorded in the notes or on the computer system. Missing details also reduce the quality of patient care by disrupting communication between the patients, their families and health staff, causing missed outpatient appointments and losing potentially critical information about the patient. It is important to check details with patients to ensure that personal information is up to date.

Records need to be communicated

Your records are a crucial means of communicating with colleagues. It is essential for effective patient care that records are used and communicated. Where tragedy occurs in health settings, the resulting inquiry report repeatedly cites a failure of communication as a cause. It is a recurring theme in mental health inquiries (Anderson, 2003) and in child death inquiries (DH, 2003a). Records are not a paper exercise. Nurses must communicate the contents and findings of their records to other members of the care team to ensure that concerns and risks are monitored and minimised.

Case study 11.13: The consequences of a failure to communicate a record entry

In Gauntlett v Northampton HA *[1985], a patient gave her visiting husband a box of matches saying, 'Take these because I'll set fire to myself'. Her husband handed the matches to the charge nurse, who failed to record or communicate the concern. Four days later the patient set fire to the tee shirt she was wearing, burning herself badly.*

Keeping records secure

All NHS records are public records under the provisions of the Public Records Act 1958 (sections 3(1)–(2)). The Secretary of State for Health and all NHS organisations have a duty under this Act to make arrangements for the safe keeping and eventual disposal of all records. Chief executives and senior managers of all NHS organisations are personally accountable for the safe keeping of records.

Activity 11.4 — *Critical thinking*

Security of patient records

What measures must you take to ensure the safety and security of patient records?

Now read below for further information.

Under the Public Records Act, nurses are accountable for any records that they create or use in the course of their duties. You have a duty to ensure that records are kept safe and secure by:

- ensuring the physical security of such records, keeping them locked away when not required;
- ensuring that records and their binders are in a good state so that information is held securely, loose-leaf information such as test results is properly secured, and information cannot be lost or mislaid from the records;
- maintaining security of access to information within the records by ensuring that they cannot be inadvertently read by others;
- maintaining a written log of incoming/outgoing records through the use of a tracing system that allows for the physical tracking of records.

Putting the record straight

The Audit Commission (2002) found that subjecting records to a regular audit is the best way to ensure high-quality record keeping.

Activity 11.5 **Reflection**

Audit of records

Having read this chapter, if you were to audit your record entries, what key standards would you wish to meet?

Now read below for further information.

In their advice sheet on record keeping, the NMC (2007) recommends the following content for nursing records. The information in patient records must:

- be factual, consistent and accurate;
- be written in such a way that the meaning is clear;
- be recorded as soon as possible after an event has occurred;
- be recorded clearly and indelibly;
- be recorded so that any justifiable alterations or additions are dated, timed and signed in such a way that the original entry can still be read clearly;

- be accurately dated, timed and signed, with the signature printed alongside the first entry, where this is a written record, and attributed to a named person in an identifiable role for electronic records;
- not include abbreviations, jargon, meaningless phrases, irrelevant speculation or offensive or subjective statements;
- be readable when photocopied or scanned;
- be recorded, wherever possible, with the involvement of the patient;
- be recorded in terms that the patient can understand;
- be in chronological order;
- identify risks or problems that have arisen and the action taken to rectify them;
- give a full account of the assessment and the care that has been planned and provided;
- provide relevant information about the condition of the patient;
- provide evidence that you have discharged your duty of care;
- provide a record of any arrangements that have been made for the continuing care of a patient.

You are also required to make more frequent entries for patients who:

- have complex problems;
- are vulnerable or at risk of harm or abuse;
- require more intensive care than normal;
- are confused and disoriented or generally give cause for concern.

The five-minute audit

To ensure that your record entries meet the requirements of the NMC standards and the law, ask a colleague or mentor to conduct a five-minute audit on your most recent entry, and highlight:

1. **Incomplete tasking**
    - Is the entry complete?
    - Have you shown that you have discharged your duty of care?
    - Often only describe half of what you did. The examples below do not give sufficient detail:
        - Consent taken
        - Vaccination given
        - Risks explained.

2. **Fact or supposition**
   - Wherever an opinion or conclusion is expressed it should have a factual basis.
   - Need to recognise what is a fact and what is a supposition; the examples below are all suppositions that need the facts underpinning them to be included:
     - Mrs Jones is immature
     - The child understands the treatment
     - The bruise and swelling are consistent with hitting his head on the door.
3. **Communication**
   - Failure of communication underpins litigation:
     - Will the record entry be clearly understood by those who read it?
     - Do you need to expand entries so that everyone understands what you mean?
     - Have you avoided the use of abbreviations?

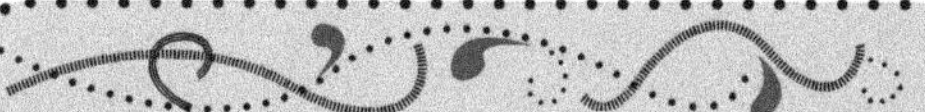

Chapter summary

- Record keeping is a basic nursing duty.
- Records provide evidence of involvement with patients.
- Records provide a plan of care for a patient and are crucial in monitoring progress and communicating concerns.
- Records also have a vital role in protecting nurses from litigation.
- If it is not written down it is difficult to prove it happened.
- Records must be thorough, contemporaneous and clear.
- Expressions of dissent must be recorded.
- Records must corroborate discussions with colleagues.
- Records must be communicated to be effective.
- Records subject to audit have a higher standard of record keeping.
- Good record keeping will demonstrate that you have met your legal and professional obligations and discharged your duty of care.

Activity: Brief outline answer

Activity 11.3: Team working (page 247)

The temptation to use jargon and abbreviations as a form of professional shorthand is compelling for busy, overworked health staff. However, as this activity demonstrates, the risk of miscommunication increases dramatically by using this shorthand.

Here are some other examples:

- UBI: unexplained beer injury;
- NQR: not quite right;
- GOK: God only knows.

Further reading

For key advice on record keeping in the context of healthcare we recommend:

Department of Health (2006) *Records Management: NHS Code of Practice.* London: The Stationery Office.

Nursing and Midwifery Council (2007) *NMC Record Keeping Guidance.* London: NMC.

For a consideration of the common problems associated with poor records we recommend you read:

Audit Commission (1999) *Setting the Record Straight: A review of progress in health records services.* London: The Stationery Office.

Useful website

NHS Evidence is an excellent website that has a searchable database of guidelines and standards including those for record keeping:

www.library.nhs.uk

Chapter 12
Confidentiality

NMC Standards for Pre-registration Nursing Education

This chapter will address the following competencies:

Domain 1: Professional values

6. All nurses must understand the roles and responsibilities of other health and social care professionals, and seek to work with them collaboratively for the benefit of all who need care.

Domain 2: Communication and interpersonal skills

8. All nurses must respect individual rights to confidentiality and keep information secure and confidential in accordance with the law and relevant ethical and regulatory frameworks, taking account of local protocols. They must also actively share personal information with others when the interests of safety and protection override the need for confidentiality.

Chapter aims

By the end of this chapter you will be able to:

- discuss the rationale for imposing a duty of confidence on registered nurses and midwives;
- outline three spheres of the duty of confidence that registered nurses and midwives are subject to;
- compare the scope of the legal, professional and contractual obligation of confidence;
- describe the circumstances that would allow you to disclose confidential patient information;
- explain three ways in which the duty of confidence may be modified by statute;
- discuss the measures nurses must take to ensure that confidential patient information is disclosed with appropriate care.

Introduction

This chapter explores confidentiality in the context of nursing and healthcare. It considers the scope and sources of a nurse's duty of confidentiality before discussing the circumstances that would allow you to disclose information about a patient. Leading on from that the chapter highlights the measures you must take to ensure that any disclosure of information is done with appropriate care.

Maintaining the confidentiality of a patient's health information is a fundamental element of professional conduct and ethical practice for all registered nurses. The relationship between nurse and patient is essential for proper assessment and care that is largely based on a patient's personal history of their health problem. Patients pass on sensitive information relating to their health and other matters as part of their desire to receive treatment. They do so in confidence and expect you to respect their privacy by ensuring the confidentiality of the information they give.

To ensure the highest standard of conduct and ethical practice in relation to the protection of health information, a duty of confidence is imposed on all staff, volunteers and contractors within the NHS.

Activity 12.1 *Reflection*

Defining confidentiality

Before you begin reading about the nurse's duty of confidence to the patient, write down what you consider the term confidentiality means.

An outline answer is given at the end of the chapter.

Duty of confidence

A duty of confidence arises when one person discloses information to another in circumstances where it is reasonable to expect that the information will be held in confidence.

For nurses, there are three key spheres to the duty that come together to reassure patients that the confidentiality of their health information will be respected (see Figure 12.1).

1. A duty to respect patient confidentiality that is a specific requirement linked to disciplinary procedures in all NHS employment contracts and underpinned by the NHS code of practice on confidentiality (DH, 2003c).
2. A legal duty that is derived from case law and supplemented by statute law (*Cornelius v De Taranto* [2001]).
3. A professional duty established by *The Code: Professional standards of practice and behaviour for nurses and midwives* (NMC, 2015a).

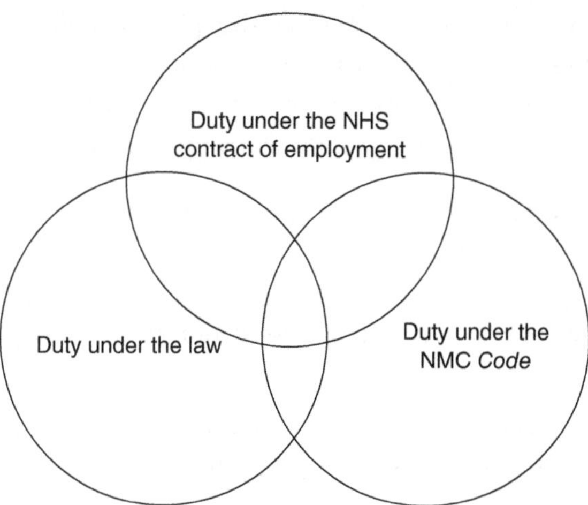

Figure 12.1: The three spheres of the duty of confidence owed by registered nurses and midwives.

However, the duty of confidence is not absolute. There will be occasions when confidential information about a patient will need to be disclosed to others. Such a disclosure must be to an appropriate person and comply with the requirements of your contractual, professional and legal duty of confidence, or you will be called to account and face sanctions for breaching confidentiality.

It is essential, therefore, that you:

- understand the scope of the duty of confidence owed to the patients in your care; and
- only disclose information given in confidence where it is right and proper to do so.

Activity 12.2 *Critical thinking*

The need for a duty of confidence

You have seen that a duty of confidence is imposed on nurses requiring them to respect the confidentiality of patient information. Write down why you think it is necessary for nurses to be subject to a legal, professional and contractual duty of confidence to their patients.

An outline answer is given at the end of the chapter.

The scope of the duty

The contractual duty of confidence

In recognition of the need to protect patient information and maintain the confidentiality of health information, all contracts of employment in the NHS must contain a clause that imposes a duty of confidence on all staff and stresses that disciplinary action will result if that duty is breached (DH, 2003c). Similarly, all contracts with outside agencies and arrangements with volunteers and others – including student nurses – who undertake work or placements with the NHS must also include a clause imposing a duty of confidence.

In order to discharge this duty, all staff and students will need to show that they have fulfilled their responsibilities by ensuring that:

- they do not disclose confidential patient information through inappropriate means, such as gossiping;
- when they seek advice about a patient's care and treatment with a colleague, they do so in private so that confidentiality is not inadvertently breached;
- they accurately record information received from and about their patients;
- they keep patient information and records private and physically secure;
- they only access information for the patients in their care;
- they only disclose patient information to an appropriate source in accordance with the NHS code of practice on confidentiality, the requirements of the law and the NMC *Code*.

Case study 12.1: Jailed for breaching confidentiality

A healthcare nursing assistant was jailed for eight months for selling stories to The Sun *newspaper about notorious patients at Broadmoor Hospital, including the Yorkshire Ripper. Some 14 tips were passed on to the newspaper for a total payment of £7,125. The judge said the nursing assistant was well aware of his duty of confidentiality and the articles generated as a consequence of the information provided were significantly detrimental to the patients' well-being.*

(O'Carroll, 2015)

The duty extends to all patients, both past and present. Although there is no specific legal or professional requirement that states that a duty of confidence extends to deceased patients, the contractual duty imposed by the NHS extends confidentiality beyond the grave and includes those who have died.

The professional duty of confidence

The professional requirement for confidentiality is stipulated in the NMC's *Code* (2015a) which states that a registered nurse must respect people's right to confidentiality.

Activity 12.3 *Evidence-based practice and research*

The professional duty of confidence

Download and read the NMC's explanatory note on confidentiality (at **www.nmc-uk.org**), then:

- outline the extent of a nurse's professional duty of confidence to patients;
- list the exceptions to that duty that would allow you to disclose information about a patient.

An outline answer is given at the end of the chapter.

This clause imposes on nurses a duty not to voluntarily disclose information gained in a professional capacity to a third party, and this is enforced by the threat of professional discipline. An explanatory paper by the NMC on professional conduct highlights a breach of confidentiality as a form of misconduct likely to result in removal from the register (NMC, 2004).

Case study 12.2: Inappropriate disclosure of patient information in breach of a nurse's professional duty of confidence

A specialist community public health nurse who had an affair with an ex-patient told him of an abortion his partner had undergone 19 years earlier (Evening Gazette, 2006). When asked where she had got the information from, she revealed that it had come from the woman's health record. The nurse admitted breaching confidentiality and was found guilty by a Conduct and Competence Committee of the NMC, who removed her name from the professional register.

Confidence and the law

As well as the professional duty of confidence there is a legal obligation on nurses to respect patients' confidences. The law relating to confidence is dealt with largely at common law. The obligation arises out of a general duty on everyone to keep confidential information secret (*Prince Albert v Strange* [1849]). That is, there is a public interest in keeping confidential information secret.

In order to establish a breach of confidence, three elements must be satisfied, as stated by Lord Keith in *Attorney General v Guardian Newspapers Ltd* [1987].

1. The information must have the necessary quality of confidence. That is, the information is not generally available or known. Information of a personal or intimate nature qualifies (*Stephens v Avery* [1988]) and this is very much the type of information nurses receive from their patients.
2. The information has been imparted in circumstances giving rise to an obligation of confidence. The law has long recognised that particular relationships gave rise to a duty of confidence. These include priest and penitent, solicitor and client, and the nurse–patient relationship. The courts, however, have gone further and have extended the obligation to include situations where an obviously confidential document is wafted by an electric fan out of a window into a crowded street, or a private diary is dropped in a public place (or these days an email goes astray).
3. The information has been divulged to a third person without the permission and to the detriment of the person originally communicating the information. An invasion of personal privacy will suffice (*Margaret, Duchess of Argyll v Duke of Argyll* [1967]). As it is in the public interest that medical confidences are kept secret, the court will regard an unwarranted disclosure of patient information as detrimental.

It can be seen that the very private nature of the information nurses are given by their patients and the trust generated by the nature of the nurse–patient relationship give rise to an obligation of confidence that the law seeks to protect. Consequently, the court will consider that an inappropriate disclosure of this information is bound to be detrimental to the patient and find that a breach of confidence has occurred.

Case study 12.3: Breaching the common law duty of confidence to a patient

In X v Y and Others *[1988], a health authority employee passed on to a newspaper information obtained from medical records of two patients who were HIV positive. The patients worked as doctors in the area and the newspaper wished to publish the details. The court granted the doctors an injunction preventing publication, holding that the public interest in preserving the confidentiality of hospital records outweighed any public interest in the freedom of the press, because victims of the disease ought not to be deterred by fear of discovery from going to hospital for treatment.*

It can be seen from the case study above that disclosure of health information to a newspaper without the agreement of the patient is an unjustified breach of confidence. The same would be true where a nurse discloses information that identifies a patient in their care on social networking sites or micro-blogging sites such as Facebook and Twitter. For example, a nurse who uploaded pictures of a patient undergoing surgery to Facebook was suspended by her trust. The photographs were taken with a camera phone without the patient's knowledge while she was in the operating theatre. The room and hospital are identifiable from the insignia on the wall. In another case five nurses from Broadmoor Hospital were sacked for discussing patients on social networking sites. As student nurses you must be very careful that any information you put on social networking sites does not breach patient confidentiality or the NMC's *Code*. A student who commented that she was going to 'mess about with dead bodies' on Facebook was given a final warning by her university for unprofessional conduct.

There is a range of statutory provisions that limit or prohibit the use and disclosure of information in specific circumstances.

Data Protection Act 1998

The Data Protection Act 1998 implements a European Union directive on the protection of individuals with regard to the processing of personal data and on the free movement of such data (Directive 95/46/EC). The 1998 Act provides a framework that governs the so-called processing of personal data.

Personal data is defined under the Data Protection Act 1998 as data that relates to a living individual who can be identified:

- from that data; or
- from data and other information that may be in your possession.

This includes any expression of opinion about the individual and any indications of your intentions to the individual.

'Processing' is an umbrella term and includes:

- holding information about patients;
- obtaining information from patients or others about a patient;
- recording patient information;
- using the information;
- disclosing patient information.

The 1998 Act applies to all forms of media, including paper records, electronic records and images. All processing of patient information must be fair and lawful and this will usually be the case where:

- the common law of confidentiality and any other applicable statutory restrictions on the use of information are complied with;
- the patient, known as the data subject, was not misled or deceived into giving the information;
- the patient is given basic information about who will process the data and for what purpose;
- in the case of personal health information, the conditions of schedules 2 and 3 of the Data Protection Act 1998 concerning sensitive data are met by ensuring that the information is necessary for medical purposes.

Human Rights Act 1998

Article 8 of the European Convention on Fundamental Rights and Freedoms establishes a right to respect for private and family life. This right emphasises the duty to protect the privacy of individuals and preserve the confidentiality of their health records. Article 8 is broad in scope and covers the collection, use and exchange of personal data as well as issues such as telephone tapping, parental access and the custody of children, the right to be free from noise and environmental pollution, and a person's right to express their identity and sexuality. Public authorities must preserve the individual's confidence when collecting and using personal data.

In *R (Robertson) v City of Wakefield Metropolitan Council* [2002], a man complained that his right to respect for a private life under article 8 of the European Convention on Human Rights was being infringed by his local council as they were selling to commercial companies personal details that he was required to provide for inclusion on the electoral roll. These companies were using the information for direct marketing.

The court held that article 8 was breached by the council. In determining whether article 8 was engaged it was necessary to take into account not just the information that was disclosed, but also the use to which it would be put. Where names and addresses were to be passed on to commercial companies for direct marketing purposes, this amounted to an interference with the right to private life.

Exceptions to the obligation of confidence

Neither the professional nor legal duties of confidentiality are absolute and they are subject to a range of exceptions that justify disclosure. It is important that nurses are aware of these exceptions in order to avoid a charge of professional misconduct and liability for breach of confidence.

The NMC, in clause 5 of *The Code* (2015a), leaves the decision to divulge a confidence with the registered nurse by viewing it as a matter of professional judgement. Yet little specific guidance is given on circumstances in which disclosure is justified. No guidance is given on the difference between a power to disclose, where a nurse can consider all the circumstances and decide if it is appropriate to divulge information, and a duty to disclose, where, regardless of circumstances, the law requires disclosure.

Activity 12.4 — *Reflection*

Disclosing information about patients

The duty of confidence owed by a nurse is not absolute. There will be times when it will be appropriate to disclose information about a patient.

Consider circumstances where you would think it was appropriate to divulge information about patients in your care.

An outline answer is given at the end of the chapter.

Consent of the patient

Permission to disclose confidential information from the person who originally imparted it is the starting presumption in law and an obvious exception. The courts generally require this consent to disclosure be in the form of an explicit consent, preferably signed by the patient (*Cornelius v De Taranto* [2001]). This ruling also reflects the requirements of the Data Protection Act 1998. The consent exception is only valid if the person knows exactly what information is to be disclosed and who is to receive the information.

The requirements for obtaining explicit consent from patients for the disclosure of personal health information are:

- be honest and clear about the information to be disclosed and the reason for disclosure, allowing patients to seek as much detail as they require to make a free choice;
- give patients an opportunity to talk to someone they trust and ask questions;
- allow the patient reasonable time to reach a decision;
- be prepared to explain any form that the patient may be required to sign;
- explain that consent can be refused or withdrawn at any time;
- ensure that you note that consent has been received in a patient's health record or by using a consent form signed by the patient.

Disclosure for care and treatment purposes

An area where a nurse might exercise professional judgement and disclose confidential information is with those directly involved in the care of the patient.

Confidentiality is allowed to be breached where information is shared with other nurses concerned with the clinical care of the patient. This exception also covers doctors and others for whom the information provided is necessary for the performance of their duties. These professionals are also bound by a duty of confidentiality. To require an express consent from a patient each time a patient's case was discussed would be impractical and even detrimental to the patient.

Where patients have consented to healthcare, research has consistently shown that they are content for information to be disclosed in order to provide that healthcare (NHS IA, 2002).

It is still essential that you ensure that patients understand how their information is to be used to support their healthcare and that they have no objections. To ensure this, you must:

- check where practicable that information leaflets on patient confidentiality and information disclosure have been read and understood by the patient;
- make it clear to patients why personal health information is recorded and why health records need to be accessed by other health professionals;
- make it clear to patients why you need to share their health information with others;

- ensure that patients have no concerns about how you will use their personal information;
- answer any questions the patient may have or direct the patient to someone who can answer their questions;
- respect the rights of patients to request access to their health records.

Where the patient has no objections, consent can be implied, provided that the information is shared no more widely than with those directly concerned with the care and treatment of the individual. Wide disclosure to any doctor or nurse is not justified.

Case study 12.4: The limit to the clinical family

In Cornelius v De Taranto *[2001], a teacher who claimed to be suffering from work-related stress saw a psychiatrist privately as part of gathering evidence against her employer. The psychiatrist sent a copy of her medico-legal report to the teacher's GP and a general consultant psychiatrist, as well as to her solicitor. Mrs Cornelius sued for breach of confidence. The Court of Appeal held that there was a breach of confidence and that Mrs Cornelius had not expressly consented to the dissemination of the report. The report had nothing to do with her treatment, so dissemination to other health professionals could not be justified on therapeutic grounds. The doctor could not rely on an implied consent in these circumstances.*

Patients who refuse consent to disclose treatment information

Patients have the right to be informed that they can object to the disclosure of confidential information that identifies them.

Where a patient refuses to allow information to be disclosed to other health professionals involved in providing care, it could mean that the care that can be provided is limited and in some circumstances it might not be possible to offer treatment.

Patients must be told if their decisions to refuse to allow disclosure of treatment information will have implications for the provision of care or treatment. Health professionals cannot treat patients safely or provide continuity of care without having relevant information about a patient's condition and medical history.

Disclosing information when a patient specifically asks you to do so

When a health professional is asked by a patient to pass on confidential information about them, the court regards this as a binding obligation. In *C v C* [1946], Justice Lewis considered the refusal of a sexually transmitted disease clinic to divulge information about a patient despite his request for disclosure. The judge held that, while it was important that proper secrecy be observed in sexually transmitted disease clinics, those considerations did not justify a health professional refusing to divulge confidential information to a named person when asked by the patient to do so. In the circumstances of this case the information should have been given, and in all cases where the circumstances are similar there is no breach of confidence in giving the information asked for.

Activity 12.5 *Evidence-based practice and research*

Share with Care

Download a copy of *Share with Care: People's views on consent and confidentiality of patient information* (NHS IA, 2002) by following the link on the book's website. Read and consider what the report discovered about patients' views on health professionals disclosing their personal information.

An outline answer is given at the end of the chapter.

Disclosing information without specific consent

The Department of Health advises that there are a number of exceptions allowing disclosure to appropriate sources without the consent of the patient (DH, 2003c). These exceptions act as a useful aid to nurses when making a judgement about disclosing information concerning a patient.

Where a patient is incapable of receiving information or of consenting to disclosure, disclosure of care and treatment information to the client's relative or main carer may be judged to be appropriate. Similarly, disclosure to appropriate sources would be allowed in cases of the suspected abuse of dependent elderly people and children under vulnerable adult and child protection procedures (DH, 1999, 2000).

Disclosure in the public interest

A major defence used by individuals who have had to justify the disclosure of confidential information has been that disclosure was necessary in the public interest. The courts accept that, when a case concerning the disclosure of confidential information comes before them, they are required to strike a balance between two competing interests:

- the public interest in keeping confidential information secret; and
- the public interest in allowing disclosure.

The public interest exception covers a broad range of situations that allow for confidential information to be disclosed without the consent of the patient. These situations include:

- disclosure in the interests of justice;
- disclosure for the public good;
- disclosure to protect a third party;
- disclosure to prevent or detect a serious crime.

Disclosure in the interests of justice

Unlike lawyers, nurses do not have a privileged relationship with their patients. A court has the power to order disclosure of confidential matters if it is in the interest of justice, and refusing to do so would result in conviction for contempt of court. For example, in *Attorney General v Mulholland* [1963], two journalists refused before a tribunal to name or describe the sources of information in articles written by them, which the chairman of the tribunal certified were relevant to the inquiry. One of the journalists was sentenced to six and the other to three months' imprisonment for contempt. On appeal, the court confirmed that the questions were relevant and necessary to the tribunal's inquiry; thus there was no privilege and the sentences would stand.

In exercising this power the court must be satisfied that disclosure will satisfy the interests of justice. Where this is not the case they can refuse to order disclosure. For example, in *D v National Society for the Prevention of Cruelty to Children* [1977], the NSPCC received a complaint from an informant about the alleged maltreatment of a girl aged 14 months. That evening an inspector from the society called at the parents' home and enquired about the baby. The mother, who was very upset, called the family doctor, who found the baby to be healthy and unharmed. The family demanded to be told the name of the informant. When the inspector refused to give it, the family brought legal proceedings to reveal the identity of the informant. The House of Lords held that the importance of preserving confidentiality for the protection of children overrode the requirement that the mother should be given the information she sought in order to pursue her claim.

Nurses, therefore, could be required by the courts to disclose information about their patients both in the form of written statements and as oral evidence, where this is necessary in the interests of justice.

Disclosure for the public good

There may be circumstances where the public interest is served by disclosing information even though no crime has been committed or court action taken. This might include disclosing information to a regulatory body such as the NMC. For example, in *Woolgar v Chief Constable of Sussex* [2000], a nurse was interviewed under caution by the police following a patient's death over alleged drug misuse. The information obtained was insufficient to bring charges. The police passed the tapes to the nursing regulatory body, which was investigating the nurse, and she claimed a breach of confidence. The Court of Appeal held that comments made in police interviews were confidential and remained so even if not used in criminal proceedings. However, disclosure to a regulatory body could be justified in the absence of consent if it was necessary for the public good to allow the regulatory body to properly investigate the allegations against the nurse.

Disclosure to protect a third party

The law accepts that there may be circumstances where disclosure of confidential information is necessary in order to protect a third party, particularly where this concerns a vulnerable adult or child.

The nurse would need to consider all the circumstances and use their professional judgement, informed by reference to the common law, to decide if the public interest in protecting the third party outweighed the public interest in keeping confidential information secret.

For example, in *Re L (Care Proceedings: Disclosure to Third Party)* [2000], a paediatric nurse sought an injunction preventing a local authority passing information about her mental health problem to the nursing regulatory body following care proceedings concerning her and her child. The court allowed the disclosure, holding that the right of the nurse and her child to confidentiality had to be balanced against the public interests in protecting others from a nurse whose fitness to practise had been called into doubt.

Disclosure to prevent or detect a serious crime

There may be circumstances where a nurse is made aware that a patient has committed or intends to commit a crime. Before disclosing such information, it will be necessary for the health professional to weigh the seriousness of the crime against the countervailing public interest in maintaining patient confidentiality.

For example, in *W v Egdell* [1990], Dr Egdell had been commissioned by W's solicitor to prepare a report for his upcoming appeal against detention under the Mental Health Act 1983. W had been an in-patient at a special hospital for ten years after he shot five people and was now seeking discharge or relocation to a less secure unit. His consultant psychiatrist supported W's appeal as he felt he had made good progress. However, Dr Egdell's report strongly opposed his relocation and pointed out W's continued interest in firearms and explosives. On receiving the report, W's solicitor withdrew the appeal, which prompted Dr Egdell to send a copy to the medical director of the hospital as he felt the patient was deceiving his doctors. W then sued for breach of confidence.

The court held that Dr Egdell's duty of confidence to W had to be weighed against the public interests in preventing crime. Dr Egdell was justified in taking this course of action as W posed a real risk to public safety, and the medical team at the hospital were entitled to full information relating to his dangerousness.

It can be seen from *Egdell* that disclosure is justified where the crime represents a real risk to public safety. That is, there must be a need to prevent or detect a serious crime to justify breaching patient confidentiality, as the countervailing public interest in maintaining sensitive health information would generally outweigh disclosure.

It is very interesting to contrast the disclosure in *W v Egdell* [1990] with the earlier case of *X v Y and Others* [1988], where two doctors in general practice had their HIV status revealed to a national newspaper by employees of a health authority. Here, the court held that there was a breach of confidentiality, as there was no public interest to justify overriding the duty of confidence owed to the doctors.

Where a nurse believes they are justified in disclosing information about a patient, that disclosure must be to an appropriate source. Indeed, Lord Justice Bingham, in *W v Egdell* [1990], stressed that while the doctor was right to pass on information to other doctors in Broadmoor about W's dangerousness, he could not lawfully sell the contents of his report to a newspaper. Nor could he, without a breach of the law as well as professional etiquette, discuss the case in a learned article or in his memoirs or in gossiping with friends, unless he took steps to conceal the identity of the patient.

Is there a duty to warn of risk of physical harm?

In one American case, the concept of disclosure in the public interest was taken a stage further when a counsellor was successfully sued for failing to disclose information about a serious risk of physical harm to a client's ex-girlfriend on the grounds of client confidentiality. In *Tarasoff v Regents of the University of California* [1976], Tatiana Tarasoff was killed by her ex-boyfriend and the University of California was sued by her parents. The California Supreme Court heard the case twice and extended the duty to warn on each occasion.

In the first trial they held that privilege ends where public peril begins. In the second, that a therapist has a duty to use reasonable care to protect potential victims. The *Tarasoff* case created a new cause of action in negligence in the United States.

Such has been the impact of the case in America that so-called *Tarasoff* warnings are routinely issued by psychiatrists and psychologists, warning potential victims of the threat towards them.

There is yet to be a similar case before the British courts. Little authoritative guidance is available on whether *Tarasoff* warnings are required to avoid liability in negligence by nurses and others in the UK. Any trial on the issue would largely depend on the legal proximity of the potential victim to the nurse. If the person is another patient of the nurse's, then a duty to warn is probably owed. If the person is a close relative of the patient and the nurse adopts a holistic or family-centred approach to care, it is argued that a duty would also exist. However, if the potential victim is an unidentified member of the public or someone the nurse does not know, no duty to warn will arise.

This was certainly held to be the case in *Palmer v Tees HA* [2000]. Here, it was claimed that the health authority had been negligent in failing to diagnose the real and substantial risk that an outpatient in their care would sexually abuse children. The patient abducted and murdered a child and her mother sued the health authority for failing to warn the public of the risk he posed.

However, the judge held that, where it was alleged that a defendant was responsible for the action of a third party, then that required a special class of person at risk, not an unidentified category.

Therefore, as the identity of the victim was not known to the health authority, it did not owe a duty of care. In seeking to expand on his judgment, the judge added that a health authority had no general immunity from an action of this sort if the case demanded it. If there had been any identifiable special factors that could have put the victim above other members of the public, the outcome may well have been different. Hence, if a person known to a health professional is identified as being at risk of harm from the criminal act of another patient, there probably exists a duty to warn.

Activity 12.6 — *Critical thinking*

Breach of confidentiality

You are working in a busy A&E department when, at about 2 a.m., a man presents himself with a wound to his left leg. He has apparently driven to the hospital on his own. He will not give any information about how he sustained this injury and he smells strongly of alcohol. He wants to be treated as soon as possible and then go home. Following an examination by the casualty officer, it becomes apparent that he has sustained a gunshot wound.

On your way to the reception area, you are approached by a police officer. He asks you if you have had a patient admitted with injuries to his leg. No one else is available to speak to the officer as they are all busy with a victim of a serious road traffic collision.

Discuss whether you would be justified in disclosing the name of the patient to the police officer.

An outline answer is given at the end of the chapter.

Disclosing anonymised information

Information is provided by patients in confidence and must be treated as such, as long as it remains capable of identifying the individual it relates to. However, anonymised information is not considered confidential and may be used with few constraints. Information that does not identify an individual directly and that cannot reasonably be used to determine identity is considered to be anonymous information.

Case study 12.5: Disclosing anonymised information

In R v Department of Health Ex p. Source Informatics Ltd (No. 1) *[2001], Source Informatics appealed against a policy of the Department of Health, which advised that the practice of GPs and pharmacists selling anonymous prescription details was a breach of confidence. The company argued that the collection of data concerning the prescribing habits of a GP was useful for those seeking to assess prescribing patterns. Although the individual GP, whose consent would be required, was identified, the patient would remain anonymous. The Court of Appeal allowed the appeal as the law was concerned with protecting the right to privacy, but that had not been breached because all the patients' personal details had been expunged.*

Effective anonymisation requires more than just the removal of names and addresses. A full postcode, NHS number or even the name of the ward with the date of admission to hospital can be strong identifiers, along with other information such as a date of birth, particularly if looked at in combination with other data items.

Anonymised patient information can be used for a range of purposes, such as audit, effective planning of services, research, education and even inclusion in assignments and journal articles. As Lord Justice Bingham held in *W v Egdell* [1990], if a health professional discloses information about a patient to a newspaper or makes a comment in a journal article or while gossiping with friends, this would be a breach of the duty of confidence unless they took appropriate steps to conceal the identity of the patient.

Disclosing information with appropriate care

The general duty of confidence imposed on registered nurses requires that patient information is kept confidential and must not be disclosed.

However, this duty is not absolute and there will be occasions where confidential information will need to be disclosed.

Given that registered nurses will face sanctions from their employer, professional regulatory body and the law for an unwarranted breach of confidence, it is essential that any disclosure of information is done appropriately within the requirements of the duty owed to the patient.

Where you are unclear as to whether a disclosure of information is justified, you should seek advice from a senior colleague or manager. You must also follow the policies on the use and disclosure of patient information that all NHS establishments are required to have, along with the advice given in *Confidentiality: NHS code of practice* (DH, 2003c). In addition, you must consider the requirements of your *Code* and the law of confidence.

Where a patient has been told that patient information will be recorded and used for the purpose of delivering effective healthcare, you may share information with other members of the clinical team caring for that individual. Disclosure must be restricted to the clinical team only.

Your duty of confidence to the patient generally requires that disclosure of confidential information for purposes other than care and treatment must only be done with the explicit consent of the patient, unless an exception to that duty applies or the information can be disclosed in an anonymised form (NMC, 2015a). Anonymous information is information from which all identifying particulars have been removed.

Where you intend to disclose confidential information without the explicit consent of the patient, you will need to consider carefully whether an exception to the general duty of confidence applies.

Human Rights Act 1998

Article 8 of the European Convention on Human Rights may be engaged if the information to be disclosed interferes with the right to respect for private and family life, home and correspondence.

Where the information is disclosed with the consent of the patient, article 8 will not be engaged. If article 8 is engaged, you will need to demonstrate that disclosure is:

- in accordance with the law;
- in pursuit of a legitimate aim; and
- necessary in a democratic society.

Where the disclosure complies with both the Data Protection Act 1998 and the common law of confidentiality, human rights requirements will generally be satisfied.

Common law of confidence

Under the common law, information is confidential where:

- it has the necessary quality of confidence; and
- it has been communicated in circumstances giving rise to an obligation of confidence.

This would apply to information obtained in the course of the nurse–patient relationship. This information may be shared with other members of the clinical team for purposes relating to care and treatment. Disclosure for any other purpose must only be made with the explicit consent of the patient, unless an exception to the duty arises.

Before disclosing confidential information without consent you will need to consider whether:

- the common law duty has been modified by statute; or
- there is an overriding public interest that justifies disclosure.

Data Protection Act 1998

The Data Protection Act 1998 applies to personal information held on computer or as part of a relevant filing system. This definition would include health records. Under the provisions of the Act a decision to disclose personal health information must be fair and lawful.

To be lawful, the disclosure of personal health information must meet the requirements of the common law duty of confidence and be justified under the requirements of schedules 2 and 3 of the Data Protection Act 1998, which deal with the processing, including disclosure, of personal information and sensitive personal information respectively.

Caldicott guardians

Each NHS organisation has a guardian of person-based clinical information who oversees the arrangements for its use and sharing.

They ensure that patient-identifiable information is only shared for justified purposes and that only the minimum necessary information is shared in each case.

Every use or flow of patient-identifiable information must be regularly justified and routinely tested against the principles developed in the Caldicott report.

- Justify the purpose(s) for using confidential information.
- Only use it when absolutely necessary.
- Use the minimum that is required.
- Access should be on a strict need-to-know basis.
- Everyone must understand his or her responsibilities.
- Understand and comply with the law.

The Caldicott guardian plays a key role in ensuring that the NHS satisfies the highest practical standards for handling patient-identifiable information. The guardian should actively support work to facilitate and enable information sharing and advise on options for the lawful and ethical processing of information to ensure that such sharing is appropriate.

Activity 12.7 *Critical thinking*

Appropriate disclosure of patient information

Outline how you would ensure the appropriate disclosure of information regarding a patient in your care in the following circumstances:

1. Information about the condition of a celebrity admitted to hospital for surgery to the media waiting outside the hospital.
2. Information about a large quantity of ecstasy found on a patient admitted to ICU following a road traffic collision.
3. Information to managers undertaking an audit of care on the ward.
4. Information about a patient's condition to a friend who is enquiring on the telephone.
5. Information to a court about a patient's whereabouts on a particular time and day.
6. Information about a patient's condition to the doctor in charge of his care.

(Hint: use *Confidentiality: NHS code of practice* (DH, 2003c) as a resource in completing this activity.)

An outline answer is given at the end of the chapter.

In exercising their professional duty, nurses and midwives will both seek and receive information of a confidential nature from their patients. Generally, they will be required to keep this information to themselves and respect the right of the patient not to have their health information disclosed. However, when such information involves, for example, a threat of harm to others, a decision whether or not to disclose that information to others can pose a dilemma.

Nurses have to balance the legal and professional duty to maintain confidentiality against the exceptions to that duty allowing disclosure. While under certain circumstances the courts can require disclosure, it is left largely to nurses to exercise their professional judgement when deciding whether or not to reveal confidential information to others. This leaves them open to a charge of breaching both the professional and legal duty of confidence and risking sanctions that could include losing their job and professional status together with the possibility of damages for the patient. However, the common law and the decisions of the courts have provided guidance for health professionals on what information is confidential, when a duty of confidence exists, and the exceptions to that duty.

Nurses must inform their professional decision-making by adhering to the guidance of courts, their code of conduct and the NHS code of practice on confidentiality in resolving the dilemmas that arise from the burden of keeping a confidence. In this way a balance will be reached in maintaining both the patient's right to have their confidences respected and the need to share confidential information where a public interest in protecting others arises.

Social networking

Social networking sites such as Facebook, Twitter and LinkedIn have transformed how information is accessed and shared. In the United Kingdom there are some 25 million adult Facebook users and the NMC (2011b) estimates that some 355,000 registered nurses use the site.

Social networks encourage an online persona and build a personal network that connects cascading online friends to an open worldwide community (Lenhart and Madden, 2006). The average Facebook user has 130 friends, and is connected to 80 community pages, groups and events while the average Twitter user has 300 followers (Briggs, 2011). This openness and ease of access to information has been seen as a force for good in healthcare with social networking sites forming part of the strategic information sharing policies of NHS organisations. Patients also use the sites to research their conditions. Up to a third of people use them to find fellow sufferers and to engage in discussions about their health and the management of their conditions (Deloitte Centre for Health Solutions, 2010).

Confidentiality and social networks

That openness and the wide, rapid dissemination of information have raised concerns about their recreational use by nurses who often fail to realise how widely linked groups of online contacts are and how quickly information is spread through the network.

When using social networks nurses have to consider whether their remarks or photographs are in keeping with their duty of confidence.

Inappropriate dissemination of information has led to disciplinary action. A nurse was disciplined after a picture on Facebook showed her topless in her uniform in front of sleeping patients while on night duty (Welsh, 2008).

Case study 12.6: Student nurse disciplined

A student nurse was disciplined after commenting on a social network that she would be 'messing with dead bodies' and 'cutting up dead people' not realising that the assumed private interaction would be seen by others.

(Stoke Sentinel, *2009)*

Employers also ensure the reputation of their organisation is maintained by taking disciplinary action against staff who, in their view, act inappropriately through social networks. A group of A&E doctors and nurses were suspended after photographs of staff playing a lying down game 'planking' appeared on Facebook showing them on resuscitation trolleys, ward floors and a helicopter landing pad when on night shift (*Wiltshire Gazette and Herald*, 2009).

The vast majority of employers, including PCT and NHS trusts, have a policy on the use of social networking sites by staff and nurses must ensure that they adhere to that policy even when using the sites for recreational purposes. Nurses also have a legal duty of confidence with the courts willing to intervene to prevent information being disclosed (*Attorney General v Guardian Newspapers Ltd* [1987]).

As you have seen this legal duty is enforced through the Data Protection Act 1998 and the office of the Information Commissioner. A hospital worker was charged with an offence under the Data Protection Act 1998 when he accessed a hospital computer to find the details of a female outpatient he was attracted to and later contacted her on Facebook (Ward, 2011).

The Data Protection Act imposes on nurses a duty not to voluntarily disclose information gained in a professional capacity to a third party. This includes inappropriate use of information on social networking sites. The duty is enforced by the threat of professional discipline.

Case study 12.7: Nurse struck off for inappropriate use of Facebook

A nurse who started a relationship with a former patient on Facebook was struck off by the NMC who found the nurse had conducted an inappropriate relationship with the former patient by communicating with her through Facebook.

(NMC, 2010)

Advice on the use of social networks

The NMC (2011a) has issued advice to nurses on the standards expected of them when using social networks. It makes clear that *The Code* (NMC, 2015a) applies to the use of social networking sites and other forms of online communication and nurses must *uphold the reputation of [their] profession at all times.* Conduct online is judged in the same way and to the same standard as conduct in a nurse's work and private life. Fitness to practise will be impaired if a nurse acts inappropriately online including where they:

- share confidential information online;
- post inappropriate comments about colleagues or patients;
- use social networking sites to bully or intimidate colleagues;
- pursue personal relationships with patients;
- distribute sexually explicit material; or
- use social networking sites in any way which is unlawful.
  (NMC, 2011b)

The NMC recommends that nurses exercise caution when interacting online and in particular to ensure that they:

- keep their personal and professional life separate as far as possible;
- uphold the reputation of their profession even where they have not identified themselves as a nurse;
- protect privacy by adjusting privacy settings online;
- do not use social networks to build or pursue relationships with patients;
- do not accept a friendship request from a current or former patient;
- do not discuss work-related issues online even where anonymised;
- never post pictures of patients online;
- never use a mobile phone camera in the workplace;
- do not use social networks for raising and escalating concerns or whistleblowing;
- treat everything online as public, permanent and shared;
- follow workplace policy for staff and students on the use of social networking sites.

Chapter summary

- Maintaining the confidentiality of a patient's health information is a fundamental element of professional conduct and ethical practice for all registered nurses.
- Patients pass on sensitive information in confidence and expect you to respect their privacy by ensuring the confidentiality of the information they give.
- A duty of confidence is imposed on nurses to reassure patients that their health information will be respected.
- The duty is imposed by all contracts of employment in the NHS, the NMC's *Code* and the law.

continued . . .

- The duty of confidence imposed on nurses is not absolute and is subject to a range of exceptions that justify disclosure.
- Consent from the patient allowing disclosure of confidential information is the starting presumption in law.
- Consent to disclose confidential information to other members of the clinical team may be implied where the patient understands how the information is to be used and has no objections.
- Where a patient refuses to allow information to be disclosed to other health professionals involved in their care, it could result in limited care and treatment.
- There are a number of exceptions allowing disclosure to appropriate sources without the consent of the patient.
- The public interest exception covers a broad range of situations that allow for confidential information to be disclosed without the consent of the patient.
- Anonymised information is not considered confidential and may be used with few constraints.
- It is essential that any disclosure of information is done appropriately within the requirements of the duty owed to the patient.
- Each NHS organisation has a guardian of person-based clinical information, known as a Caldicott guardian, who oversees the arrangements for the use and sharing of clinical information.
- Social networks are a common form of online interaction. Nurses must consider whether the remarks and photographs they post on social networking sites are in keeping with their duty of confidence.
- The NMC (2011a) has issued advice on the standards expected when using social networks.

Activities: Brief outline answers

Activity 12.1: Reflection (page 256)

Confidentiality relates to the duty to maintain confidence and thereby respect the privacy of a patient's health information.

Activity 12.2: Critical thinking (page 257)

Imposing a duty of confidence reassures patients that their personal health information will be treated sensitively and with respect, and will not be disclosed unnecessarily.

Activity 12.3: Evidence-based practice and research (page 259)

The NMC demands that registered nurses treat a patient's health information as confidential. You are required to inform patients how and why their health information will be shared with those involved in their care. Disclosure must occur where you believe someone to be at risk of harm.

The NMC suggests that disclosure can occur:

- with the consent of the patient;
- without consent where it is necessary in the public interest to protect a person from risk of harm.

Any other disclosure is a matter for a nurse's professional judgement and they will be accountable for that decision. The NMC gives no guidance as to what circumstances might justify disclosure.

Activity 12.4: Reflection (page 262)

Your list will demonstrate that the duty of confidence is not absolute and a number of exceptions to the duty exists and include disclosure:

- with the consent of the patient;
- for care and treatment purposes;
- when a patient specifically asks you to do so;
- when a patient is incapable of receiving information;
- in cases of suspected abuse of dependent elderly and children;
- in the interests of justice;
- for the public good;
- to protect a third party;
- to prevent or detect a serious crime;
- under statutes that empower the health professional to disclose information;
- under statutes that require information to be disclosed under specific circumstances.

Activity 12.5: Evidence-based practice and research (page 265)

Below are the main findings:

- High level of trust in the NHS to protect patient confidentiality, but low awareness of how the NHS uses patient information.
- People were more concerned about who used the information and whether it was anonymous than how the information would be used.
- People were comfortable with their GP, hospital doctors and emergency services having access to their data, although they reserved the right to limit access to very sensitive information.
- People felt that all others treating them should be allowed access on a 'need to know' basis.
- People felt that information released outside the NHS, or used by the NHS for purposes other than treatment, should be anonymised or patient permission sought to use identifiable data.
- Once information was anonymised, a majority were happy not to be asked for consent to share it.
- People differed over how their consent should be obtained for using identifiable information. Some wanted to be asked for a one-off consent; others wanted their consent to be sought each time information was used other than for treatment. Some wanted to be asked every time information was used, including for treatment.

Activity 12.6: Critical thinking (page 269)

Gunshot wounds are usually the result of a serious incident and so the police should be told whenever a person has arrived at a hospital with such a wound.

In this case, it would be reasonable to confirm the existence of such a patient without disclosing identifying details, such as the patient's name and address.

Remember that the police are responsible for assessing the risk posed by members of the public who are armed. By knowing of the existence of the patient, the police can consider the risk of a further attack on the patient and also risks to staff, patients and visitors in the A&E department or elsewhere in the hospital.

Once you have confirmed the existence of the patient, the police will usually ask to see him or her. The treatment and care of the patient is your first concern, so do not allow police access to the patient if this will delay or hamper treatment or compromise the patient's recovery.

If a patient's treatment and condition allows them to speak to the police, you should ask the patient whether they are willing to do so. Patients have a right to expect that information about them will be held in confidence by their nurses. This is an important element of a relationship of trust between nurses and patients.

However, if the patient cannot give consent, or says 'no', information can still be disclosed if there are grounds for believing that this is in the public interest or that disclosure is required by law.

Disclosures in the public interest are justified where:

- a failure to disclose information would put the patient, or someone else, at risk of death or serious harm;
- a disclosure may assist in the prevention, detection or prosecution of a serious crime.

Both of these situations might apply in a case where a patient has a gunshot wound.

Remember, if there is any doubt about whether disclosure is justified, the decision to disclose information without consent should be made by, or with the agreement of, the consultant in charge, or the trust's Caldicott guardian.

Wherever practicable, patients should be told that a disclosure will be or has been made and the reasons for disclosure must be recorded in the patient's notes.

Activity 12.7: Critical thinking (page 272)

1. Normally, there is no basis for disclosure of confidential and identifiable information about patients to the media. There will be occasions, however, when NHS hospitals and staff are asked for information about individual patients, such as requests for updates on the condition of celebrity patients. Where practicable, the explicit consent of the individual patient concerned must be obtained before disclosing any information about their care and treatment, and that includes their presence in the hospital. Where consent cannot be obtained or is withheld, disclosure will only be justified if it is in the public interest. Where a patient is not competent to make a decision about disclosure, the views of family members should be sought and decisions made in the patient's best interests.
2. The police have no general right of access to health records, but there are statutes that require disclosure to them and some that permit disclosure. The Road Traffic Act 1988 requires disclosure of information that would lead to the identity of a person involved in a road traffic offence and you would be obliged to give this information if asked by a police officer. In the absence of a requirement to disclose, there must be either explicit patient consent or a robust public interest justification. In this case, the public interest in preventing or detecting a serious crime would allow disclosure. Supplying a class A drug such as ecstasy is a serious offence and you would be empowered to disclose the information to the police. Where disclosure is justified, it should be limited to the minimum necessary to meet that purpose and the patient should be informed of the disclosure unless it would defeat the purpose of the investigation, allow a potential criminal to escape or put staff at risk.

3. The evaluation of clinical performance against standards or through comparative analysis, with the aim of informing the management of services, is an essential component of modern healthcare provision and is regarded as a healthcare purpose. Disclosure of information relevant to the audit would be a justified disclosure. Every effort should be made to ensure that patients are aware that audit takes place and that it is essential if the quality of care they receive is to be monitored and improved.
4. Friends often provide valuable help and support to patients, and also act as carers. However, the explicit consent of a competent patient is needed before disclosing information to a friend. The best interests of a patient who is not competent to consent may also warrant disclosure. Where disclosure of information does go ahead, only information essential to a patient's care should be disclosed and patients should be made aware that this is the case.
5. The courts have legal powers to require disclosure of confidential patient information in the interests of justice. However, you need to take care to limit disclosure to the matter required by the court and provide only the precise information requested.
6. Disclosing information to the doctor in charge of the patient's care is a justified disclosure and necessary for the proper treatment of the patient. Patients should be made aware that information about their care will be shared with other members of the clinical team and, where this occurs, the explicit consent of the patient to such a disclosure is not necessary.

Further reading

A recommended read for general guidance on the role and application of the duty of confidence in the NHS is provided by:

Department of Health (2003) *Confidentiality: NHS code of practice.* London: DH.

For an insight into patients' views on the need for confidentiality and information sharing we recommend:

NHS Information Authority (2002) S*hare with Care: People's views on consent and confidentiality of patient information.* London: NHS IA.

Useful website

The Health and Social Care Information Centre has incorporated NHS Connecting for Health. It supports the NHS in providing better, safer care, by delivering computer systems and services that improve how patient information is stored and accessed. It has a range of sources on patient confidentiality and can be accessed at:

www.hscic.gov.uk

Chapter 13
Health and safety

NMC Standards for Pre-registration Nursing Education

This chapter will address the following competencies:

Domain 1: Professional values

4. All nurses must work in partnership with service users, carers, families, groups, communities and organisations. They must manage risk, and promote health and well being while aiming to empower choices that promote self-care and safety.
8. All nurses must practise independently, recognising the limits of their competence and knowledge. They must reflect on these limits and seek advice from, or refer to, other professionals where necessary.

Domain 4: Leadership, management and team working

6. All nurses must work independently as well as in teams. They must be able to take the lead in coordinating, delegating and supervising care safely, managing risk and remaining accountable for the care given.

Chapter aims

By the end of this chapter you will be able to:

- state why health and safety matters should concern registered nurses;
- outline the general duties owed by employers and employees under the Health and Safety at Work etc. Act 1974;
- describe the regulations governing specific health and safety requirements in the NHS;
- explain the process of health and safety management;
- discuss the requirements for the safe handling of loads;
- define the term 'reasonably practicable' in relation to manual handling.

Introduction

From your very first day as a student nurse your university and clinical placements will be concerned for your safety and the safety of the patients you care for. In this chapter you will explore the duties owed by healthcare employers and their staff under the health and safety legislation. The chapter will consider the process of safety management and in particular the requirements for the safe handling of loads. The chapter ends with a discussion of the human rights impact of health and safety laws.

Some 1.7 million people are employed by the NHS and ensuring the health and safety of employees is essential to the efficient delivery of healthcare.

Activity 13.1 *Team working*

Risks at work

In a group, list the potential risks to your health and safety that you have encountered during clinical practice. When you have completed that list, make another with the potential hazards faced by patients receiving healthcare.

Now read below for further information. An outline answer is also given at the end of the chapter.

The Health and Safety Executive (2007) estimate that absence in the NHS costs some £1 billion annually, and the following are the four main causes:

- **Musculoskeletal disorders** – along with stress, these are the biggest cause of sick leave in the NHS, accounting for some 40 per cent. A quarter of all nurses have at some time taken time off as a result of a back injury sustained at work.
- **Stress** – this is a major cause of work-related ill health and sick leave among healthcare employees. Work-related stress accounts for over a third of all new incidences of ill health and each case leads to an average of 30.2 working days lost. A total of 13.8 million working days were lost to work-related stress, depression and anxiety in 2006/7.
- **Violence** – NHS staff and other healthcare workers are four times more likely to experience work-related violence and aggression than other workers. Employers must assess the risk of verbal and physical violence to their employees and take appropriate steps to deal with this risk.
- **Slips and trips** – in 2006/7, 53 per cent (841 of 1,561) of major injuries to employees in the health services were as a result of slips or trips.

Patients are also placed at risk of injury if appropriate safety measures are not taken. The NHS Litigation Authority (2007) estimates that some £500 million is paid annually by the health service in compensation claims and fines for breaching health and safety laws. The cost in human terms can also be high. Mistakes and errors can compromise safety to the point where lives are put at risk and, sadly, fatalities occur. The risk to patients include: medication errors, treatment errors, falls, violence, poorly maintained equipment, human errors, fire and hospital acquired infections.

Case study 13.1: Patient dropped off at wrong address

Two NHS trusts were fined a total of £27,500 over the death of a 93-year-old woman, dropped off at the wrong house by an ambulance crew (Hughes and Butler, 2007). The lady, who suffered from dementia, became confused in the unfamiliar surroundings and fell, breaking her leg. She died some five weeks later in hospital.

Case study 13.2: Nurse left on his own on a ward killed by a patient

*A London trust was fined £28,000 and £14,000 costs at the Old Bailey following a prosecution brought by the Health and Safety Executive, after a nurse was killed by a psychiatric patient (*M2 Presswire*, 2005). The junior member of staff was working alone on the ward without clear procedures and with inadequate measures in place to check on his safety. He suffered multiple injuries that resulted in the loss of his life.*

Health and safety law

To prevent the avoidable loss of life and minimise the days lost to absence, the NHS as an employer has a legal duty to comply with the requirements relating to health and safety at work.

The Health and Safety at Work etc. Act 1974 is the basis of health and safety law in the UK, and sets out general duties that:

- employers have towards employees and members of the public using their service;
- employees have to themselves and to each other.

Breaching or failing to comply with these duties are criminal offences.

The employer's general duty is set out in section 2 of the Health and Safety at Work etc. Act 1974 and states that an employer has:

- a duty to ensure *so far as is reasonably practicable*, the health, safety and welfare at work of employees and any others who may be affected by the undertaking …

The legal standard imposed by the 1974 Act is *reasonably practicable* or *so far as is reasonably practicable.* The standard implies a weighing up of the risk against the cost in terms of time, money or trouble of preventing or controlling the risk.

The duty of employees at work is set out in section 7 of the Health and Safety at Work etc. Act 1974, which states that:

- it shall be the duty of every employee while at work:
  - to take reasonable care of their own health and safety and of any other person who may be affected by their acts or omissions;
  - to cooperate with their employer so far as is necessary to enable that employer to meet their requirements with regard to any statutory provisions.

Activity 13.2 *Critical thinking*

Health and safety duties owed by employees

The Health and Safety at Work etc. Act 1974 places a duty on employees to take reasonable care of their own health and safety. List reasonable measures a registered nurse could take to ensure their health and safety in the course of their work.

An outline answer is given at the end of the chapter.

The duty to report incidents

As well as a duty under the Health and Safety at Work etc. Act 1974, a registered nurse is also under a professional duty to act to identify and minimise risks to patients and clients (NMC, 2015a).

A nurse who raises an issue of health and safety with an employer, either directly or through a union, is entitled to protection from dismissal and victimisation under the Public Interest Disclosure Act 1998. Under the Act each NHS employer has a duty to establish a procedure for employees to raise concerns where:

- a criminal offence has been, is being or is likely to be committed; or
- the health or safety of an individual has been, is being or is likely to be endangered.

Case study 13.3: Concern about infant deaths

*A doctor concerned about perinatal mortality rates (stillbirths and deaths of those aged less than one week) in South Tyneside was sacked after highlighting the high infant death rate and the appalling treatment of female patients (*The Journal, *2006). She ultimately won her case for unfair dismissal and racial discrimination.*

Health and safety regulations

The Health and Safety at Work etc. Act 1974 is supplemented by a wide range of secondary legislation in the form of regulations and orders that focus on specific areas of workplace health and safety, such as manual handling. Most of this secondary legislation begins in the form of a European

Union directive that must be implemented in the law of individual member states. The directives aim to harmonise workplace health and safety throughout all countries of the European Union. Table 13.1 lists the main regulations that affect the health service and their employees.

Table 13.1: Regulations relating to health and safety in the NHS

Regulations	Scope
Management of Health and Safety at Work Regulations 1999	Sets out how employers are required to assess risk in all work activities, implement control measures if required, provide information and training, and appoint competent persons.
Manual Handling Operations Regulations 1992	Cover the moving and handling of objects, either by hand or by bodily force.
Control of Substances Hazardous to Health Regulations 2002	Relate to the assessment of hazardous substances and biological agents, and the implementation of appropriate precautions.
Reporting of Injuries, Diseases and Dangerous Occurrences Regulations 1995	Require employers to notify certain types of injury, disease and dangerous occurrences to the Health and Safety Executive.
Personal Protective Equipment at Work Regulations 1992	Cover the provision of suitable and sufficient protective clothing and equipment, such as uniforms and gloves, etc.
Workplace (Health, Safety and Welfare) Regulations 1992	Cover issues such as ventilation, temperature, flooring and workstations, etc.
Health and Safety (Display Screen Equipment) Regulations 1992	Set out requirements for the use of visual display units, workstations, seating, etc.
Provision and Use of Work Equipment Regulations 1998	Cover the safe use and maintenance of equipment, such as hoists.
Health and Safety (First Aid) Regulations 1981	Concern first aid requirements, such as the contents of first aid boxes and the number of trained first aid personnel.
Health and Safety (Safety Signs and Signals) Regulations 1996	Specify the minimum requirements for safety signs at work.
The Fire Precautions (Workplaces) Regulations 1997	Require employers to assess the risk of fire in the workplace.
Hazardous Waste (England and Wales) Regulations 2005	Specify the requirements for the classification, segregation and disposal of waste, including that which is infectious and hazardous.

It is essential that employers and staff work together to ensure effective implementation of health and safety measures. This joint approach helps to promote and raise awareness among employers and staff, thereby creating a positive safety culture.

Involving staff in workplace health and safety is a legal requirement under the provisions of the Safety Representatives and Safety Committee Regulations 1977, and the Health and Safety (Consultation with Employees) Regulations 1996, which require staff representatives to:

- consult with and be consulted by employers regarding:
  - the introduction of measures that may affect health and safety;
  - arrangements for appointing competent persons to assess risks;
  - provision of health and safety information and training;
- investigate hazards, accidents and complaints, etc.;
- make representation to the employer on health and safety matters;
- perform workplace inspections;
- be given time off to perform their duties and undertake health and safety training.

Managing health and safety

The Health and Safety Executive (2006) requires workplace health and safety to be managed methodically to ensure that risks are minimised. This includes establishing a health and safety policy to provide information on the management of work-related risks. The policy will complement the trust's policies that relate to specific requirements, such as manual handling and the control of substances hazardous to health.

It also includes demonstrating that health and safety management is organised and functioning by reference to the four Cs.

- **Cooperation:**
  - good safety performance depends on everyone cooperating and safety is everybody's business;
  - there is a legal requirement to consult with staff representatives on health and safety matters.
- **Communication:**
  - consultation with staff safety representatives;
  - performing workplace inspections at regular intervals with written reports available for staff to view;
  - setting up a workplace Safety Committee.

- **Control:**
  - there is a legal requirement to exercise control of health and safety to ensure compliance; if there is failure to comply with an identified safety rule, such as not disposing of clinical waste appropriately, and action is not taken to rectify the situation, both the employer and staff member break the law.
- **Competence:**
  - having the knowledge and skills needed to work without risk to yourself or to others who come into contact with your work;
  - managers must ensure that individuals for whom they are responsible have the appropriate skills and knowledge to work without risk to themselves or to others;
  - competence is a legal requirement imposed on employers through health and safety regulations; training in health and safety measures is a mandatory component of a health service contract.

Activity 13.3 *Team working*

Health and safety training

In a group, discuss which elements of your nursing programme might be considered to be health and safety training, for example fire training, manual handling training, etc. Make a list of the topics covered. Now compare that list with the list of hazards you identified in Activity 13.1. Does the training reflect the hazards you are likely to encounter?

An outline answer is given at the end of the chapter.

The Health and Safety Executive (2006) requirements also include:

- assessment and monitoring of risks:
  - assessment of the risks associated with performing workplace tasks and identification of any workplace precautions and risk control systems that may be required and their successful implementation;
  - monitoring through inspections and risk assessments;
- review and audit:
  - performance must be reviewed against an audit of documentation, such as workplace inspections, risk assessments, accident and incident reports, and attendance on health and safety training courses.

Workplace risk assessments

A risk assessment is the identification of hazards present in the workplace and an estimate of the risk associated with performing a task. A hazard is something that has the potential to cause harm and a risk is the likelihood of that hazard causing an accident or incident.

There is a legal duty to perform risk assessments under the provisions of the Management of Health and Safety at Work Regulations 1999.

Once a hazard has been identified, the likelihood of the risk occurring and the severity of the harm must be considered. The law requires that risks should be reduced *so far as is reasonably practicable.* That means that the degree of risk should be balanced against the time, trouble, cost and physical difficulty of taking measures to avoid it.

Activity 13.4 *Group working*

Risk assessment bed rails

Bed rails or cot sides are commonly used to prevent falls from bed but can pose a risk to patient safety.

In groups list the potential risks associated with using bed rails and how you would minimise the risks to prevent falls.

To assist you and to see what advice the Health and Safety Executive gives on the risks and safe use of bed rails, go to **www.hse.gov.uk/healthservices/bed-rails.htm**

As this is for your own observation and experience, there is no outline answer at the end of the chapter.

On identifying a risk, steps must be taken to minimise it by:

- elimination of the hazard at source; if this is not possible, the hazard must be reduced;
- taking action, if the hazard has to be reduced, to control the risk by introducing workplace precautions, such as alarms, training and information, safety cabinets, ventilation systems, etc.
- putting in place, once workplace precautions have been introduced, a system to monitor compliance with those precautions.

For example, the Control of Substances Hazardous to Health Regulations 2002 seek to control exposure to hazardous substances that arises from work under an employer's control.

The regulations require that exposure of employees to substances hazardous to health is either prevented or, where this is not reasonably practicable, adequately controlled (Control of Substances Hazardous to Health Regulations 2002, Regulation 7(1)).

Employers must, therefore, where reasonably practicable, eliminate completely the use or production of substances hazardous to health in the workplace by changing the method of work, modifying the process or substituting a non-hazardous substance.

Where prevention of exposure to substances hazardous to health is not reasonably practicable, employers must adequately control exposure.

Case study 13.4: Latex allergy

In Dugmore v Swansea NHS Trust *[2002], a nurse was awarded £345,000 from her employing trust for injuries caused by hazardous substances. The nurse was forced to abandon her career due to an allergy to latex and gave up nursing in 1997 after experiencing asthma, skin problems and anaphylactic attacks after exposure to latex.*

The trust was liable because, although they took the step of providing the nurse with latex-free products, other staff on the ward continued to use them and this was enough to trigger an allergic reaction.

Sharps injuries

Sharps injuries are a well-known risk in the health and social care sector. Sharps contaminated with an infected patient's blood can transmit more than 20 diseases, including hepatitis B, hepatitis C and human immunodeficiency virus (HIV). Because of this transmission risk, sharps injuries can cause worry and stress to the many thousands who receive them.

Sharps are the collective name for needles, blades and other medical instruments that are necessary for healthcare and cause injury by cutting or pricking the skin. Where a sharp instrument injures a person by penetrating the skin, this is called a percutaneous injury.

The Health and Safety Executive recommends that if you receive a sharps injury you should:

- encourage the wound to gently bleed, ideally holding it under running water;
- wash the wound using running water and plenty of soap;
- avoid scrubbing the wound while you are washing it;
- be sure NOT to suck the wound;
- dry the wound and cover it with a waterproof plaster or dressing;
- seek urgent medical advice from your occupational health service as effective prophylaxis is available;
- report the injury to your employer.

The main risk from a sharps injury is the potential exposure to infections such as blood-borne viruses from a blade or needle sharp contaminated with blood or a bodily fluid from a patient. The blood-borne viruses of most concern are:

- hepatitis B (HBV)
- hepatitis C (HCV)
- human immunodeficiency virus (HIV).

Health and Safety (Sharp Instruments in Healthcare) Regulations 2013

In common with other health and safety risks, the law applies as it does to other risks from work activities. However, to minimise the risk of injury from sharps, the European Union has introduced an EU Council directive 2010/32/EU on the prevention of sharps injuries in the hospital and healthcare sector. Many of the requirements contained in the directive already formed part of health and safety law in the United Kingdom. The remaining requirements were implemented in the Health and Safety (Sharp Instruments in Healthcare) Regulations 2013.

The regulations only apply to employers, contractors and workers in the healthcare sector. NHS trusts/boards, independent healthcare businesses and other employers whose main activity is the management, organisation and provision of healthcare will be subject to the regulations.

Activity 13.5 *Research*

Complying with the Health and Safety (Sharp Instruments in Healthcare) Regulations 2013

The Health and Safety Executive has produced a health services information sheet on the Health and Safety (Sharps Instruments in Healthcare) Regulations 2013 to provide guidance on how to comply with the regulations.

Download the information sheet from: **www.hse.gov.uk/pubns/hsis7.pdf**

Then in groups consider how far the placement areas you have worked on have complied with the requirements of the regulations and what, if anything, they need to do to improve compliance with the 2013 regulations.

As this is for your own observation and experience, there is no outline answer at the end of the chapter.

Reporting accidents and incidents

Reporting accidents and incidents at work is an essential component of monitoring the effectiveness of health and safety measures, and preventing the recurrence of an incident. In addition to local NHS trust accident reporting procedures, there is a legal requirement to report certain categories of accidents that occur within the workplace to the Health and Safety Executive under the Reporting of Injuries, Diseases and Dangerous Occurrences Regulations 1995.

Accidents at work are only reportable if they arise out of, or in connection with, work. There are different categories of accidents, including:

- **death or major injuries:** when a member of staff or a patient is killed or suffers a major injury (including injuries sustained as a result of physical violence) while working;
- **injuries that last over three days:** when accidents (including acts of physical violence) result in the injured person being away from work or unable to perform their normal duties for more than three days (including non-working days);
- **diseases:** where a doctor notifies the trust in writing that an employee is suffering from a disease specified in regulations and linked with a workplace activity; reportable diseases include:
  - occupational dermatitis;
  - occupational asthma or respiratory sensitisation as a result of exposure to chemical substances;
  - infections such as hepatitis, tuberculosis, legionella and tetanus;
  - infection reliably attributable to working with biological agents – exposure to blood or body fluids or any potentially infective material.

Dangerous occurrences

Dangerous occurrences or near misses must also be reported and these are events that may not result in a reportable injury, but have the potential to do significant harm. In the health service reportable occurrences would include:

- collapse, overturning or failure of load-bearing parts of lifts and lifting equipment, such as a hoist;
- explosion, collapse or bursting of any closed vessel or associated pipework, such as an autoclave;
- electrical short-circuit or overload causing fire or explosion;
- explosion or fire causing suspension of normal work for over 24 hours;
- accidental release of any substance that may damage health.

Manual handling

Musculoskeletal injury, particularly back injury, is one of the most common causes of incapacity among nurses. Secombe and Smith (1996) argue that some 3,600 nurses have to retire each year because of back injuries, with a further 80,000 estimated to have hurt their backs. The Health and Safety Executive shows that, from 1992 to 1995, some 14,000 manual handling accidents were reported in the NHS, with 60 per cent of these involving the handling of patients (Health and Safety Executive, 2002). The National Audit Office (2003) found that back injury forms a third of all reported injuries in the NHS and claims that only 42 per cent of back injury is actually reported.

Reducing the risk of injury

The Management of Health and Safety at Work Regulations 1999 require employers to make an assessment of the risks to the health and safety of their employees and others they have contact with at work. The regulations further require that protective and preventative measures be put in place to avoid such risks.

The Manual Handling Operations Regulations 1992 deal specifically with the manual handling of loads. Regulation 2(1) defines manual handling as *any transporting or supporting of a load (including the lifting, putting down, pushing, pulling, carrying or moving thereof) by hand or by bodily force.* A load is defined as including *any person and any animal.* It is clear that the scope of the regulations includes the lifting and moving of patients by nursing staff.

Regulation 4 of the 1992 regulations places a duty on employers to avoid hazardous manual handling operations so far as is reasonably practicable. Where this cannot be avoided, the regulation requires an assessment of the manual handling operation and that steps be taken to reduce the risk of injury to the lowest level that is reasonably practicable. Particular consideration should be given to the provision of mechanical assistance, such as hoists, but, where this is not reasonably practicable, employers should explore improvements to the task, the load and the working environment.

Both the general duty to protect the health and safety of employees and the specific duty to reduce risks to health due to the manual handling of loads apply to the NHS, and NHS and primary care trusts have felt the heavy cost of breaching that duty.

Case study 13.5: Compensation for breaching a statutory duty, causing back injury

In Knott v Newham Healthcare Trust *[2003], the Court of Appeal upheld an order for the award of £414,000 to a nurse who had injured her back due to the trust's inadequate arrangements for lifting. The court found that no real steps had been taken to reduce risk of injury and that the trust was in breach of its statutory duty under the 1992 regulations.*

The high cost of awards and, similarly, high legal costs have reinforced the duty of NHS trusts to protect the health and safety of their employees.

No-lift policies

The great majority of trusts now implement manual handling procedures through a no-lift policy. Tracy and Ruszala (1996) suggest that the no-lift policy is the only means of reducing injury when handling patients. This view is echoed by the RCN, which in its *Code of Practice for Patient Handling* (2002) argues that hazardous manual handling should be eliminated in all but exceptional or life-threatening situations. NHS trusts and unions representing staff in the health service see the use of a no-lift policy as the key tool in reducing manual handling injuries. Instead of lifting manually, these policies require that the great majority of patient lifting is achieved by mechanical means.

Activity 13.6 *Evidence-based practice and research*

No-lift policies

Before reading this section, read the manual handling policy of the NHS trust that you attend for clinical practice. Note the requirements of the policy. Does it allow any form of lifting or moving of patients by manual means?

An outline answer is given at the end of the chapter.

The meaning of 'reasonably practicable'

Despite the liability NHS trusts face under statutory health and safety provisions, the duty is not absolute. The Health and Safety at Work etc. Act 1974 and its regulations only require the duty to be carried out so far as is reasonably practicable.

The meaning of this phrase was considered by the Court of Appeal in *Edwards v National Coal Board* [1949]. Lord Justice Asquith held that reasonably practicable did not mean physically possible. NHS trusts are not required to spend all their funds on ensuring the safety of staff. Rather, there is a narrower requirement to balance the likelihood of the risk occurring against the cost in terms of money, time and trouble in averting the risk. In manual handling terms, this has generally been considered to be balancing the risk of injury to staff against the cost and availability of suitable equipment. The rights and preferences of patients were considered secondary to the primary duty of protecting the health and safety of staff. Under no-lift policies, patients would not be moved or lifted if manual handling was assessed as hazardous and suitable equipment was not available.

Activity 13.7 *Evidence-based practice and research*

The East Sussex case

To assist you in applying the legal concepts introduced in the next section of the chapter, download and read *R (on the application of A & Others) v East Sussex County Council and Another* [2003] from **www.bailii.org/ew/cases/EWHC/Admin/2003/167.html**. Then in a group discuss the facts of the case and whether you agree with the outcome of the case.

An outline answer is given at the end of the chapter.

Since the introduction of the Human Rights Act 1998, however, the High Court has revisited the interpretation of 'reasonably practicable' and now requires the rights of patients to be considered when assessing moving and handling needs.

Duty to the patient

At common law patients are owed a duty of care that requires that health professionals meet the needs of their patients in accordance with a standard accepted by a responsible body of professional opinion and that stands up to logical analysis (*Bolitho v City and Hackney HA* [1998]). Meeting this duty may require the manual handling of patients even where there is a risk of injury.

The common law duty of care requires that a person whose job includes lifting people accepts a greater risk than those whose handling duty is restricted to inanimate objects. When working in healthcare settings the care of patients gives rise to an inherent need for some manual handling to take place.

Case study 13.6: No compensation for back injury sustained at work

In King v Sussex Ambulance NHS Trust *[2002], an ambulance man failed in his claim for compensation for an injured back caused by lifting a patient downstairs with a colleague. The Court of Appeal held that the method to be adopted when moving and handling a person had to be appropriate. In judging what is appropriate, the court requires that account be taken of the circumstances of the case having regard not only to the medical needs of the patient but also their wishes and feelings.*

In this case, the Court of Appeal was clear that the ambulance trust's duty to the patient required that she be removed to hospital. The limited availability of suitable equipment meant there was little the trust could do other than allow the manual lifting of the patient down the stairs. This was a hazardous lift and a career-ending injury occurred. The court held, however, that there was no breach of the Manual Handling Regulations 1992 or negligence on behalf of the trust.

Chapter summary

- Some 1.7 million people are employed by the NHS and ensuring the health and safety of employees is essential to the efficient delivery of healthcare.
- The Health and Safety Executive estimates that absence in the NHS costs some £1 billion annually.
- Patients are placed at risk of injury if appropriate safety measures are not taken.
- The basis of health and safety law in the UK is the Health and Safety at Work etc. Act 1974.
- An employer has a duty to ensure, so far as is reasonably practicable, the health, safety and welfare at work of employees and any others who may be affected by the undertaking.
- An employee, while at work, has a duty to take reasonable care of their own health and safety and that of any other person who may be affected by their acts or omissions.

continued . . .

- The Health and Safety at Work etc. Act 1974 is supplemented by a wide range of secondary legislation in the form of regulations that focus on specific areas of workplace health and safety (see Table 13.1, page 284).
- Employers and staff must work together to ensure effective implementation of health and safety measures.
- The Health and Safety Executive requires workplace health and safety to be managed methodically to ensure that risks are minimised.
- There is a legal duty to perform risk assessments under the provisions of the Management of Health and Safety at Work Regulations 1999.
- The Control of Substances Hazardous to Health Regulations 2002 control exposure to hazardous substances that arise out of work.
- It is a legal requirement to report certain accidents that occur in the workplace to the Health and Safety Executive under the Reporting of Injuries, Diseases and Dangerous Occurrences Regulations 1995.
- Musculoskeletal injury, particularly back injury, is one of the most common causes of incapacity among nurses.
- The Manual Handling Operations Regulations 1992 deal specifically with the manual handling of loads.
- There will be circumstances where the risk to the patient, if not lifted, will override the nurse's ordinary health and safety concerns, even where manual handling would be considered hazardous.
- In the case of hazardous handling situations, manual handling will be the exception rather than the rule.

Activities: Brief outline answers

Activity 13.1: Team working (page 281)

Nurses

Your list should include:

- musculoskeletal disorders;
- stress;
- violence;
- slips and trips.

Patients

Your list should include:

- medication errors;
- treatment errors;
- falls;
- violence;

- poorly maintained equipment;
- human error;
- fire;
- hospital acquired infections.

Activity 13.2: Critical thinking (page 283)

Your list will include:

- wearing appropriate personal protective equipment;
- regular attendance at health and safety training;
- complying with health and safety policies for the NHS trust;
- reporting hazards and incidents promptly;
- seeking assistance when necessary;
- working with the employer to improve health and safety.

Activity 13.3: Team working (page 286)

Your list detailing the training you have received should coincide with the main hazards faced by NHS staff as identified by the Health and Safety Executive. Training should therefore include moving and handling loads, fire training, prevention of violence, and breakaway training and managing stress.

Activity 13.6: Evidence-based practice and research (page 292)

To be lawful, a no-lift policy should allow lifting or moving by manual means where the life of a patient is at risk, where a patient is likely to face inhuman or degrading treatment or where it is necessary to maintain dignity or contact with the community.

Activity 13.7: Evidence-based practice and research (page 292)

The case is an interesting analysis of health and safety in nursing and of no-lift policies in particular. It does raise questions about the rights of the nurse compared to the rights of the patient. Should you be required to put yourself at risk of injury to preserve the human rights of a patient?

Further reading

For a fuller discussion of the health and safety risks to staff we recommend:

National Audit Office (2003) *A Safer Place to Work: Improving the management of health and safety risks to staff in NHS trusts* (House of Commons Papers). London: NAO.

Useful websites

The National Patient Safety Agency leads and contributes to improved, safe patient care by informing, supporting and influencing the health sector. Its website can be found at: **www.npsa.nhs.uk**

The Health and Safety Executive's role is to prevent death, injury and ill health to those at work and those affected by work activities, including in the health service. It provides a wide range of information about health and safety at: **www.hse.gov.uk**

References

Anderson, M (2003) One flew over the psychiatric unit: mental illness and the media. *Journal of Psychiatric and Mental Health Nursing*, 10 (3): 297.

Andrews, J and Butler, M (2014) *Trusted to Care: An Independent Review of the Princess of Wales Hospital and Neath Port Talbot Hospital at Abertawe Bro Morgannwg University Health Board.* Stirling: University of Sterling.

Association of Directors of Adult Social Services (2009) Directors report extra demands being placed on adult social services. London: ADASS.

Attewill, F (2007) Jehovah's Witness mother dies after refusing blood transfusion. *The Guardian*, 5 May.

Audit Commission (2002) *Setting the Record Straight.* London: Audit Commission.

Bainham, A (1990) *Children: The new law.* London: Family Law.

Baroness Hale of Richmond (2004) *Paul Sieghart Memorial Lecture, What Can the Human Rights Act Do for My Mental Health?* London: British Institute of Human Rights.

Beauchamp, T and Childress, J (1989) *Principles of Biomedical Ethics.* Oxford: Oxford University Press.

Briggs, M (2011) *Start Spreading the News.* Cambridge, MA: Nieman Foundation for Journalism.

Brindley, M (2003) Doctors find code writing is best way to treat patients. *Western Mail*, 19 August, p8.

Butler-Sloss, E (2003) *Are We Failing the Family? Human rights, children and the meaning of family in the 21st century.* London: Department for Constitutional Affairs.

Care Quality Commission (CQC) (2009) *Care Quality Commission Regulations.* London: The Stationery Office. Available online at www.legislation.gov.uk/uksi/2009/3112/contents/made

Care Quality Commission (CQC) (2014) *Guidance for Providers on Meeting the Fundamental Standards and on CQC's Enforcement Powers.* London: CQC.

Carruthers, I and Ormondroyd, J (2009) *Achieving Age Equality in Health and Social Care.* London: Central Office of Information.

Council of Europe (1950) *European Convention on Fundamental Human Rights and Freedoms.* Rome: Council of Europe.

Creighton, S (2006) *Child Protection Statistics.* London: NSPCC Research Department.

Crown Prosecution Service (2004) *Code for Crown Prosecutors.* London: CPS.

Daily Mail (2010) Care home manager guilty of killing resident 'will be jailed'. April.

Deloitte Centre for Health Solutions (2010) *Social Networks in Health Care: Communication, collaboration and insights.* London: Deloitte Centre for Health Solutions.

Department for Constitutional Affairs (2007) *Mental Capacity Act 2005 Code of Practice.* London: The Stationery Office.

Department for Education (DfE), Department of Health and Home Office (2011) *Vetting and Barring Scheme Remodelling Review: Reports and recommendations.* London: The Stationery Office.

Department of Health (DH) (1997) *Children Act 1989: Guidance and regulations.* London: HMSO.

Department of Health (DH) (1999) *Working Together to Safeguard Children.* London: The Stationery Office.

Department of Health (DH) (2000) *No Secrets: Guidance on developing and implementing multi-agency policies and procedures to protect vulnerable adults from abuse.* London: The Stationery Office.

Department of Health (DH) (2003a) *The Investigation of Events that Followed the Death of Cyril Mark Isaacs.* London: The Stationery Office.

Department of Health (DH) (2003b) *The Victoria Climbié Inquiry (Lord Laming CM 5730).* London: The Stationery Office.

Department of Health (DH) (2003c) *Confidentiality: NHS code of practice.* London: Department of Health.

Department of Health (DH) (2003d) *Every Child Matters (Cm 5860).* London: The Stationery Office.

Department of Health (DH) (2004) *Independent Investigation into How the NHS Handled Allegations About the Conduct of Clifford Ayling (Chair: The Honourable Mrs Justice Pauffley) (Cmd 6298).* London: Department of Health.

Department of Health (DH) (2009) *Reference Guide to Consent for Examination or Treatment,* 2nd edn. London: DH.

Department of Health (DH) (2012a) *Liberating the NHS: No decision about me without me. Further consultation on proposals to secure shared decision making.* London: Crown Copyright.

Department of Health (DH) (2012b) *Transforming Care: A national response to Winterbourne View Hospital Department of Health Review: Final Report.* London: TSO.

Department of Health (DH) (2014) *Hard Truths: The journey to putting patients first. Government response to the Mid Staffordshire NHS Foundation Trust Public Inquiry CM 8777.* London: Department of Health.

Director of Public Prosecutions (DPP) (2010) *Policy for Prosecutors in Respect of Cases of Encouraging or Assisting Suicide.* London: Crown Prosecution Service.

Edwards, S (2009) *Nursing Ethics: A principle based approach,* 2nd edn. London: Palgrave.

Evening Gazette (2006) Struck off. 31 January, p5.

Fleming, N (2007) Sex assaults and abuse uncovered at care homes. People with learning difficulties sacrificed to the needs of institutions, says report on NHS Trust. *Daily Telegraph,* 17 January, p10.

General Chiropractic Council, General Dental Council, General Medical Council, General Optical Council, General Osteopathic Council, General Pharmaceutical Council, Nursing and Midwifery Council and Pharmaceutical Society of Northern Ireland Department of Health Social Services and Public Safety (2014) The professional duty of candour. Available online at www.gmc-uk.org/joint statement_on_the_professional_duty_of_candour_FINAL.pdf_58140142.pdf

General Medical Council (GMC) (2010) *Treatment and Care Towards the End of Life: Good practice in decision making.* London: GMC.

Gillon, R (1994) Medical ethics: four principles plus attention to scope. *BMJ* 309: 184.

Griffith, R and Tengnah, C (2009) Understanding the Safeguarding Vulnerable Groups Act 2006. *British Journal of Community Nursing,* 14 (7): 309–13.

Hampshire and Isle of Wight Counter Fraud Team (2007) Student midwife starts jail sentence. *Fraud Matters,* June, p1.

Health and Safety Executive (2002) *Health and Safety Statistics.* London: HSE.

Health and Safety Executive (2006) *Five Steps to Risk Assessment.* London: HSE.

Health and Safety Executive (2007) *Health and Safety in Health and Social Care Services.* London: HSE.

Health Service Commissioner (1999) *Inappropriate Response to Deterioration in the Condition of a Patient over the Weekend against Hastings and Rother NHS Trust – Case No. E.2291/98–99.*

Health Service Journal (2012) CQC criticises poor discharges at Lincoln. 30 May.

Health and Social Care Information Centre (2015) *Mental Capacity Act 2005: Deprivation of Liberty Safeguards (England) 2015.* London: HSCIC.

HM Government (2006) *Working Together to Safeguard Children.* London: The Stationery Office.

Home Office (2011) *A Review of Criminal Records Regime in England and Wales: Report on Phase 2.* London: The Stationery Office.

Home Office (2012a) *Changes to Disclosure and Barring: What you need to know.* London: Crown Copyright.

Home Office (2012b) *Domestic Violence Disclosure Scheme Guidance.* London: Home Office.

House of Commons (2013) *Report of the Mid Staffordshire NHS Foundation Trust Public Inquiry (Chair Robert Francis QC) HC947.* London: The Stationery Office.

House of Commons Health Committee (2004) *Elder Abuse: Report of session 2003–4, vol 1.* London: The Stationery Office.

Hughes, G and Butler, C (2007) Ambulances 'must improve to stop another tragedy'; report paints damning picture. *Daily Post,* 29 January, p5.

The Journal (2006) Trust faces £2 million legal bill. 17 May, p15.

Kennedy, I and Grubb, A (1998) *Principles of Medical Law.* Oxford: Oxford University Press.

Kirby, D (2004) Care boss and a box of teeth. *Manchester Evening News,* 16 March, p22.

Lancashire Telegraph (2013) Accrington nurse struck off after botched catheter fitting. 24 January.

Law Commission (1993) *Consultation Paper 130: Mentally Incapacitated and Other Vulnerable Adults: Public law protection.* London: The Stationery Office.

Lenhart, A and Madden, M (2006) *Social Networking Websites and Teens: An overview.* Washington: Pew Internet and American Life Project.

Lewis, F and Batey, M (1982) Clarifying autonomy and accountability in nursing services. *Journal of Nursing Administration,* 12 (9): 13–18.

McNicoll, A (2014) Man 'left in squalor' after errors assessing his mental capacity, ombudsman finds. *Community Care,* 12 June, p3.

Marsden, S (2014) Daughter who helped parents in suicide pact stood in stunned silence watching them die, inquest hears. *Telegraph,* 15 January, p13.

Marsh, B and Narain, J (2003) Patient died because of GP's bad handwriting. *Daily Mail,* 4 February, p4.

Ministry of Justice (2008a) *Deprivation of Liberty: Code of Practice to supplement the main Mental Capacity Act 2005 Code of Practice.* London: TSO.

Ministry of Justice (2008b) *Mental Capacity Act 2005: Deprivation of liberty safeguards; Code of Practice to supplement the main Mental Capacity Act 2005 Code of Practice.* London: TSO.

M2 Presswire (2005) Fine following death of nurse at NHS mental health trust. 5 May.

Nathan, H (1957) *Medical Negligence.* London: Butterworths.

National Advisory Group on the Safety of Patients in England (2013) *A Promise To Learn – A Committment to Act: Improving the safety of patients in England.* London: Department of Health.

National Audit Office (2003) *A Safer Place to Work.* London: NAO.

National Health Service Information Authority (NHS IA) (2002) *Share with Care: People's views on consent and confidentiality of patient information.* London: NHS IA.

National Health Service Litigation Authority (NHS LA) (2007) *Annual Report and Accounts 2007* (HC 908). London: The Stationery Office.

National Health Service Litigation Authority (NHS LA) (2013) *Reports and Accounts 2012–2013.* London: The Stationery Office.

National Health Service Litigation Authority (NHS LA) (2015) *Factsheet 3 Claims Information.* London: NHS LA.

National Patient Safety Agency (2004) *Seven Steps to Patient Safety.* London: NPSA.

Nursing and Midwifery Council (NMC) (2002) *Practitioner–Client Relationships and the Prevention of Abuse.* (First published by the UKCC in 1999.) London: NMC.

Nursing and Midwifery Council (NMC) (2004) *Complaints about Unfitness to Practise: A guide for members of the public.* London: NMC.

Nursing and Midwifery Council (NMC) (2007) *NMC Record Keeping Guidance.* London: NMC.

Nursing and Midwifery Council (NMC) (2010) *Reasons for the Substantive Hearing of the Conduct and Competence Committee Panel.* Held at MWB Business Exchange, 77 Oxford Street, London on 6 September 2010. London: NMC.

Nursing and Midwifery Council (NMC) (2011a) *Social Networking Sites.* London: NMC. Available online at www.nmc-uk.org/Nurses-and-midwives/Advice-by-topic/A/Advice/Social-networking-sites

Nursing and Midwifery Council (NMC) (2011b) *Conduct and Competence Committee Substantive Hearing.* 4, 5 and 6 July 2011, Nursing and Midwifery Council, 61 Aldwych, London, WC2B 4AE, and resuming on: 17 and 18 November 2011. London: NMC.

Nursing and Midwifery Council (2015a) *The Code: Professional standards of practice and behaviour for nurses and midwives.* London: NMC.

Nursing and Midwifery Council (2015b) *Conduct and Competence Committee Substantive Hearing.* Monday 3 August 2015, Nursing and Midwifery Council, 2 Stratford Place, London, E20 1EJ. London: NMC.

Nursing and Midwifery Council (2015c) *Annual Fitness To Practise Report 2014–15.* London: NMC.

Nursing and Midwifery Council (2016) *Reasons for the Substantive Hearing of the Conduct and Competence Committee.* 29 June–1 July 2016 at the NMC, 2 Stratford Place, London, E20 1EJ. London: NMC.

Nursing and Midwifery Council and General Medical Council (2015) Openness and honesty when things go wrong: the professional duty of candour. Available online at www.gmc-uk.org/static/documents/content/DoC_guidance_englsih.pdf

O'Carroll, L (2015) Ex-Broadmoor worker jailed for selling stories to the Sun. *The Guardian,* 26 November, p23.

O'Keefe, M, Hills, A, Doyle, M, McCreadie, C, Scholes, S, Constantine, R, Tinker, A, Manthorpe, J, Biggs, S and Erens, B (2007) *UK Study of Abuse and Neglect of Older People: Prevalence survey report.* London: National Centre for Social Research.

Rideout, RW (1983) *Principles of Labour Law.* London: Sweet and Maxwell.

Royal College of Nursing (RCN) (2002) *Code of Practice for Patient Handling.* London: RCN.

Rudgard, O (2015) Nurse who helped herself to patient's chips and curry sauce struck off nursing register. *Liverpool Echo,* 25 February, p7.

Scottish Star (2013) Insulin nurse is barred. 18 April.

Secombe, I and Smith, G (1996) Voting with their feet. *Nursing Standard,* 11 (1): 22–3.

South Wales Argus (2013) Health board pays out over Newport gran negligence claim. 4 February.

Steinbock, B (1980) *Killing and Letting Die.* New Jersey: Prentice Hall.

Stoke Sentinel (2009) Facebook comment lands nurse in hot water. 23 February.

Strokes, P (2005) GP cleared of three murders faces 12 further inquiries. *Telegraph,* 16 December, p3.

Sunday Mercury (2013) Nurse forgot to give child medication. 12 May.

The Shipman Inquiry (2004) *Fifth Report: Safeguarding Patients: Lessons from the Past – Proposals for the Future (Cm 6394).* London: The Stationery Office.

This is Worcestershire (2004) Care assistant loses unfair sacking claim. 17 June, p3.

Thompson, I, Melia, K and Boyd, K (2000) *Nursing Ethics.* London: Churchill Livingstone.

Tracy, M and Ruszala, S (1996) *Introducing a Safer Handling Policy.* London: National Back Pain Association.

United Nations (1948) *Universal Declaration of Human Rights: Adopted by General Assembly Resolution 217 A(III).* New York: United Nations General Assembly.

United Nations Children's Fund (2003) *A League Table of Child Maltreatment Deaths in Rich Nations* (Innocenti Report Card No. 5). Florence: Unicef.

Unsworth, C (1987) *The Politics of Mental Health Legislation.* Oxford: Clarendon Press.

Ward, P (2011) Man on hospital data breach charge. *UKPA,* 30 November.

Welsh, S (2008) Think before you post. *Aberdeen Press and Journal,* 5 December.

Western Mail (2008) Neglectful husband left epileptic wife stranded with pies and water. 29 November, p13.

Wheeler, R (2006) Gillick or Fraser? A plea for consistency over competence in children. *British Medical Journal,* 332 (7545): 807.

Williams, R (2009) Equality bill takes aim at 'institutional ageism' in NHS. *The Guardian,* 23 October.

Wiltshire Gazette and Herald (2009) Wiltshire hospital staff suspended over Facebook picture game. 9 September.

Wright, O (2003) Doctors taught art of writing clearer notes. *The Times* (London), p10.

Index